External Fixation in Orthopedic Traumatology

Frontispiece

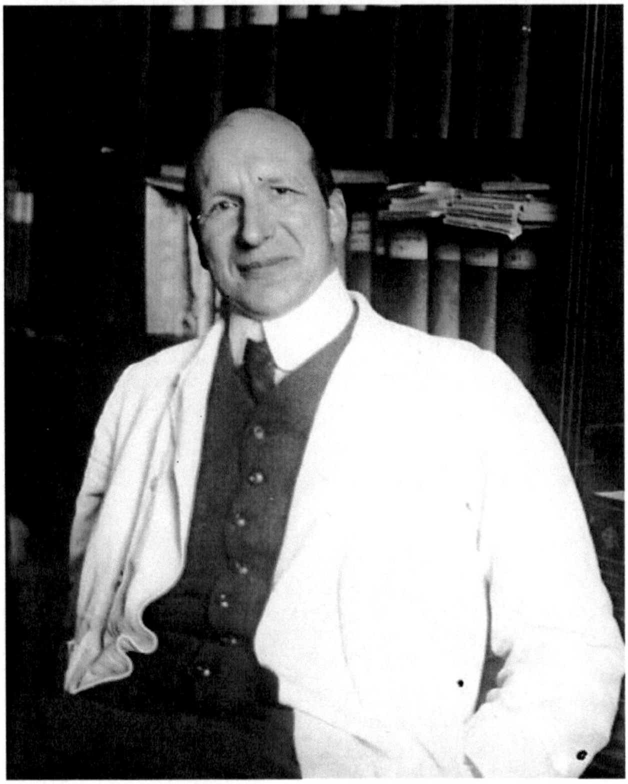

Raoul Hoffmann in 1922

Photograph courtesy of Dr. Anne-Christine Hoffmann and the Hoffmann Family, Geneva, Switzerland

Hoffmann is external fixation. This book is in tribute to Dr. Hoffmann, a private practitioner of surgery who worked in Geneva, Switzerland, and in his mature years developed the technique, improved the equipment and established the indications for external skeletal fixation. Hoffmann actualized fixateurs. Born in Berlin the son of a Lutheran minister, Hoffmann was brought up in French Geneva and trained first as a theologian and then as a physician. He met his wife Elsa in Sweden and served as a Christian missionary in Kashmir. He raised his family in Tramelan, a small watchmaking town in Swiss Jura. Hoffmann was a doctor, minister, family man and outdoorsman. He reestablished his practice in Geneva where he not only made external fixation work but also promoted abstinence from drink. Hoffmann lived from 1881–1972, a great man of the last century.

Schwechter EM, Swan KG. Raoul Hoffmann and his external fixateur. JBJS. 2007;89:672–8.

David Seligson • Cyril Mauffrey
Craig S. Roberts
Editors

External Fixation in Orthopedic Traumatology

Springer

Editors
Dr. David Seligson
Department of Orthopaedics
University Hospital Louisville
Louisville,
KY, USA
seligson@louisville.edu

Dr. Craig S. Roberts
Department of Orthopaedics
University Hospital Louisville
Louisville,
KY, USA
craig.roberts@louisville.edu

Dr. Cyril Mauffrey
Department of Orthopaedics
University Hospital Louisville
Louisville,
KY, USA
cmauffrey@yahoo.com

ISBN 978-1-4471-2199-2 e-ISBN 978-1-4471-2197-8
DOI 10.1007/978-1-4471-2197-8
Springer London Dordrecht Heidelberg New York

British Library Cataloguing in Publication Data
A catalogue record for this book is available from the British Library

Library of Congress Control Number: 2011941601

Printed on acid-free paper

Springer is part of Springer Science+Business Media (www.springer.com)

This book is dedicated to family, friends and all significant others.

David Seligson

I dedicate this book to my parents, my three daughters Oceane, Manon, Chiara and my wife Marzia, for all their patience and love.

Cyril Mauffrey

This work goes to my wife Theresa, my daughter Stephanie and my son John.

Craig S. Roberts

Foreword

The history of external fixation goes back to the ancient times when Hippocrates in about 400 BC wrote about a simple external fixator. Hippocrates described a form of external fixation to splint a fracture of the tibia with the device consisting of closely fitting proximal and distal Egyptian leather rings connected by four wooden rods from a cornel tree.

Malgaigne in 1840 has been credited with the first use of "pins" when he created a simple metal pin in a leather strap for the percutaneous pin treatment of a tibial fracture.

In the early twentieth century, Lambotte, a Belgian surgeon, designed a device for external fixation that allowed the placement of pins in any needed direction while the pins were connected to a rod by adjustable clamps.

More recently, several surgeons such as Shanz, Reidel, Stader and Anderson, with their work, have been credited for the evolution of external fixation design systems. In 1938, it was Dr. Hoffmann from Switzerland, who realized that major improvements were desirable to make the external fixator more clinically applicable. He developed a technique based on closed reduction with guided percutaneous pin placement. One could argue that Hoffmann's technique represented the first application of minimally invasive orthopedic surgery.

Despite all the good intentions of the surgeons to apply the concept of external fixator in the clinical setting, during the Second World War, several studies were published describing complications of the technique, including pin infections, pin breakage or loosening, nerve or tendon damage from pin insertion, and loss of reduction. As a result of these reports, external fixation developed a bad reputation and its popularity declined.

More recently, however, external fixation underwent many changes allowing for the various previous complications to be addressed. Overall, improvements in fixator configurations and the skill and judgment of surgeons led to the current acceptance of the method.

Nowadays, external fixation is considered as a valuable clinical treatment option, providing surgeons with the ability to affect the spatial relationship of tissues, both statically and dynamically, utilising minimally invasive techniques. The simplicity and speed of application, the adjustability of the frame configuration and the minimal blood loss with the negligible interference of the blood supply at the cutaneous and osseous levels are some of the advantages of the external fixation technique.

Currently, external fixation has many applications in the care of the trauma patient. Open fractures with severe soft tissue injuries and/or massive contamination are ideally suited to this technique. External fixation is also a versatile salvage technique for the complications arising from extremity trauma. The management of residual fracture deformity, bone loss, and infections are often simplified by external fixation. It can also be used as a salvage tool in cases associated with major complications after nailing or plating. It can be applied as a temporarily treatment of long bone fractures in patients with multiple injuries until the physiological state has been optimised so that conversion of the external fixator to a nailing/plating procedure can be performed. In cases of persisting infection or ongoing problems with soft tissue coverage, external fixation can be considered as the definitive stabilisation method in this group of patients. Moreover, in complex periarticular fractures, where the concept of damage control for the extremities is applied, external fixation can span the affected joint, allowing adequate resuscitation of the surrounding soft tissues, temporarily restoration of the mechanical axis and rotation until definitive reconstruction can be performed with open reduction internal fixation techniques.

The textbook of external fixation in orthopedic traumatology is a superb volume on the current state of the art. All the anatomical sites of the skeleton where external fixation can be applied in simple and complex clinical situations are included. All relevant chapters have been prepared by contributors who have a deep understanding of the subject.

This book is a testament to the present concepts of application of external fixation techniques. It will find a special place in the reading rooms of both junior and senior surgeons.

The editors are to be congratulated for putting together a superb textbook on external fixation for the trauma and orthopedic surgeon.

Leeds, UK Peter V. Giannoudis

Preface

"External fixation in Orthopedic traumatology" focuses on the use of external fixation in the acute management of patients with serious orthopedic injuries. The book highlights the indications for external fixation and provides an evidenced based guide to both the specialist orthopedic surgeon and the trainee. The manuscript is organized in 14 chapters covering the indications and surgical techniques for pelvis, lower limb and upper limb injuries, including detailed illustrations and clinical photographs that will enable the reader to rapidly visualize the structure of the construct and to plan for surgery accordingly. More general topics such as damage control orthopedics, biomechanics of external fixation and medico-legal considerations surrounding the injured patients are also included to provide an overall picture of the Orthopedic trauma patient. The Combined experience of the editors and authors, their involvement in a number of external fixation system designs and their international reputation in the field contribute to making this textbook an essential tool that should be available to all orthopedic surgeons dealing with injured patients.

David Seligson
Cyril Mauffrey
Craig S. Roberts

Contents

Contributors

Dennis Beck, M.D. Orthopaedics Associates, Evansville, IN, USA

Charles Daniel Benson, M.D. Department of Orthopedic Surgery, Resident in Orthopedic Surgery, University of Kansas Medical Center, Kansas City, Kansas, USA

Thomas De Coster Division of Trauma, Department of Orthopaedics, University of New Mexico, Albuquerque, NM, USA

Thomas Dienstknecht Department of Orthopaedic Trauma, University of Aachen Medical Center, Aachen, Germany

Paul J. Dougherty Department of Orthopaedics, University of Michigan, Ann Arbor, MI, USA

Peter V. Giannoudis Department of Trauma & Orthopaedic Surgery, School of Medicine, University of Leeds, Leeds, UK

Jessica Heinsen, M.D. Department of Orthopaedics, University Hospital Louisville, Louisville, KY, USA

Kimberly M. Kesling Department of Orthopaedics, Clinical Services, Darnall Army Medical Center, Ft Hood, TX, USA

N.S. Laud, M.D. Department of Orthopaedics, Laud Clinic, Mumbai, Maharashtra, India

Cyril Mauffrey, M.D., FRCS Department of Orthopaedics, University Hospital Louisville, Louisville, KY, USA

Janet Macphaden Department of Orthopaedics, Nurse Practitioner, University Hospital Louisville, Louisville, KY, USA

Alfredo Aybar Montoya, M.D. Department of Orthopaedics, Av. San Felipe, Jesus Maria, Lima 14, Peru

Hans-Christoph Pape Department of Orthopaedic Trauma, University of Aachen Medical Center, Aachen, Germany

V. Manakavala Perumal, M.D. PWD Road, Chettikulam Junction, Nagercoil, Tamil Nadu, India

Craig S. Roberts, M.D., M.B.A. Department of Orthopaedics, University Hospital Louisville, Louisville, KY, USA

Laura Ruhala, M.D. Department of Engineering, University of Southern Indiana, Evansville, IN, USA

David Seligson, M.D. Department of Orthopaedics, University Hospital Louisville, Louisville, KY, USA

Madhusudhan Yakkanti Department of Orthopaedic Surgery, University Hospital Louisville, Louisville, KY, USA

Jonathan Yerasimides Department of Orthopaedics, University Hospital Louisville, Louisville, KY, USA

G. Zych Department of Orthopaedic Trauma, University of Miami Leonard M Miller School of Medicine, Miami, FL, USA

Chapter 1
Damage Control Orthopedics in the Polytrauma Patient

Hans-Christoph Pape, Thomas Dienstknecht, and Peter V. Giannoudis

1.1 Introduction

Trauma continues to represent the major cause of death in patients under the age of 40. Especially road traffic injuries are the leading cause of death in high-income countries among young people aged 5–29 years [1]. The severity of consequent illness and the resulting disability is high compared with other disease processes [2, 3]. In 1998, about 5.8 million people died worldwide from accidental injuries [4]. In the United States, 12,400 people die each month following trauma [5].

Early mortality after severe trauma is either due to head trauma or exsanguination due to uncontrolled hemorrhage or late from multiple organ dysfunction syndrome (MODS). Once multiple systems are altered, the mortality rates may exceed 50%, the morbidity in survivors is severe, and the health care costs are enormous [2, 6].

1.2 Definition of Polytrauma

Polytrauma is defined as injury to at least two organ systems that cause a potentially life-threatening condition. Oftentimes, patients with an injury severity score (ISS) greater than or equal to 16 have been classified as polytraumatized, and it has been proposed that all such patients should be cared for in a designated trauma center [7].

H.-C. Pape (✉) • T. Dienstknecht
Department of Orthopaedic Trauma, University of Aachen Medical Center, Aachen, Germany
e-mail: hpape@ukaachen.de

P.V. Giannoudis
Department of Trauma & Orthopaedic Surgery, School of Medicine, University of Leeds, Leeds, UK

D. Seligson et al. (eds.), *External Fixation in Orthopedic Traumatology*,
DOI 10.1007/978-1-4471-2197-8_1,

1.3 Evolution of Care of the Multiply Injured Trauma Patient

Surgical stabilization of long bone fractures was not routinely performed before the 1950s. The patient with multiple fractures was not considered physiologically stable enough to withstand a prolonged surgical procedure because of the assumption that early manipulation of long bone fractures would release fat and intramedullary contents into the peripheral circulation and result in fat embolism syndrome [8, 9].

The splinting of femoral fractures with the use of Thomas splint, however, illustrated the importance and benefits of skeletal stabilization resulting in improved patient survival [10]. The positive effect of skeletal stabilization became even more apparent with the implementation of standardized techniques of internal fixation by the AO group [11]. Despite these early observations, operative techniques were not universally adopted and for several years the philosophy prevailed that the injured patient was "too sick to operate on." Instead, the patient was kept in skeletal traction with enforced recumbency. In addition, the reports that fracture healing would be promoted faster if the operation was not performed acutely led to the recommendations to delay surgery up to 14 days after the injury [12, 13].

In the 1970s, pioneering studies showed that early skeletal stabilization of femoral fractures dramatically reduced the incidence of traumatic pulmonary failure and postoperative complications [14, 15]. Evidence of the beneficial effects of early operative fracture stabilization (within 24 h of injury) was further supported by other studies that followed. Not surprisingly, the greatest benefits of early fracture stabilization were shown in patients who had sustained the most severe injuries [16, 17].

Despite this gathering evidence, the orthopedic mindset did not change until the late 1980s when Bone et al. showed the beneficial effect of early fracture stabilization on both morbidity and length of hospital stay [18]. This study firmly established the early surgical stabilization of long bone fractures. This new philosophy in the management of the patient with multiple injuries was named Early Total Care (ETC). The previously held belief among surgeons that the patient was "too sick to operate on" was now replaced with the opposite belief that the patient was "too sick *not* to operate on."

Early total care became the gold standard treatment in orthopedic trauma surgery. Developments in intensive care medicine supported this more aggressive surgical approach to the injured patient. Early total care represented a giant step forward in the management of the multiply injured patient. The advantages for countless patients who were able to ambulate early and be discharged from hospital more quickly avoiding the complications associated with prolonged bed rest have been well documented in several studies [19–21].

In the early 1990s, a variety of unexpected complications related to the early stabilization of long bone fractures appeared in the literature. The dogma of the benefits of early total care was increasingly questioned. It was suggested that the operative procedure used to stabilize the long bones, in most cases a reamed intramedullary nail, could provoke pulmonary complications rather than protect against them. The findings of a multicenter study by the AO foundation reinforced this concern [22]. An unexpectedly high rate of pulmonary complications was reported in young patients after reamed femoral intramedullary nailing without suffering thoracic trauma [22]. The authors concluded that the method of stabilization and the timing of surgery may have played a major role in the development of these complications.

An increasing number of reports continued to appear in the literature describing an adverse outcome after ETC including an increased incidence of adult respiratory distress syndrome (ARDS) and multiple organ dysfunction syndrome (MODS) [23, 24]. These complications most often were developed in selected patient groups, particularly those with severe chest injuries and following severe hemodynamic shock states [25–27]. The findings of these studies created a lot of controversy and the belief that ETC was not the answer for all multiply injured patients and that there was a particular subgroup of patients in whom it was actually detrimental to their outcome to be managed by this approach. The clinical difficulty in judging the acute setting in which patients could safely undergo early total care stimulated the creation of a specific subgroup of patients who were at high risk of deterioration after extensive surgery. On the basis of both clinical and laboratory findings, these patients were described as the "borderline patient" or the "patient at risk" [28]. This terminology reflects the treating physician's awareness of the potential for the development of unexpected complications.

Today it is clear that both the type and severity of injury (first hit phenomenon) predisposes the borderline patient to deterioration after surgery. Furthermore, the type of surgery (second hit phenomenon) poses a varying burden on the patient's biological reserve (individual biological response) and may predispose them to an adverse outcome. Clearly, only one of the above factors can be currently modulated by medical treatment (second hit phenomenon – type of surgical treatment). This entails that the impact of inappropriate clinical decisions may have a detrimental effect on the well-being of the patient. This predicament creates a dilemma for the surgeon. The patient was "too sick not to operate on" to provide skeletal stabilization, but when should this fracture fixation be performed and what procedure should be used?

Rapidly it became evident that the inability to quantify not only the biological impact of the initial injury but also the additional impact of the surgical procedure is important. The crude clinical parameters used did not reflect the impact of the surgical load on the inflammatory system. Recently, advances in molecular medicine allow the measurement of pro-inflammatory cascades during surgery and highlight the importance of inflammatory mediators in the response to trauma [29–32]. Numerous reports were able to demonstrate that surgery in fact caused a variety of subclinical changes in the inflammatory system that could become clinically relevant and have a cumulative effect if several impacts were added [33–35].

The concept of damage control orthopedics (DCO) for the management of the polytraumatized patient was born in trying to answer the questions of when to operate and how in the severely injured patient and through a better understanding of the inflammatory response to trauma [36]. The era of damage control orthopedics started in the mid 1990s, with reports of temporary external fixation of femoral shaft fractures in multiply injured patients, and continues over 10 years later [37–39].

Table 1.1 Definition of the borderline patient

• ISS > 40
• Hypothermia below 35°C
• Initial mean pulmonary arterial pressure >24 mmHg or a >6 mmHg rise in pulmonary artery pressure during intramedullary nailing or other operative intervention
• Multiple injuries (ISS > 20) in association with thoracic trauma (AIS > 2)
• Multiple injuries in association with severe abdominal or pelvic injury and hemorrhagic shock at presentation (systolic BP < 90 mmHg)
• Radiographic evidence of pulmonary contusion
• Patients with bilateral femoral fracture
• Patients with moderate or severe head injuries (AIS 3 or greater)

1.4 Grading of Patient's Condition

Knowledge of treatment algorithms is of paramount importance to avoid distraction from occult life-threatening problems. An example of this is missed intra-abdominal exsanguination while managing severe extremity injuries. The trauma team has to quickly ascertain the extent of the injury as well as assess the pulmonary status and overall hemodynamic status of the patient. Standardized diagnostic and operative tactics should be applied and coordinated to avoid mistakes that could impact negatively on the patient's prognosis. During the treatment course, the clinical scenario can change rapidly and management plans must be able to adapt accordingly. Therefore, the clinical judgment of the patient's condition is crucial. All patients should be placed into one of four categories (stable, borderline, unstable, in extremis) in order to guide the subsequent approach to their care. This is done on the basis of overall injury severity, the presence of specific injuries, and current hemodynamic status as described before [40].

a. Stable condition
   Stable patients have no immediately life-threatening injuries, respond to initial fluid therapy, and are hemodynamically stable without isotropic support. They are not hypothermic. There is no evidence of physiological disturbance such as coagulopathy or respiratory distress nor ongoing occult hypo-perfusion manifested as abnormalities of acid base status.
b. Borderline condition
   Borderline patients have stabilized in response to initial resuscitative attempts but have clinical features or combinations of injury, which have been associated with poor outcome and at risk of rapid deterioration. The borderline patient is well-defined (Table 1.1).
c. Unstable condition
   Patients who are hemodynamically unstable despite initial intervention are at greatly increased risk of rapid deterioration, subsequent multiple organ failure,

and death. Treatment in these cases utilizes a "damage control" approach. This entails rapid life-saving surgery only as absolutely necessitated and timely transfer to the intensive care unit for further stabilization and monitoring. Temporary stabilization of fractures using external fixation, hemorrhage control, and exteriorization of gastrointestinal injuries when possible is advocated. Complex reconstructive procedures should be delayed until stability is achieved and the acute immuno-inflammatory response to injury has subsided. This rationale is intended to reduce the magnitude of the "second hit" of operative intervention, or at least delay it until the patient is physiologically equipped to cope.

d. In extremis
Patients in extremis are very close to death having suffered severe injuries, and often have ongoing uncontrolled blood loss. They remain severely unstable despite ongoing resuscitative efforts and are usually suffering the effects of the "deadly triad" of hypothermia, acidosis, and coagulopathy. In these patients, life-threatening injuries are treated first, and definitive surgical repair is delayed and performed later if the patient survives.

1.5 Molecular Aspects of Damage Control Orthopedics

In the early 1970s, Tilney et al. were given credit for first describing sequential failure of multiple organs in 18 consecutive patients with ruptured abdominal aortic aneurysm who required postoperative hemodialysis [41]. These authors concluded that this was the result of a combination of pre-existing disease and hemorrhagic shock. Eisman et al. introduced the term "multiple organ failure" to describe the clinical course of 42 patients with progressive organ failure; half of these patients had an intra-abdominal abscess implicated as the inciting event [42]. Thus, sepsis was added to the list of risk factors for MODS. Subsequently, Fry et al. retrospectively reviewed 553 patients who required emergency operations; two-thirds had sustained major trauma. Thirty-eight (7%) patients developed MODS; 90% were septic. The authors proposed that MODS was a fatal expression of uncontrolled infection. This led to an aggressive policy of mandatory laparotomy to rule out intra-abdominal abscess [43].

Faist et al. published a review of 433 trauma patients who required emergency operations (99% blunt mechanism); 50 (12%) developed ARDS and 34 (8%) developed MODS [44]. The authors described two distinct patterns of MODS: rapid single-phase MODS due to massive tissue injury and shock or delayed two-phase MODS due to moderate trauma and shock followed by delayed sepsis. Goris et al. reviewed 92 MODS patients who had clinical signs of sepsis [45]. They separated these patients into two groups: 55 trauma patients (all blunt mechanism) versus 37 non-trauma patients who had undergone emergency laparotomy. Bacterial sepsis was confirmed in only 33% of the trauma-related MODS patients, compared with 65% of the non-trauma patients [45]. At the same time, Norton showed that drainage of an abdominal abscess reverses MODS in a disappointingly small proportion of patients [46]. Thus, the above clinical observations suggested that MODS frequently may occur in the absence of infection; the inflammatory system was implicated as a causative factor.

It is known today that the activation of the inflammatory system is the norm after traumatic injury and leads to the development of the systemic inflammatory response syndrome (SIRS). This is followed by a period of recovery mediated by counter-regulatory anti-inflammatory response (CARS) [47]. It appears that the key players in this host inflammatory response are the cytokines, the leukocytes, the endothelium, and subsequent leukocyte–endothelial cell interactions. Reactive oxygen species, eicosanoids, and microcirculatory disturbances also play pivotal roles [48].

Within this inflammatory process, a fine balance exists between the beneficial effects of inflammation and the potential for the process itself to cause and aggravate tissue injury leading to ARDS and MODS. If this inflammatory response is exaggerated or perpetuated, patients enter a state of malignant systemic inflammation (moderate or severe SIRS) that can evolve into overt ARDS/MODS. In these patients, pulmonary failure occurs first, then the other organs fail because the lungs are either more vulnerable or our clinical tools to detect lung failure are more sensitive. Proposed mechanisms for the non-septic (inflammatory) development of MODS include:

(a) The macrophage theory (increased production of cytokines and other inflammatory mediators by activated macrophages).
(b) Microcirculatory theory (prolonged hypovolemic shock promotes MODS through inadequate global oxygen delivery, ischemia reperfusion phenomena).
(c) Endothelial cell–leukocyte interactions leading to remote organ injury.
(d) Gut hypothesis (gut origin bacteria or their products contribute to MODS. It has been used to explain why no obvious site of infection can be found in as many as 30% of the bacteremic patients who die from MODS).
(e) One- and two-hit theory.

In the one-hit model, the initial injury and shock give rise to an intense systemic inflammatory response with the potential for remote organ injury. In the two-hit model, the initial stimulus is less intense and normally resolves but the patient is vulnerable to a secondary inflammatory insult that can reactivate the systemic inflammatory response and precipitate late multiple organ dysfunction. Secondary insults to the inflammatory system in the two-hit model can be caused by surgical procedures and sepsis.

Significant overlap exists in the different inflammatory theories for the development of MODS. In most patients, irrespective of the triggering event, MODS follows a predictable course, generally beginning with the lungs and progressing to liver, gastrointestinal tract, and kidney. The mortality rate progressively rises from 20% with one failed organ system to 100% when four systems fail [43].

As a result of the popularity of the above theories and the availability of techniques to measure inflammatory mediators, many researchers designed studies searching for inflammatory markers that could detect patients in the "borderline condition" being at risk of developing post-traumatic complications and thus by altering the treatment plan to be able to prevent the onset of adverse sequelae. Numerous studies have demonstrated that stimulation of a variety of inflammatory mediators takes place in the immediate aftermath following trauma [30, 34, 35, 49].

Table 1.2 Classification of serum inflammatory markers

Group	Serum inflammatory markers
Acute phase reactants	LBP, CRP, Procalcitonin
Mediator activity	TNF, IL-1, IL-6, IL-10, IL-18
Cellular activity	TNF-RI, TNF-RII, IL-1RI, IL-1RII, sIL-6R, mIL-6R, ICAM-1 Eselectin, CD11b, Elastase, HLA-DR class II antigens, DNA

This response initially corresponds to the first-hit phenomenon. Several investigators have also highlighted the issue of secondary surgical procedures acting as additional inflammatory insults, second-hit phenomenon [50, 51]. These models (first and second hit) of biological response to different stimuli have now become the basis of our treatment plans and investigations.

At the molecular level, a variety of inflammatory mediators have been implicated in the pathogenesis of organ dysfunction. Serum markers of immune reactivity can be selectively grouped into markers of a) acute phase reactants, b) markers of mediator activity, and c) markers of cellular activity (Table 1.2).

Currently, only two markers, IL-6 and HLA-DR class II molecules, can accurately predict the clinical course and outcome of the traumatized patient. Although measurement of IL-6 is routinely used in several trauma centers, the HLA-DR class II marker has not gained great acceptance because of the laboratory processing required [52, 53]. Regarding the risk of septic complications in trauma patients, procalcitonin can serve as a prognostic parameter [53].

1.6 Patient Selection for Damage Control Orthopedics Based on Physiological Parameters

As outlined above, the patient's condition may range from clinically stable to a state named "in extremis," where there is imminent danger of death. Patients in extremis have been well-classified by general surgeons (early blood loss of 4–5 L, a core temperature of 34°C, and a pH of less than 7.25) [54]. The primary goal in the unstable and in extremis situations is to prevent the lethal triad (hypothermia, coagulopathy, and acidosis).

Definitions of the patient's condition following the initial ATLS assessment would dictate the early pathway of the patient (Fig. 1.1). However, this pathway is governed by the physiological state of the patient in terms of hemodynamic stability.

Several conventional markers exist to assist the clinician to stratify the patient to one of the four groups previously mentioned (stable, unstable, borderline, in extremis).

In addition to those parameters described for the borderline patient (Table 1.1), the following clinical parameters define the status of the patient in the emergency room:

(i) *Shock*: Patients presenting with a systolic blood pressure <90 mmHg have to be regarded as volume depleted. Likewise, vasopressor dependency and low urinary

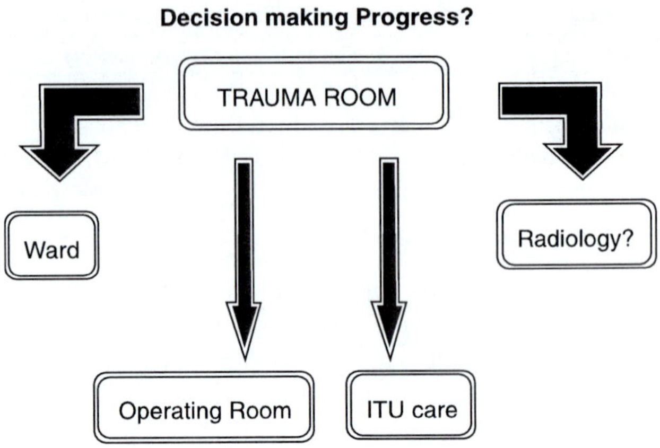

Fig. 1.1 Dispensation pathway of the traumatized patient

output are important. In young patients who have excellent compensatory mechanisms, an increased heart rate may be an important sign if the systolic pressure is about 100 mmHg. These patients may temporarily compensate a low cardiac output by a tachycardia for some time and then deteriorate acutely.

(ii) *Hypothermia*: Decreased body temperature has long been known as a signal for various complications (cardiac arrhythmias, cardiac arrest, coagulopathy). The most important lower limit is a core temperature of <33°C.

(iii) *Coagulopathy*: In addition, the hemostatic response can be of value. The most simple and rapidly available parameter in the emergency room is the platelet count. Initial platelet values <90,000 are a sign of impending disseminated intravascular coagulopathy (DIC), if no other cause of coagulopathy is present.

(iv) *Soft tissue injuries*: The effects of severe extremity soft tissue lesions usually do not become evident until days after injury. The same holds true for lung contusions. Quantification of soft tissue injury to the extremities and the lungs continues to be a challenge.

The initial patient assessment can be structured according to the four categories described above. The parameters of these four cascades to be remembered are summarized in the following phrase: soft tissue injuries (major extremity fractures, crush injuries, severe pelvic fractures, lung contusions, AIS > 2), coagulopathy (platelets < 90,000), and shock (systolic BP < 90 mmHg, requirement of vasopressors) contribute to hypothermia (core temperature < 33°C), and are dangerous (Table 1.3). Fortunately, the majority of patients belong to the group classified as "stable" or to the "borderline" patient group (grade I or II if stable after resuscitation) who can be safely stabilized during the course of the emergency treatment. These patients should be submitted to early fracture stabilization in order to benefit from the advantages of this approach. If patients are in an unstable condition or do not respond to resuscitation at all (grade II if uncertain after resuscitation, III, IV), they should not undergo prolonged surgical therapy and their fractures should be treated by early temporary measures, such as external fixation. Arbitrary threshold values are documented that indicate a high risk situation on admission and during the further course with regard to the development of organ dysfunction (Table 1.4).

Table 1.3 Parameters for evaluation of patient's condition

	Parameter indicative of high risk patients		Parameter indicative of high risk patients	
Patho-physiology	Admission (day 1)	Time to normalization in case of an uneventful course	Clinical course (>day 2)	Comment
Shock	BP < 90 mmHg >5 blood Units/2 h Lactate >2.5 mmol/l Base excess >8 mmol/L	<1 day	Catecholamine dependency >2 days	Irrelevant after resuscitation
Coagulation	Platelet count <90,000	1–2 days	>3 days below 100,000 or failure to increase	Simple parameter, good indicator
Core temperature	<33°C	Hours	Irrelevant after rewarming	Irrelevant after rewarming
Soft tissue injuries	$PaO_2/FiO_2 < 300$ Lung contusions, AIS > 2 Chest trauma score; TTS > II Abd. trauma (Moore > II) Complex pelvic trauma	<2–4 days	$PaO_2/FiO_2 < 300$ for >2 days Pathological extravascular lung water (>10 mL/kg BW)	Lung function often close to normal for 2–3 days (PaO_2/FiO_2 > 300)

1.7 Patient Selection for Damage Control Orthopedics Based on Injury Complexes

Specific orthopedic injury complexes are considered today as appropriate to damage control orthopedics in a patient with polytrauma including the presence of pelvic fractures associated with hemorrhage, femoral fractures, multiple long bone fractures, mangled extremities, traumatic brain injury, and severe chest trauma.

The geriatric, multiply injured patient with compromised biological reserve is also another indication for application of the damage control principle.

1.7.1 Pelvic Fractures

The overall prevalence of pelvic fractures presenting with hemodynamic instability has been reported to range from 2% to 20% [55–60]. Errors in early management may lead to significant increases in mortality. Early recognition and appropriate

Table 1.4 Parameters indicative of high-risk patients

	Parameter	Stable (grade I)	Borderline (grade II)	Unstable (grade III)	In extremis (grade IV)
Shock	• Blood pressure (mmHg)	100 or more	80–100	60–90	<50–60
	• Blood units (2 h)	0–2	2–8	5–15	>15
	• Lactate levels	Normal range	Around 2.5	>2.5	Severe acidosis
	• Base deficit mmol/l	Normal range	No data	No data	>6–8
	• ATLS classification	I	II–III	III–IV	IV
Coagulation	• Platelet count (μg/ml)	>110,000	90,000–110,000	<70,000–90,000	<70,000
	• Factor II and V (%)	90–100	70–80	50–70	<50
	• Fibrinogen (g/dl)	>1	Around 1	<1	DIC
	• D-Dimer	Normal range	Abnormal	Abnormal	DIC
Temperature		>34°C	33–35°C	30–32°C	30°C or less
Soft tissue injuries	• Lung function; PaO_2/FiO_2	350–400	300–350	200–300	<200
	• Chest trauma scores; AIS	AIS I or II	AIS 2 or more	AIS 2 or more	AIS 3 or more
	• Chest trauma score; TTS	0	I–II	II–III	IV
	• Abdominal trauma (Moore)	<II	<III	III	III or >III
	• Pelvic trauma (AO class.)	A type (AO)	B or C	C	C (crush, rollover abd.)
	• Extremities	AIS I–II	AIS II–III	AIS III–IV	Crush, rollover extrem.
Surgical strategy	Damage control (DCO) or Definitive surgery (ETC)	ETC	DCO if uncertain ETC if stable	DCO	DCO

management of patients within this group can therefore offer significant improvements in outcome.

Patients with pelvic fractures in an "unstable" or "in extremis" clinical condition who undergo prolonged operative interventions could initiate a series of reactions at the molecular level, predisposing the patient to an adverse outcome. Any surgical intervention here must be considered immediately life saving and should therefore be simple, quick, and well performed. Protocols designed to reduce mortality should stop bleeding, detect and control associated injuries, and restore hemodynamics. A staged diagnostic and therapeutic approach is required. During the first 24 h, death from exsanguination has been identified as a major cause of mortality. The severity of bleeding is a crucial hallmark for survival during the early period after injury. In young patients who are able to compensate for extensive blood loss for several hours, underestimation of the true hemodynamic status can lead to fatal outcome. Because of the disastrous hemodynamic conditions of these patients, only external devices that are easy to apply can be used effectively. These devices, by external compression, reduce the intrapelvic volume and create a tamponade effect against ongoing bleeding. They also restore stability and bone contact to the posterior elements of the pelvis and contribute to blood clotting. Pelvic packing should be considered in cases where, despite the application of the external fixator, ongoing bleeding is encountered. In this situation, angiographic embolization is both time consuming and inhibitive to dynamic assessment and further treatment. Pelvic packing allows the simultaneous assessment and treatment of abdominal injuries. In the presence of multiple massive bleeding points, tamponade of the areas or temporary aortic compression should be considered. Complex reconstructive procedures in the abdomen should be avoided in the presence of pelvic hemorrhage. A major splenic rupture usually necessitates splenectomy. In liver injuries, attention is paid only to major vessels and hepatic tamponade is applied. Bowel injuries are clamped and covered and definitive treatment performed after the hemodynamic situation is stabilized [61–64].

Angiographic embolization is not usually indicated in this patient population. However, in cases where hemodynamic stability with volume replacement can be achieved but ongoing pelvic hemorrhage is suspected (expanding hematoma), then angiography could be considered as an adjunct to the treatment protocol [65, 66].

Damage control orthopedics is the current treatment of choice for the severely injured patient with an unstable pelvic ring injury and hemodynamic instability.

1.7.2 Lower Extremity Injuries (Bilateral Femoral Shaft Fractures – Intra-articular Fractures – Mangled Extremity)

Certain injuries have been observed to occur more frequently in patients who go on to develop systemic complications. Among the long bone injuries, femoral shaft fracture has been associated with an increased risk of adverse outcome. This appears to be based on the fact that the femoral shaft fracture is the most frequent long bone fracture in polytrauma patients and is associated with high velocity impact and soft tissue damage and blood loss (the femoral shaft is surrounded by the largest soft tissue envelope of any long bone).

All extremity fractures must be considered with the associated hemorrhage and local soft tissue injuries [67]. The injury initiates a local inflammatory response with increased systemic concentrations of pro-inflammatory cytokines. Cytokine levels correlate with the degree of tissue damage and the incidence of osseous fractures. This suggests that injury plays a major role in determining the release of these pro-inflammatory mediators [67]. Concentrations of inflammatory cytokines in injured tissue have been measured at many times supporting our understanding that they are locally generated [68, 69].

The importance of these entities is supported by the fact that patients with bilateral femoral shaft fractures have demonstrated a compound higher morbidity and mortality rate (16% vs. 4% for isolated femoral injuries) (Fig. 1.2) [70]. A quantitative event in terms of local and systemic cytokine release and fat embolization has been suggested [71], although Copeland et al. reported that the increase in mortality may be related to associated injuries rather than to bilateral femoral fracture itself [72].

With these facts in mind, it seems clear that multiply injured patients with extremity injuries should also benefit from a damage control strategy. The associated soft tissue injury rather than acute hemorrhage appears to be most important in initiation of the systemic response. Prolonged fracture manipulation in the presence of severe soft tissue injury may cause further damage and increase systemic delivery of inflammatory mediators [67].

Another indication for application of the damage control principle is the case where a complex intra-articular injury is present either in isolation or in a polytrauma setting. Injuries that are amenable to this approach are fragmented proximal and distal tibial fractures, distal femoral fractures, and supracondylar distal humeral fractures. The application of a spanning external fixator is useful for preventing further soft tissue damage and organizing CT scanning where appropriate to assist the surgeon with the preoperative planning (Fig. 1.3).

The mangled extremity is a special entity for consideration for DCO. Advances in microvascular techniques allowed for reliable repair of vascular and nerve injuries, which usually accompany severe open fractures of the lower limbs. The introduction of free-flap transfer with microvascular techniques in the early 1970s constituted a major breakthrough in the treatment of open fractures with severe soft-tissue defects and limb ischemia [73]. Nevertheless, certain concerns have been posed as to whether a salvaged limb can always function better than a prosthesis [74, 75]. Hence, various scoring systems have been developed in an effort to reliably determine which limbs are salvageable or not [76, 77]. The most commonly used grading system is the Mangled Extremity Severity Score (MESS) [78]. In a study by Helfet et al., a MESS score of 7 or higher had a 100% predictive value for amputation [79]. The predictive value of MESS, though, was challenged in a study, as it was found that it lacked sensitivity [80]. It is thus obvious that, even with the use of the available scoring systems, the decision as to whether to perform a limb salvage operation over amputation, in severe open fractures, is not an easy one. Scoring systems can help in the decision-making process;

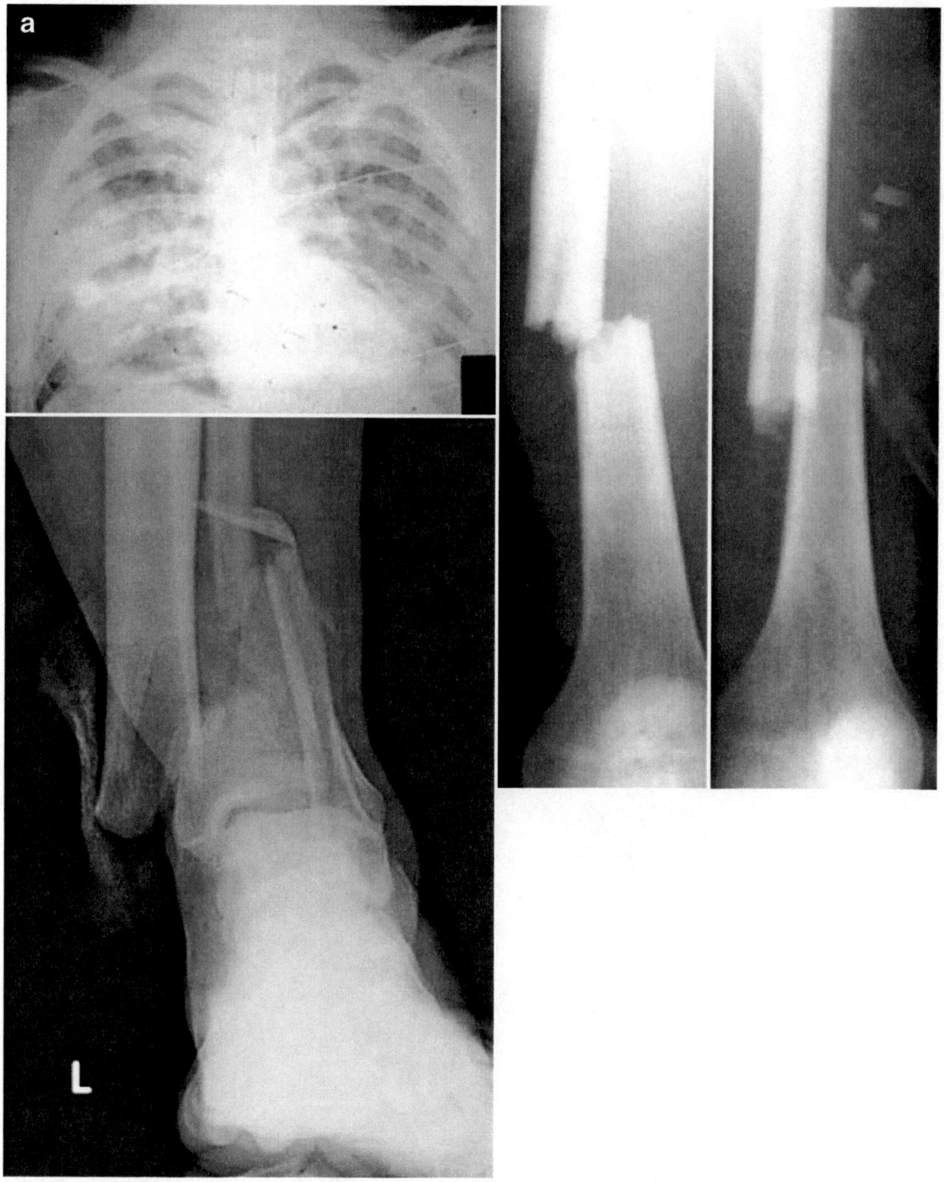

Fig. 1.2 (**a**) Polytraumatized patient with bilateral femoral shaft fracture, chest injury, and left distal tibial pilon fracture. (**b**) Temporary stabilization of fractures with external fixators. (**c**) Definitive reconstruction was performed and physiological state of the patient was normalized: at day 5 of the femur and day 10 of the pilon fracture

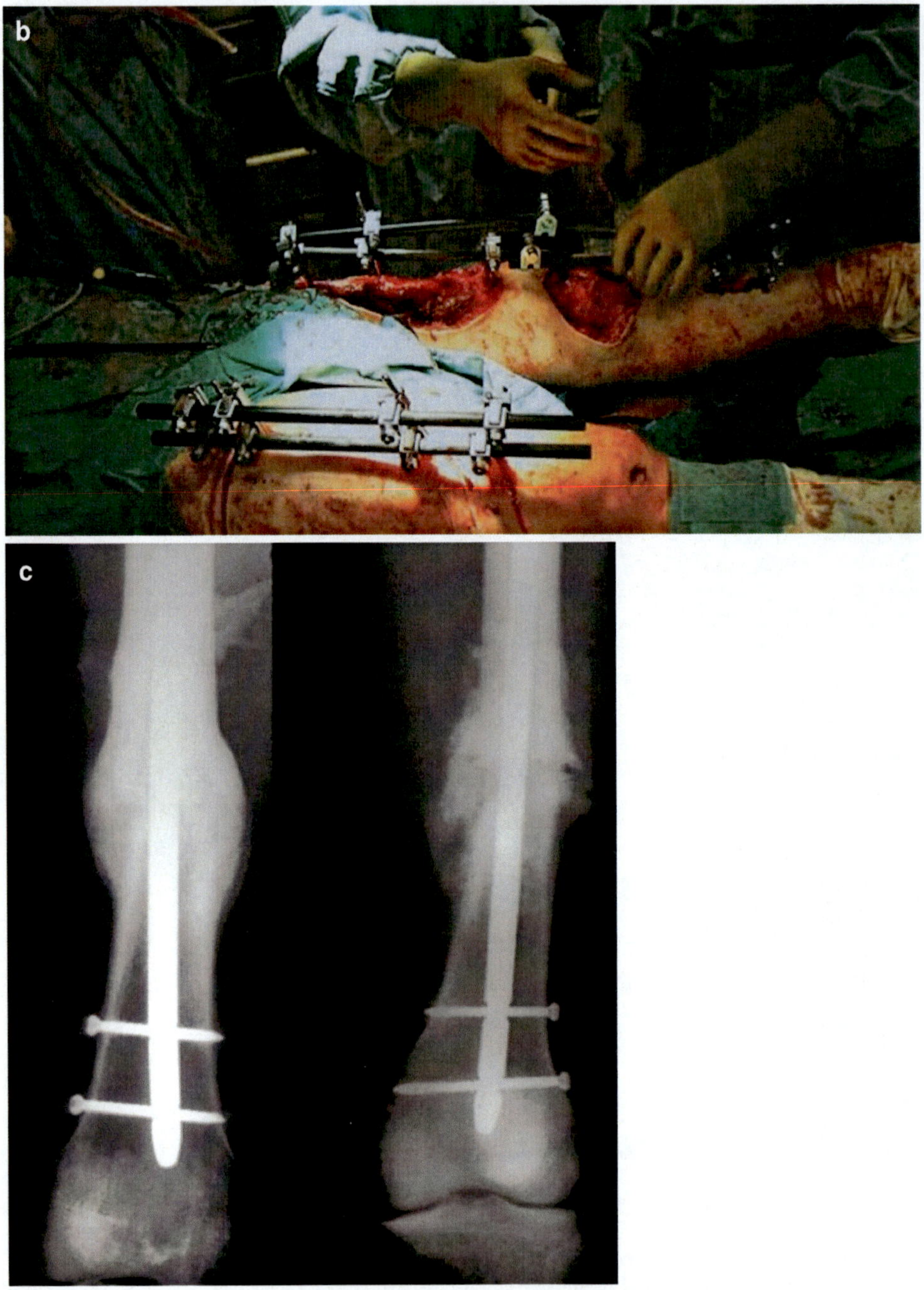

Fig. 1.2 (continued)

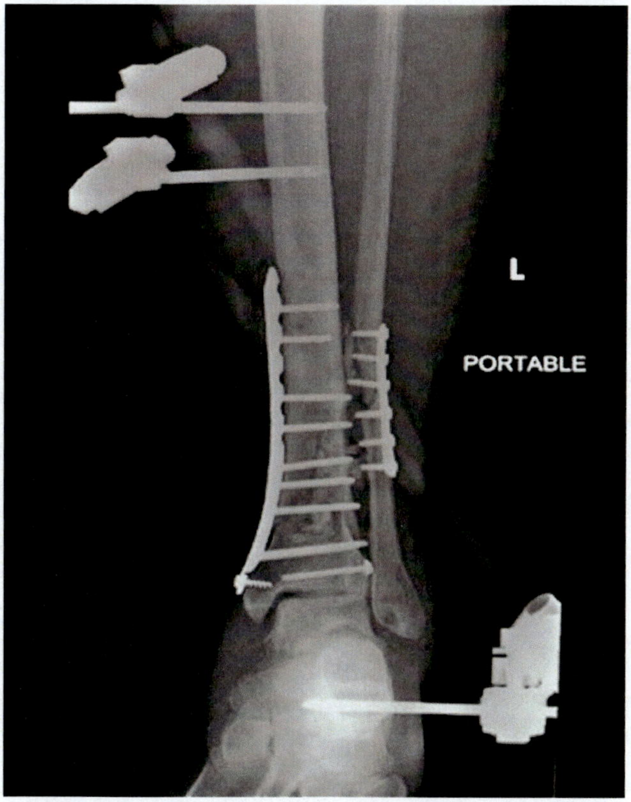

Fig. 1.2 (continued)

however, the decision about the surgical treatment should involve at least two senior surgeons experienced in modern limb salvage techniques [81, 82]. The Lower Extremity Assessment Project (LEAP) study, a multicenter, prospective, observational study, found that reconstruction and limb salvage typically results in 2-year outcomes equivalent to those of amputation for high energy (Gustilo grade IIIB and IIIC and selected IIIA fractures) below the distal femur [83]. Interestingly, there was no significant difference in the scores on the Sickness Impact Profile (SIP) between the patients treated with above-the-knee and those treated with below-the-knee amputation. Patients treated with a through-the-knee amputation had worse regression-adjusted SIP scores and slower self-selected walking speeds than either a below-the-knee amputation or an above-the-knee amputation. It appears that the disability persists in these cases. At 7-year follow-up, MacKenzie and Bosse [84] reported that patients that reported low self-efficacy, weak social support, and high levels of depression, anxiety, and pain were significantly more likely to have poor outcomes.

A damage control orthopedics approach to saving the limb could assist in terms of making it possible to improve the surgeon-controlled variables relating to better outcomes. The efficacy of the protocol of spanning external fixation, antibiotic bead pouches, and the vacuum-assisted wound closure technique has been well described providing stage reconstruction in difficult clinical scenarios [85–87].

1.7.3 Brain – Chest Injury – Geriatric Patient

The timing of stabilization of long bone fractures in trauma patients with associated severe traumatic brain injury has been a topic of ongoing discussion for several years. In patients with a significant closed head injury, the treatment and protection of the central nervous system is a priority due to the sensitivity and vulnerability of the injured brain to further insult (primary and secondary brain damage). On the one hand, early definitive fracture stabilization could be beneficial in the head-injured patient by reducing pain at the fracture site, thereby minimizing involuntary movements of the unconscious patient, which could cause further pain and autonomic disturbances. Fracture stabilization has a positive effect on the patient's metabolism, muscle tone, body temperature, and therefore cerebral function. On the other hand, unstabilized fractures

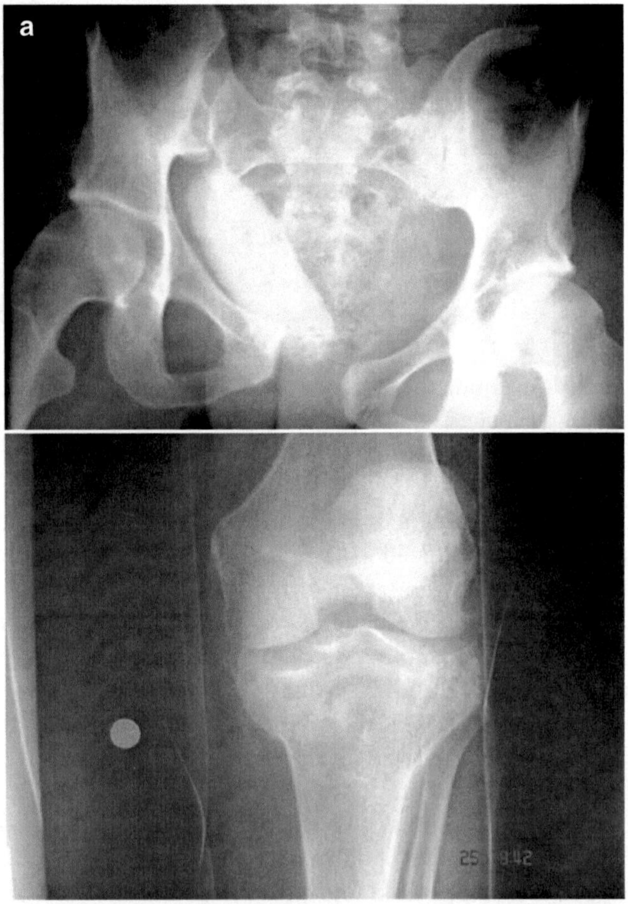

Fig. 1.3 (**a**) Polytraumatized patient with vertical shear pelvis fracture and left tibial plateau fracture. (**b**) Application of external fixator to pelvis and tibial plateau fracture. (**c**) Definitive reconstruction of the pelvic ring with plating of pubis symphysis and SI screws and double plating of the tibial plateau at days 5 and 8, respectively

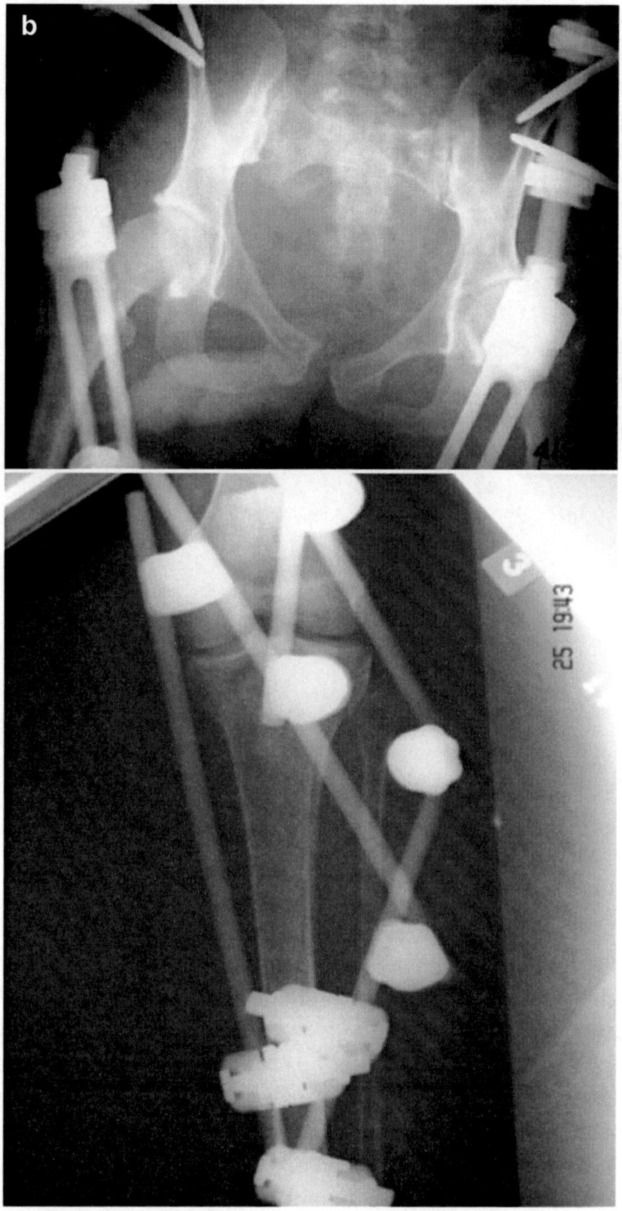

Fig. 1.3 (continued)

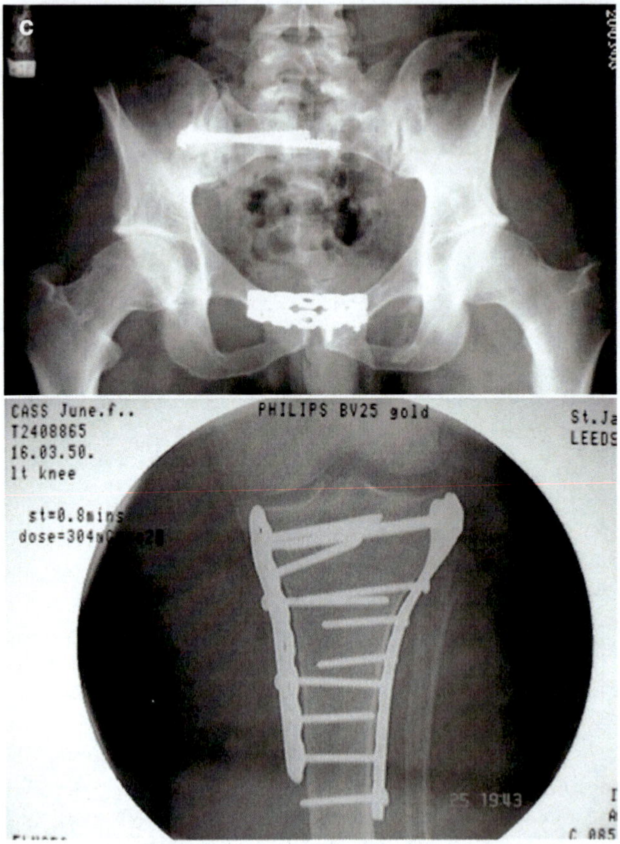

Fig. 1.3 (continued)

may cause deterioration in the patient's condition by exacerbating soft tissue damage, or the development of fat embolism and respiratory insufficiency [15, 25, 88].

By contrast, several authors have suggested that early fixation of fractures in patients with traumatic brain injury may be deleterious to the eventual neurological outcome and be associated with secondary brain injury [89, 90]. Numerous pathogenic mechanisms have been described for secondary brain injury [91, 92]. All are known to have the common final pathway of hypovolemia and hypoxia [93]. These factors can be exacerbated, in the short term, by injudicious fracture fixation, when intra-operative blood loss and hypoxia can compound the effects of inadequate resuscitation [94, 95].

In general terms, the management for unstable patients with traumatic brain injury should be based on the individual clinical assessment and treatment requirements, and in these cases damage control orthopedics can be beneficial by providing temporary fracture stabilization to an injured extremity followed by staged definitive osteosynthesis without compromising the patient's head injury. The following recommendations were recently made [96].

1. The initial management of the head-injured patient should be similar to that of the polytrauma patient without head injury, focusing on the rapid control of hemorrhage and the restoration of vital signs and tissue perfusion.

2. Initially, the severity of the head injury should be assessed by the Glasgow Coma Scale prior to administration of analgesia and sedation. Guidelines published by NICE should be followed to select patients for cranial CT scanning, with subsequent decisions based on these criteria.
3. Secondary brain damage should be avoided at all times. It may follow inadequate resuscitation or decreased MAP/increased ICP during operative interventions, such as long bone fixation.
4. In physiologically unstable patients, the treatment protocol should be based on individual clinical assessment and treatment requirements, rather than rigid, mandatory time policies in respect to fixation of long bone fractures. In such cases, the "damage control" approach should be considered.
5. ICP monitoring should be used according to the most recent guidelines.
6. ICP monitoring should be used not only on the intensive care unit, but also during operative procedures, since aggressive ICP management in these patients appears to be related to improved outcomes.
7. Maintenance of CPP > 60–70 mmHg and ICP <20 mmHg is mandatory before, during, and after the surgical procedures.
8. Musculoskeletal injuries should be managed aggressively, with the assumption that full neurological recovery will occur.

Also in polytraumatized patients, concerns have been raised about patients with associated chest trauma and extremity fractures. The lung seems to be the primary target for fat embolization and for mediated effects by inflammatory reactions. The latter are initiated in the immediate aftermath after injury, and femoral nailing can amplify these responses. The role of reaming in the context of early femoral fracture fixation in the patient with chest trauma is debatable. The dynamic nature of parenchymal lung injuries and the difficulty in early determination of injury severity are still significant problems in the decision-making process for the timing of fracture stabilization. Unexpected complications after ETC were observed in those patients whose injury severity was initially underestimated. The strict application of ETC, even in patients with a high ISS, or severe chest trauma, limited discussion of best management for these polytraumatized patients. Patients submitted to ETC during the last three decades have demonstrated a progressively lower ISS. It could be concluded that a more cautious approach regarding surgical treatment has been chosen. In some studies, favoring the concept of ETC, it is observed that primary fracture stabilization was only performed in multiply injured patients with a lower Injury Severity Score [97–99].

A selective approach should be used for patients with multiple injuries (long bone fractures) and a chest injury. The management of these patients should be individualized, and when early nailing is considered to increase the risk of complications the principle of damage control orthopedics should be applied with temporary external fixation of the femur followed by staged conversation within a week after the injury.

Finally, the treatment of the geriatric patient, being at high risk of early complications and mortality should also be considered within the framework of damage control orthopedics.

1.8 Efficacy of DCO and Timing of Secondary Procedures

The practice of delaying the definitive surgery in damage control orthopedics is an attempt to reduce the biological load of surgical trauma on the already traumatized patient (Fig. 1.4). In applying this approach to the management of multiple trauma, two of the most important issues is the efficacy of DCO and when is the right time to perform the secondary definitive surgery.

With regard to the efficacy of this approach, two studies have reported on the success of this approach in the management of multiply injured patients. Scalea et al. compared 43 patients treated initially with an external fixator to 284 patients treated with primary intramedullary nailing of the femur [37]. The patients treated with an external fixator were more severely injured than those treated with an intramedullary nail. They had a significantly higher Injury Severity Score (26.8 vs. 16.8) and lower Glasgow Coma Scale (11 vs. 14.2) and required significantly more fluid (11.9 vs. 6.2 L) and blood (1.5 vs. 1.0 L) administration in the initial 24 h. The median operation time was 35 min with an estimated blood loss of 90 mL versus 130 min and 400 mL blood loss in the external fixation and intramedullary nailing groups, respectively. Four patients in the external fixation group died (three from head injuries and one from acute organ failure) and one from the intramedullary nailing group. The authors concluded that external fixation was a safe, viable procedure to attain temporary rigid stabilization in patients with multiple injuries at risk of adverse outcome. In another study, Nowotarski et al. reported that the damage control orthopedics approach was a safe treatment method for fractures of the shaft of the femur in selected multiply injured patients [38].

Pape et al. has provided guidance with regard to the time interval that should be left between primary stabilization with an external fixator and definitive surgery [100]. The authors compared two groups of patients who had similar Injury Severity Score and Glasgow Coma Scale. In the first group early definitive surgery was performed, between 2 and 4 days, while in the second group late definitive surgery was performed, between 5 and 8 days, from the time of injury. Early definitive surgery was shown to have a higher incidence of multiple organ dysfunction as 46% of patients showed evidence of multiple organ dysfunction compared to 15.7% in the late surgery group ($p=0.01$). In the same study, further evidence on the optimal timing of surgery is provided from the assessment of the biological load of trauma and surgery, measured by the release of inflammatory mediators. The levels of the pro-inflammatory, cytokine interleukin 6 (IL-6) were measured on admission and at regular time intervals throughout treatment. Early secondary surgery was associated with an increased release of IL-6 when compared to late secondary surgery ($p=0.02$), and an admission IL-6 level of >500 pg/dL and early secondary surgery correlated positively with the development of multiple organ dysfunction ($p<0.001$). From these results, the conclusion was drawn that definitive surgery should be delayed until after the fourth day from initial injury.

In another study, this group sought to quantify the inflammatory response to initial surgery and conversion and link this to subsequent organ dysfunction and complications [101]. The authors reported that despite having significantly more severe injuries,

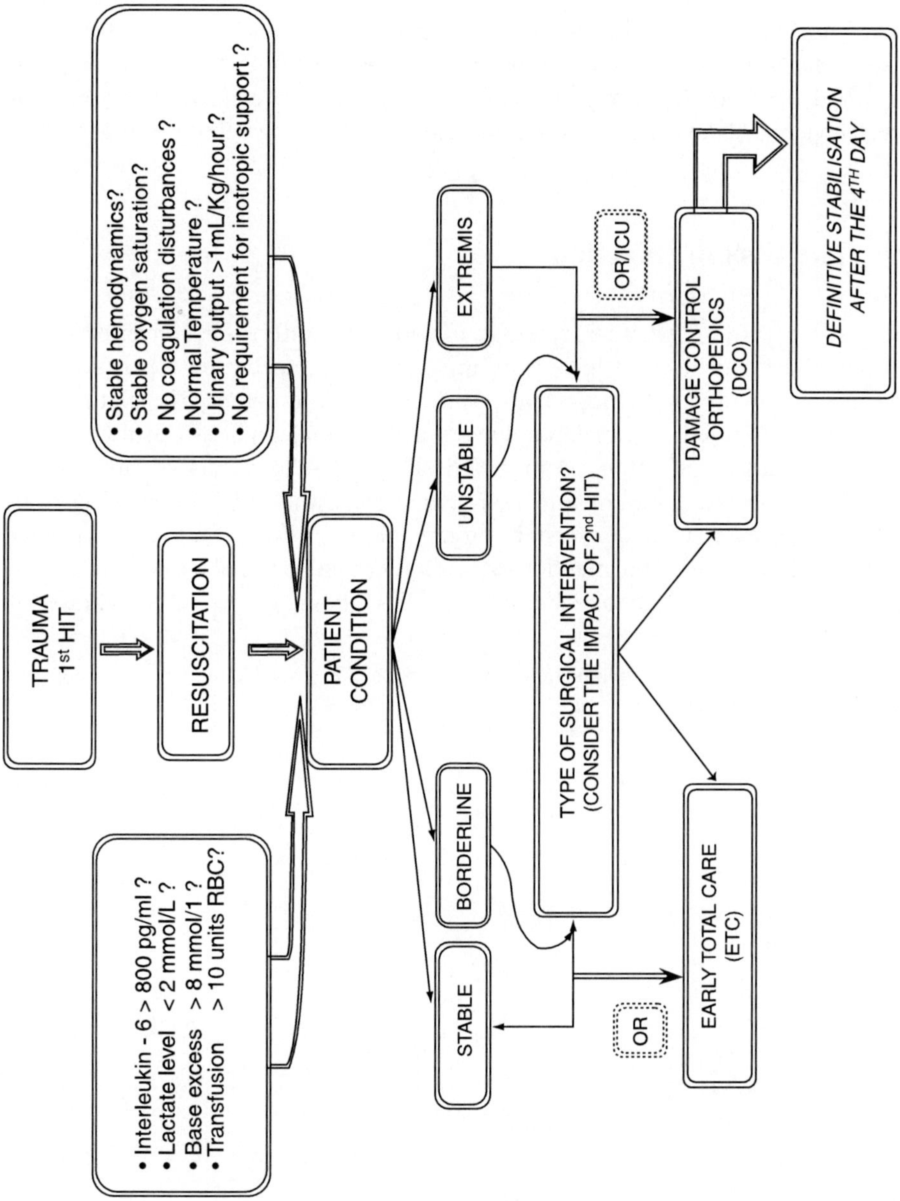

Fig. 1.4 Flowchart illustrating the concept of damage control orthopedics

patients in the DCO group had a smaller, shorter postoperative systemic inflammatory response and did not suffer significantly more pronounced organ failure than the IMN group. DCO patients undergoing conversion while their SIRS score was raised suffered the most pronounced subsequent inflammatory response and rise in organ failure score. The authors concluded that it would appear that to maximize the benefit of DCO, exchange procedures should be delayed until the patient's inflammatory response has subsided, where this is appropriate [101]. The available evidence therefore supports the view that days 2, 3, and 4 are not safe for performing definitive surgery.

1.9 The Risk of Infection

The issue regarding whether external fixation can safely be converted to an intramedullary nail without increasing infection rates has been a topic of debate for some time with conflicting results available in the literature. The first pioneer studies were focused on tibial fractures and the initial reported results showed quite high rates of infection, up to 44% [102, 103]. The results of later studies showed a much lower rate of infection after conversion with rates ranging from 4.8% to 6%, even with conversion surgery being delayed for up to 57 days (Table 1.5) [104–107]. The infection rates after femoral external fixator conversion are comparable with the two recent tibial studies, showing deep infection rates of

Table 1.5 The incidence of deep infection after conversion of external fixator to an intramedullary nail in the tibia and femur

Author and journal	Bone studied	Average length of time to conversion to IM nail (days)	Deep infection rate (%)
McGraw et al., JBJS 1988;70A:900–911 [102]	Tibia	59.5	44
Maurer et al., JBJS 1989; 71A:835–838 [103]	Tibia	65	25
Blachut et al., JBJS 1990; 72A:729–734 [104]	Tibia	17	5
Wheelwright et al., Injury 1993;23:373–375 [105]	Tibia	57	4.8
Antich et al., JBJS 1997; 79B:433–437 [106]	Tibia	14	6
Nowotarski et al., JBJS 2002;82A:781–788 [38]	Femur	7	1.7
Scalea et al., J Trauma 2000;48:613–623 [37]	Femur	5	3
Paderni et al., Chir Org Mov 2001;86:183–190 [107]	Tibia	92	5.3

1.7% and 3% [37, 38]. These results for femoral fractures are similar to the infection rates published for primary intramedullary nailing of the femur [108, 109]. The conclusion that can be drawn from these studies is that conversion of an external fixator to an intramedullary nail can be performed safely and that infection rates are not unacceptably high.

1.10 Conclusion

In attempting to reduce the biological load of trauma, surgeons are utilizing their increased knowledge of the inflammatory response to trauma and applying it in the operating room. In focusing on the effects surgery can have on the inflammatory system and the potential for some treatments to worsen the patients' overall condition, damage control orthopedics serves as a useful reminder to surgeons of the age-old importance of the medical dogma of "primum non nocere" or "do no further harm." Damage control orthopedics is a new and evolving practice, and although the available preliminary results are encouraging with regard to the efficacy and safety of this approach, further work is required to fully assess its effectiveness. In particular, research needs to be undertaken to establish whether using this approach improves the rates of morbidity and mortality and reduces the incidence of acute respiratory distress syndrome and multiple organ failure after multiple trauma.

References

1. Peden M, McGee K, Krug E, editors. Injury: a leading cause of the global burden of disease, 2000. Geneva: World Health Organization; 2002.
2. Holbrook TL, Anderson JP, Sieber WJ, Browner D, Hoyt DB. Outcome after major trauma: 12-month and 18-month follow-up results from the Trauma Recovery Project. J Trauma. 1999;46–5:765–71; discussion 71–3.
3. Gwinnutt CL, Driscoll PA, Whittaker J. Trauma systems – state of the art. Resuscitation. 2001;48–1:17–23.
4. Krug E. Injury: a leading cause of the global burden of disease. Geneva: World Health Organisation; 1999:WHO/HSC/P VI/99.11.
5. MacKenzie EJ, Fowler CJ. Epidemiology. In: Mattox KL, Feliciano DV, Moore EE, editors. Trauma 4th emergency department. New York: McGraw-Hill; 2000. p. 21.
6. Zhou Y, Baker TD, Rao K, Li G. Productivity losses from injury in China. Inj Prev. 2003;9–2:124–7.
7. Long WB, Bachulius BL, Hynes GD. Accuracy and relationship of mechanism of injury, trauma score and injury severity in identifying major trauma. Am J Surg. 1986;151:581–4.
8. Bradford DS, Foster RR, Nossel HL. Coagulation alterations, hypoxemia, and fat embolism in fracture patients. J Trauma. 1970;10:307–21.
9. Renne J, Wuthier R, House E, Cancro JC, Hoaglund FT. Fat macroglobulemia caused by fractures or total hip replacement. J Bone Joint Surg. 1978;60-A:613–8.
10. Henry BJ, Vrahas MS. The Thomas splint. Questionable boast of an indispensable tool. Am J Orthop (Belle Mead NJ). 1996;25(9):602–4.

11. Mueller ME, Allgower M, Schneider R, Willenegger H. Manual of osteosynthesis. Berlin, Heidelberg, New York: Springer; 1970.
12. Wickstrom J, Corban MS. Intramedullary fixation of fractures of the femoral shaft. J Trauma. 1967;7:551–83.
13. Smith JEM. The results of early and delayed internal fixation of fractures of the shaft of the femur. J Bone Joint Surg. 1964;46B:28–32.
14. Riska EB, Bonsdorff Hvon, Hakkinen S, Jaroma H, Kiviluoto O, Paavilainen T. Primary operative fixation of long bone fractures in patients with multiple injuries. J Trauma. 1977;17:111–21.
15. Goris RJ, Gimbrere JSF, Niekerk JLMvan, Shoots FJ, Booy LH. Early osteosynthesis and prophylactic mechanical ventilation in the multitrauma patient. J Trauma. 1982;22: 895–903.
16. Talucci RC, Manning J, Lampard S. Early intramedullary nailing of femoral shaft fractures: a cause of fat embolism syndrome. Am J Surg. 1983;146:107–11.
17. Seibel R, LaDuca J, Hassett JM, et al. Blunt multiple trauma (ISS 36), femur traction, and the pulmonary failure-septic state. Ann Surg. 1985;202:283–95.
18. Bone LB, Johnson KD, Weigelt J, Scheinberg R. Early versus delayed stabilization of fractures. A prospective randomized study. J Bone Joint Surg. 1989;71A:336–40.
19. Johnson KD, Cadambi A, Seibert GB. Incidence of adult respiratory distress syndrome in patients with multiple musculoskeletal injuries: effect of early operative stabilization of fractures. J Trauma. 1985;25:375–84.
20. Behrman SW, Fabian TC, Kudsk KA. Improved outcome with femur fractures: early vs delayed fixation. J Trauma. 1990;30:792–8.
21. van Os JP, Roumen RMH, Schoots FJ, Heystraten FM, Goris RJ. Is early osteo-synthesis safe in multiple trauma patients with severe thoracic trauma and pulmonary contusion. J Trauma. 1994;36:495–9.
22. Ecke H, Faupel L, Quoika P. Gedanken zum zeitpunkt der operation bei frakturen des oberschenkelknochens. Unfallchirurgie. 1985;11:89–93.
23. Sturm JA, Wisner HD, Oestern HJ, Kant CJ, Tscherne H, Creutzig H. Increased lung capillary permeability after trauma: a prospective clinical study. J Trauma. 1986;26:409–15.
24. Boulanger BR, Stephen D, Brennemann FD. Thoracic trauma and early intramedullary nailing of femur fractures: are we doing harm? J Trauma. 1997;43:24–9.
25. Pape HC, Auf'm'Kolk M, Paffrath T, Regel G, Sturm JA, Tscherne H. Primary intramedullary femur fixation in multiple trauma patients with associated lung contusion: a cause of post-traumatic ARDS? J Trauma. 1993;34:540–8.
26. Giannoudis PV, Abbott C, Stone M, Bellamy MC, Smith RM. Fatal systemic inflammatory response syndrome following early bilateral femoral nailing. Intensive Care Med. 1998;24:641–2.
27. Giannoudis PV, Smith RM, Bellamy MC, Morrison JF, Dickson RA, Guillou PJ. Stimulation of the inflammatory system by reamed and unreamed nailing of femoral fractures: an analysis of the second hit. J Bone Joint Surg. 1999;81B:356–61.
28. Pape HC, Giannoudis P, Krettek C. The timing of fracture treatment in polytrauma patients: relevance of damage control orthopaedic surgery. Am J Surg. 2002;183:622–9.
29. Smith RM, Giannoudis PV. Trauma and immune response. J R Soc Med. 1998;91:417–20.
30. Giannoudis PV, Smith RM, Windsor AJ, Bellamy MC, Guillou PJ. Monocyte HLA-DR expression correlates with intrapulmonary shunting after major trauma. Am J Surg. 1999; 177:454–9.
31. Giannoudis PV, Smith RM, Windsor AJ, Perry SL, Dickson RA, Bellamy MC. Immediate IL-10 expression following major orthopaedic trauma: relationship to anti-inflammatory response and subsequent development of sepsis. Int Care Med. 2000;26:1076–81.
32. Menzel CL, Pfeifer R, Darwiche SS, Kobbe P, Gill R, Shapiro RA, et al. Models of lower extremity damage in mice: time course of organ damage and immune response. J Surg Res. 2011;166(2):e149–56.

33. Bone RC. Toward a theory regarding the pathogenesis of the systemic inflammatory response syndrome: what we do and do not know about cytokine regulation. Crit Care Med. 1996;24:162–72.
34. Giannoudis PV, Smith RM, Banks RE, Windsor AR, Dickson RA, Guillou PJ. Stimulation of inflammatory markers after blunt trauma. Br J Surg. 1998;85:986–90.
35. Giannoudis PV, Smith RM, Ramsden CW, Sharples D, Dickson RA, Guillou PJ. Molecular mediators and trauma: effects of accidental trauma on the production of plasma elastase, IL-6, sICAM-1 and sE-selectin. Injury. 1996;27:376–7.
36. Giannoudis PV, Pape HC. Damage control orthopaedics in unstable pelvic ring injuries. Injury. 2004;35(7):671–7.
37. Scalea TM, Boswell SA, Scott JD, Mitchell KA, Kramer ME, Pollak AN. External fixation as a bridge to intramedullary nailing for patients with multiple injuries and with femur fractures: damage control orthopedics. J Trauma. 2000;48:613–21.
38. Nowotarski PJ, Turen CH, Brumback RJ, Scarboro JM. Conversion of external fixation to intramedullary nailing for fractures of the shaft of the femur in multiply injured patients. J Bone Joint Surg Am. 2000;82:781–8.
39. Pape HC, Hildebrand F, Pertschy S, Zelle B, Garapati R, Grimme K, et al. Changes in the management of femoral shaft fractures in polytrauma patients: from early total care to damage control orthopedic surgery. J Trauma. 2002;53(3):452–61.
40. Meregalli A, Oliveira RP, Friedman G. Occult hypoperfusion is associated with increased mortality in hemodynamically stable, high risk, surgical patients. Crit Care. 2004; 8–2:R60–5.
41. Tilney NL, Bailey GL, Morgan AP. Sequential system failure after rupture of abdominal aortic aneurysms: an unsolved problem in postoperative care. Ann Surg. 1973;178:117–22.
42. Eisman B, Beart R, Norton L. Multiple organ failure. Surgery Gynaecology Obstetrics. 1977;144:323–5.
43. Fry DE, Pearlstein L, Fulton RL, Polk Jr HC. Multiple system organ failure. The role of uncontrolled infection. Arch Surg. 1980;115:136–40.
44. Faist E, Baue AE, Dittmer H, Heberer G. Multiple organ failure in polytrauma patients. J Trauma. 1983;23:775–87.
45. Goris JA, Boekhoerst TP, Nuytinck JK, Gimbrere JS. Multiple organ failure. Arch Surg. 1985;120:1109–15.
46. Norton LW. Does drainage of intra-abdominal pus reverse multiple organ failure? Am J Surg. 1985;149:347–50.
47. Giannoudis PV. Current concepts of the inflammatory response after major trauma: an update. Injury. 2003;34:397–404.
48. Cipolle MD, Pasquale MD, Cerra FB. Secondary organ dysfunction: from clinical perspectives to molecular mediators. Crit Care Clin. 1993;9:261–97.
49. DeLong Jr WG, Born CT. Cytokines in patients with polytrauma. Clin Orthop Relat Res. 2004;422:57–65.
50. Maekawa K, Futami S, Nishida M, Terada T, Inagawa H, Suzuki S, et al. Effects of trauma and sepsis on soluble L-selectin and cell surface expression of L-selectin and CD11b. J Trauma. 1998;44:460–8.
51. Pape HC, Schmidt RE, Rice J, et al. Biochemical changes following trauma and skeletal surgery of the lower extremity – quantification of the operative burden. Crit Care Med. 2000;28:3441–8.
52. Frink M, van Griensven M, Kobbe P, Brin T, Zeckey C, Vaske B, et al. IL-6 predicts organ dysfunction and mortality in patients with multiple injuries. Scand J Trauma Resusc Emerg Med. 2009;17:49.
53. Castelli GP, Pognani C, Cita M, Paladini R. Procalcitonin as a prognostic and diagnostic toll for septic complications after major trauma. Crit Care Med. 2009;37(6):1845–9.
54. Carillo C, Fogler RJ, Shaftan GW. Delayed gastrointestinal reconstruction following massive abdominal trauma. J Trauma. 1993;34:233–5.

55. Buckle R, Browner B, Morandi M. Emergency reduction for pelvic ring disruptions and control of associated hemorrhage using the pelvic stabilizer. Tech Orthop. 1995;9:258–66.
56. Gansslen A, Pohlemann T, Paul C, et al. Epidemiology of pelvic ring injuries. Injury. 1996;27:S-A13–9.
57. Kellam J. The role of external fixation in pelvic disruptions. Clin Orthop. 1989;241:66–82.
58. Musemeche CA, Fischer RP, Cotler HB, Andrassy RJ. Selective management of pediatric pelvic fractures: a conservative approach. J Pediatr Surg. 1987;22:538–40.
59. Poka A, Libby E. Indications and techniques for external fixation of the pelvis. Clin Orthop. 1996;329:54–9.
60. Riska E, von Bonsdorf H, Hakkinen S, et al. External fixation of unstable pelvic fractures. Int Orthop. 1997;3:183–8.
61. Krige JE, Bornman PC, Terblanche J. Therapeutic perihepatic packing in complex liver trauma. Br J Surg. 1992;79:43–6.
62. Little JM, Fernandes A, Tait N. Liver trauma. Aust NZJ Surg. 1986;56:613–9.
63. Parreira JG, Solda S, Rasslan S. Damage control. A tactical alternative for the management of exsanguinating trauma patients. Arq Gastroenterol. 2002;39:188–97.
64. Shapiro MB, Jenkins DH, Schwab CW, et al. Damage control: collective review. J Trauma. 2000;49:969–78.
65. Frevert S, Dahl B, Lönn L. Update on the role of angiography and embolisation in pelvic fracture. Injury. 2008;39(11):1290–4.
66. Constantini TW, Bosarge PL, Fortlage D, Bansal V, Coimbra R. Arterial embolization for pelvic fractures after blunt trauma: are we all talk? Am J Surg. 2010;200(6):752–7.
67. Hauser CJ, Zhou X, Joshi P, Cuchens MA, et al. The immune microenvironment of human fracture/soft-tissue haematomas and its relationship to systemic immunity. J Trauma. 1997;42:895–903.
68. Hauser CJ, Joshi P, Zhou X, et al. Production of interleukin-10 in human fracture soft-tissue haematomas. Shock. 1996;6:3–6.
69. Perl M, Gebhard F, Knöferl MW, et al. The pattern of preformed cytokines in tissue frequently affected by blunt trauma. Shock. 2003;19:299–304.
70. Giannoudis PV, Cohen A, Hinsche A, et al. Simultaneous bilateral femoral fractures: systemic complications in 14 cases. Int Orthop. 2000;24:264–7.
71. Raman R, Sidhom S, Pape HC, Giannoudis PV. Systemic effects of bilateral tibial versus bilateral femoral shaft fractures. Is there a difference? Acta Orthop Belg. 2004;70:134–41.
72. Copeland CE, Mitchell KA, Brumback RJ, et al. Mortality in patients with bilateral femoral fractures. J Orthop Trauma. 1998;12:315–9.
73. Daniel RK, Taylor GI. Distant transfer of an island flap by microvascular anastomoses. A clinical technique. Plast Reconstr Surg. 1973;52:111–7.
74. Lange RH, Bach AW, Hansen ST, Johansen KH. Open tibial fractures with associated vascular injuries: prognosis for limb salvage. J Trauma. 1985;25:203–8.
75. Georgiadis GM, Behrens FF, Joyce MJ, Earle AS, Simmons AL. Open tibial fractures with severe soft-tissue loss. Limb salvage compared with below-the-knee amputation. J Bone Joint Surg Am. 1993;75-A:1431–41.
76. Gregory RT, Gould RJ, Peclet M, et al. The mangled extremity syndrome (M.E.S.): A severity grading system for multisystem injury of the extremity. J Trauma. 1985;22:1147–50.
77. Johansen K, Daines M, Howey T, Helfet D, Hansen ST. Objective criteria accurately predict amputation following lower extremity trauma. J Trauma. 1990;30:568–73.
78. Bhandari M, Guyatt GH, Swiontkowski MF, Schemitsch EH. Treatment of open fractures of the shaft of the tibia. A systematic overview and meta-analysis. J Bone Joint Surg Br. 2001;83-B:62–8.
79. Helfet DL, Howey T, Sanders R, et al. Limb salvage versus amputation: preliminary results of the Mangled Extremity Severity Score. Clin Orthop. 1990;256:80–6.
80. Robertson PA. Prediction of amputation after severe lower limb trauma. J Bone Joint Surg Br. 1991;73-B:816–8.

81. Smith RM, Gopal S. Mini-symposium: tibial fractures. Open fractures: principles of management. Curr Orthop. 1999;13:87–91.
82. Durrant CA, Mackey SP. Orthoplastic classification systems: the good, the bad, and the ungainly. Ann Plast Surg. 2011;66(1):9–12.
83. Bosse MJ, MacKenzie EJ, Kellam JF, et al. An analysis of outcomes of reconstruction or amputation of leg-threatening injuries. New Engl J Med. 2002;347:1924–31.
84. MacKenzie EJ, Bosse MJ, The LEAP Study Group. Disability persists long term following severe lower limb trauma. Paper #68 presented at the Orthopaedic Trauma Association Annual Meeting, Hollywood; October 10, 2004.
85. Goodell JA, Flick AB, Herbet JC, Howe JG. Preparation and release characteristics of tobramycin-impregnated polymethylmethacrylate beads. Am J Hosp Pharm. 1986;43:1454–61.
86. Webb LX. New techniques in wound management: vacuum-assisted wound closure. I Am Acad Orthop Surg. 2002;10:303–11.
87. Zalavras CG, Patzakis MJ, Holtom P. Local antibiotic therapy in the treatment of open fractures and osteomyelitis. Clin Orthop Relat Res. 2004;427:86–93.
88. Beck JP, Colins JA. Theoretical and clinical aspects of post-traumatic fat embolism syndrome. AAOS ICL. 1973;22:38–44.
89. Chestnut RM. Secondary brain insults after head injury: clinical perspectives. New Horiz. 1995;3:366–9.
90. Lehmann U, Reif W, Hobbensiefken G, et al. Effect of primary fracture management on craniocerebral trauma in polytrauma. An animal experiment study. Unfallchirurg. 1995;98:437–41.
91. Chan PH, Schmidley JW, Fishman RA, et al. Brain injury, edema and vascular permeability changes induced by oxygen-derived free radicals. Neurology. 1984;34:315–8.
92. Schoettle RJ, Kochanek PM, Nemoto EM, et al. Granulocyte accumulation and edema after cerebral trauma. Crit Care Med. 1989;17:71–5.
93. Schmoker JD, Zhuang J, Shackford SR. Hemorrhagic hypotension after brain injury causes an early sustained reduction in cerebral oxygen delivery despite normalisation of systemic oxygen delivery. J Trauma. 1992;32:714–8.
94. Pietropaoli JA, Rodgers FB, Shackford SM, et al. The deleterious effect of intraoperative hypotension on outcome in patients with severe head injuries. J Trauma. 1992;33:403–7.
95. Price JE, Murray A. The influence of hypoxia and hypotension on recovery from head injury. Injury. 1972;3:218–21.
96. Grotz MR, Giannoudis PV, Pape HC, et al. Traumatic brain injury and stabilisation of long bone fractures. An update. Injury. 2004;35:1077–86.
97. Boulanger BR, Stephen D, Brenneman FD. Thoracic trauma and early intramedullary nailing of femur fractures: are we doing harm? J Trauma. 1997;43:24–8.
98. Charash WE, Fabian TC, Croce MA. Delayed surgical fixation of femur fractures is a risk factor for pulmonary failure independent of thoracic trauma. J Trauma. 1994;37:667–72.
99. Nicholas B, Toth L, van Wessem K, Evans J, Enninghorst N, Balogh ZJ. Borderline femur fracture patients: early total care or damage control orthopaedics? ANZ J Surg. 2011;81(3):148–53.
100. Pape HC, van Griensen M, Rice J, et al. Major secondary surgery in blunt trauma patients and peri-operative cytokine liberation: determination of the clinical relevance of biochemical markers. J Trauma. 2001;50:989–1000.
101. Harwood PJ, Giannoudis PV, van Griensven M, Krettek C, Pape HC. Alterations in the systemic inflammatory response after early total care and damage control procedures for femoral shaft fracture in severely injured patients. J Trauma. 2005;58:446–52.
102. McGraw JM, Lim EV. Treatment of open tibial shaft fracture. External fixation and secondary intramedullary nailing. J Bone Joint Surg. 1988;70A:900–11.
103. Maurer DJ, Merkow RL, Gustilo RB. Infection after intramedullary nailing of severe open tibial fractures initially treated with external fixation. J Bone Joint Surg. 1989;71A:835–8.

104. Blachut PA, Meek RN, O'Brien PJ. External fixation and delayed intramedullary nailing of open fractures of the tibial shaft. J Bone Joint Surg. 1990;72A:729–34.
105. Wheelwright EF, Court-Brown CM. Primary external fixation and secondary intramedullary nailing in the treatment of tibial fractures. Injury. 1993;23:373–5.
106. Antich-Adrover P, Marti-Garin D, Murias-Alvarez J, Peunte-Alonso C. External fixation and secondary intramedullary nailing of open tibial fractures. J Bone Joint Surg. 1997;79B:433–7.
107. Paderni S, Trentani P, Grippo G, et al. Intramedullary osteosynthesis after external fixation. Chir Organi Mov. 2001;86:183–90.
108. Wolinsky PR, McCarty E, Shyr Y, Johnson K. Reamed intramedullary nailing of the femur: 551 cases. J Trauma. 1999;46:392–9.
109. Bhandari M, Guyatt GH, Tong D, Adili A, Shaughnessy SA. Reamed versus nonreamed intramedullary nailing of lower extremity long bone fractures: a systematic overview and meta-analysis. J Orthop Trauma. 2000;14:2–9.

Chapter 2
Limb Damage Control Orthopedics

Madhusudhan Yakkanti, Cyril Mauffrey, and Craig S. Roberts

2.1 Introduction

The damage control (DCO) approach to the injured limb requires the application of damage control orthopedic principles to an extremity. Like the overall DCO approach to the polytrauma patient, limb damage control corrects local metabolic disturbances (e.g., acidosis, contamination, etc.), corrects local hypothermia (e.g., warming the limb, ensuring adequate perfusion, etc.), and reverses coagulopathy (e.g., controlling profound bleeding, etc.). Along with fixing local metabolic disturbances, controlling bleeding, and ensuring adequate perfusion, provisional skeletal stability with external fixation is achieved.

The most important type of extremity injury that benefits from a limb damage control approach is the mangled leg. In addition, a limited limb damage control approach can be applied to complex periarticular/articular injuries. Furthermore, the British Orthopedic Association, in its *Standards for the Management of Open Fractures of the Lower Limb: Short Guide*, has described the use of primary amputation as a "damage control procedure" when there is uncontrollable hemorrhage from an open tibial injury (multiple levels of arterial/venous damage in blast injuries), or for crush injuries exceeding a warm ischemic period of 6 h [1].

The mangled limb is defined as a limb with injury to three of four extremity systems [2] with the systems defined as the soft tissues, nerves, blood supply, and bone

M. Yakkanti (✉)
Department of Orthopaedics Surgery, University Hospital Louisville, Louisville, KY, USA
e-mail: madhuyakkanti@gmail.com

C. Mauffrey • C.S. Roberts
Department of Orthopaedics, University Hospital Louisville, Louisville, KY, USA
e-mail: cmauffrey@yahoo.com; craig.roberts@louisville.edu

D. Seligson et al. (eds.), *External Fixation in Orthopedic Traumatology*,
DOI 10.1007/978-1-4471-2197-8_2, © Springer-Verlag London Limited 2012

[3]. The initial treatment decision is between immediate limb salvage or amputation. With limb salvage, these limb injuries require methods of soft tissue injury management techniques such as antibiotic bead pouches and negative pressure dressings (e.g., VAC, etc.) in addition to external fixation. The various applications of damage control external fixation to specific periarticular/articular injuries in the non-mangled limb will be addressed elsewhere in this book.

The clinical decision whether to perform limb salvage or immediate amputation is best made in the context of the contemporary data from the Lower Extremity Assessment Project (LEAP) study. The LEAP data suggests that patient and social factors are the primary determinants of outcome after severe limb trauma rather than the nature of the orthopedic injury itself [4]. The traditional belief that amputation led to superior outcomes following severe lower extremity injury is not supported by the LEAP study [4]. The LEAP data also suggested that plantar sensation and injury scoring systems are not accurate predictors of functional outcome after these injuries. More than 40% of patients had severe functional impairment according to the Sickness Impact Profile, and only 51% were able to return to work. At average follow-up of 7 years for the LEAP study patients, there was a persistence of disability and a lower SIP Score at 24 months across all treatment groups [5]. Only 34% of patients had a normal physical SIP Subscore (≤5). Variables associated with a better outcome included male gender, younger age at the time of injury, higher socioeconomic status, being a nonsmoker, and having better self-efficacy (confidence to perform certain tasks). There was a fairly high incidence of rehospitalization between 2 and 7 years: 39% of limb salvage patients and 33% of amputees.

This chapter will review general principles of limb assessment, various external fixator montages for injuries of the lower extremity as well as the techniques of antibiotic bead pouches, negative pressure wound therapy, and antibiotic nails.

2.2 General Principles

Determining the adequacy of limb perfusion and the neurological status is part of the initial steps in the assessment of patients with a mangled limb. Doppler or conventional angiography assessment can be helpful, as well as the newer option of Computerized Tomographic Angiography (CTA), which requires additional expertise for its performance and interpretation. Specific bony injuries that carry a higher risk of an associated vascular injury include complex fractures of the proximal tibial plateau, often the result of a fracture-dislocation of the knee. The clinical assessment must be repeated at regular intervals and documented especially after reduction or application of splint. Conditions that will require immediate surgery include: vascular impairment (restoration of the circulation with shunts ideally within 3–4 h with a maximum of 6 h of warm ischemia time), compartment syndrome (for the lower leg, 4 compartments should be decompressed with a 2 incision technique), and finally in some multiply injured patients with open fractures or if the wound is heavily contaminated by marine, agricultural, or sewage matter. In any case, both the orthopedic trauma team and the plastic surgeons should agree and document early on a manage-

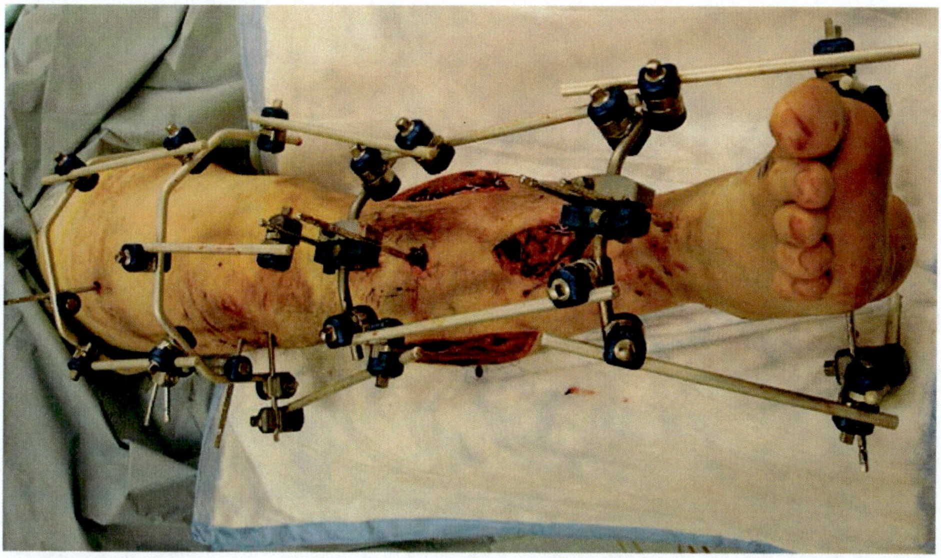

Fig. 2.1 Photograph of a full-length external fixator for a complex, segmental leg injury

ment plan and have in their minds the acute and less acute options. In the emergency room, the wound and soft tissues should only be handled to remove gross contamination, a picture should be taken for documentation purposes (and to prevent multiple handling of the wound), and the size and contamination of the skin defect should be estimated and noted. A saline-soaked dressing should be applied and covered with an impermeable film to prevent dessication before the application of a splint. Intravenous antibiotics should be started as early as possible and should consist of Co-Amoxiclav 1.2 g or Cefuroxime 1.5 g every 8 h continued until the first wound debridement. In case of Penicillin allergy, this can be replaced by Clindamycin 600 mg every 6 h. At the first debridement, patients should receive Co-Amoxiclav 1.2 g and Gentamicin 1.5 mg/kg, and these should be continued for 72 h post debridement or until definitive wound closure and fracture fixation, whichever comes first. Gentamicin 1.5 mg/kg and either Vancomycin 1 g or Teicoplanin 800 mg should be administered on induction of anesthesia at the time of skeletal stabilization and definitive soft tissue closure. These should not be continued postoperatively. The Vancomycin infusion should be started at least 90 min prior to surgery [1].

2.3 Specific Montages

2.3.1 Full-Length Fixator

Indications include segmental leg injury, multilevel fractures of the proximal and distal segments of the leg, or an ischemic leg with vascular compromise. Components

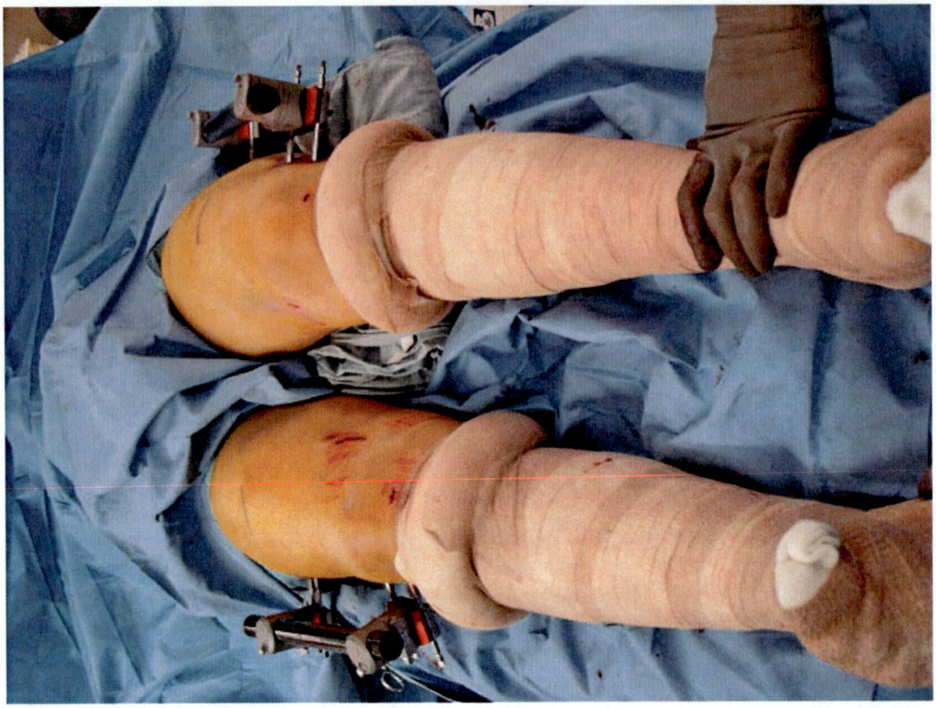

Fig. 2.2 Photograph of bilateral femoral external fixators for bilateral femoral shaft fractures

include multiple long bars and multiple pin clamps (minimum one per segment). Options are separate pin clamp cluster per fracture segment, or pin clamp in end segments only with floating middle segment. This montage of external fixation spans the whole leg from the hip to the foot (Fig. 2.1). Pitfalls include too much traction on the entire limb, creating excessive soft tissue tension with possible soft tissue swelling, sciatic nerve palsy, and thigh or calf compartment syndrome.

2.3.2 Femoral Shaft External Fixators

Indications for the application of a femoral external fixator include femoral shaft fractures in the unstable polytrauma patient, patient with a significant chest or head injury in addition to a femur fracture, an open femur fracture unsuitable for immediate femoral nailing, or a femur fracture with a thigh compartment syndrome. Components of the frame include one large bar for a one bar frame (Fig. 2.2), or two smaller bars for a delta-type frame, two pin clamps (for a frame with one bar), or four single pin-bar clamps and bar-bar clamps for a delta-type triangular frame. Options include a unilateral straight anterolateral frame with uniplanar pins or a straight lateral frame with multiplanar pins. Pitfalls include iatrogenic damage to the bulk of the quadriceps muscle anteriorly, quadriceps atrophy, pin sepsis, and neurovascular damage medially or posteriorly to the femoral shaft. The risk of local infection after external fixation of femur fractures (damage control orthopedics) is comparable to those after primary intramedullary nailing of femur fractures [6].

2.3.3 Knee Bridging External Fixators

The across-the-knee application of external fixation is useful for unstable bony segments around the knee. Indications include tibial plateau fractures, knee dislocations, knee fracture-dislocations, or the floating knee segment ("floating knee injuries"). Components include two bars with a bar-to-bar clamp (or alternatively one long bar) and two pin clamps (Fig. 2.3). Options include pin clusters with either one double-pin clamp on either the joint or, for a larger leg, one double clamp plus a single-pin clamp on either side of the joint for multiplanar fixation. In addition to neurovascular damage, other complications of pin insertion include iatrogenic joint capsule penetration, and resultant theoretical risk of joint sepsis from pin tract infections. We have found that this theoretical risk is only a problem in the subgroup of patients who are diabetic or immunocompromised [7]. We suggest avoiding pin insertion at the potential sites of future incisions.

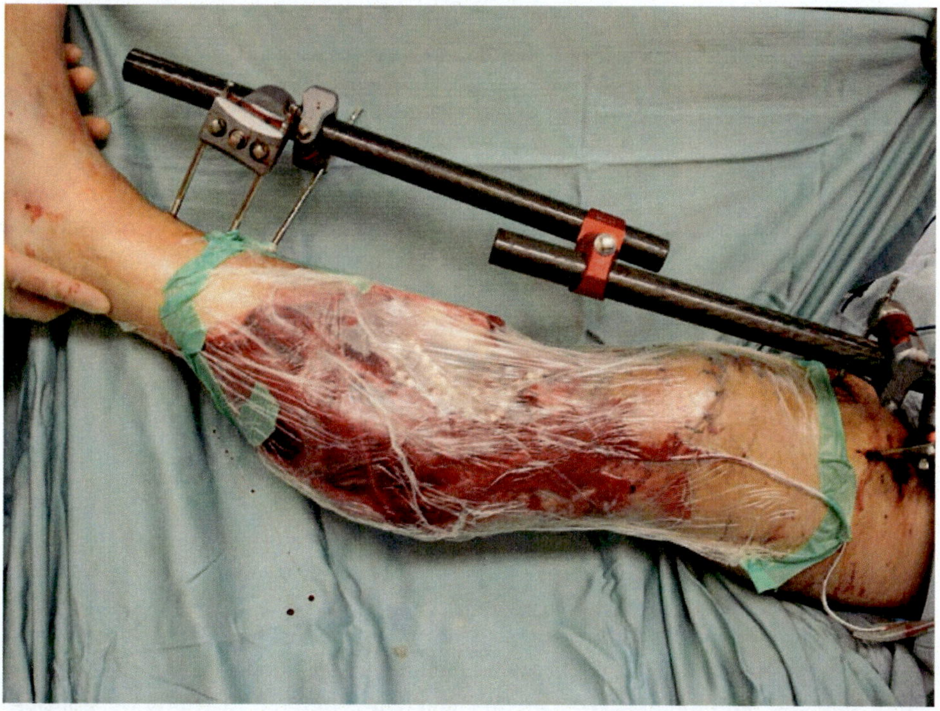

Fig. 2.3 Photograph of an across-the-knee external fixator with an antibiotic bead pouch for a complex tibial fracture with a nearly circumferential soft tissue injury

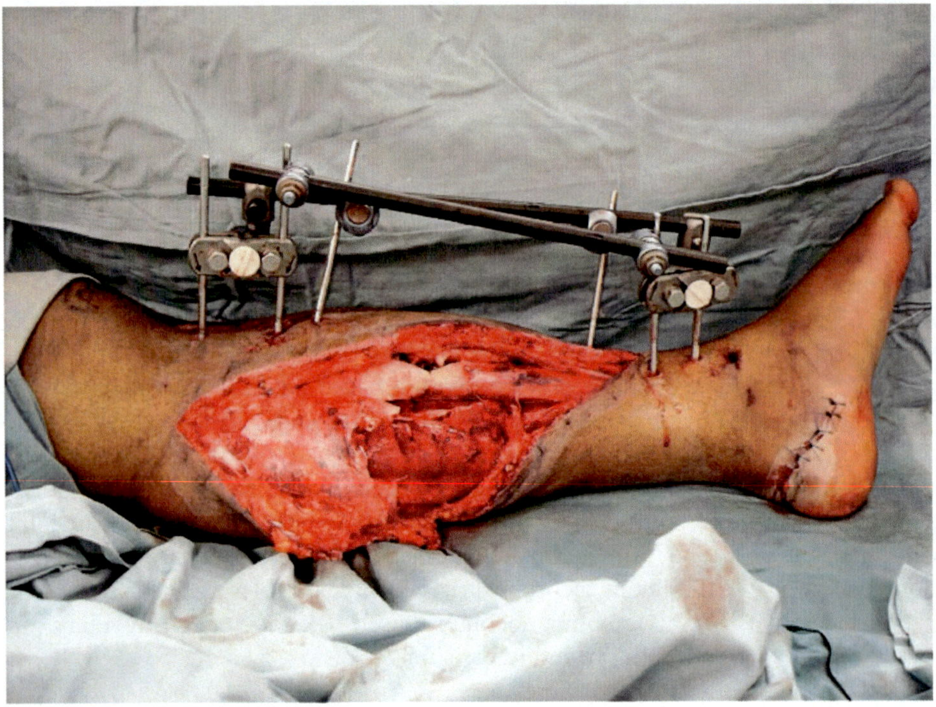

Fig. 2.4 Photograph of an external fixator for an open tibia-fibula fracture

2.3.4 Tibial Shaft External Fixators

Indications for the application of a tibial shaft external fixator are open tibial fractures with gross contamination, especially with a soft tissue injury preventing coverage of bone. Options include simple anterior frame with two double-pin clamps for more stable fractures; more complex frames with multiplanar pin (one double-pin clamp and one single-pin clamp) on either side of the fracture site (Fig. 2.4) can also be useful. Pitfalls include iatrogenic injury to the saphenous neurovascular bundle, the peroneal nerve (common or superficial branch), or the tibial nerve and artery.

2.3.5 External Fixators Across the Ankle Including the Hindfoot

The application of external fixation across the ankle is useful for complex, segmental injuries of the foot and ankle. Indications include damage control frame spanning a pilon fracture, comminuted bi- or tri-malleolar fracture, or midfoot injuries. Components include a partial hexagonal ring for the hindfoot and a partial hexagonal ring for the forefoot, a double-pin clamp with posts for the tibial pins, short rods to

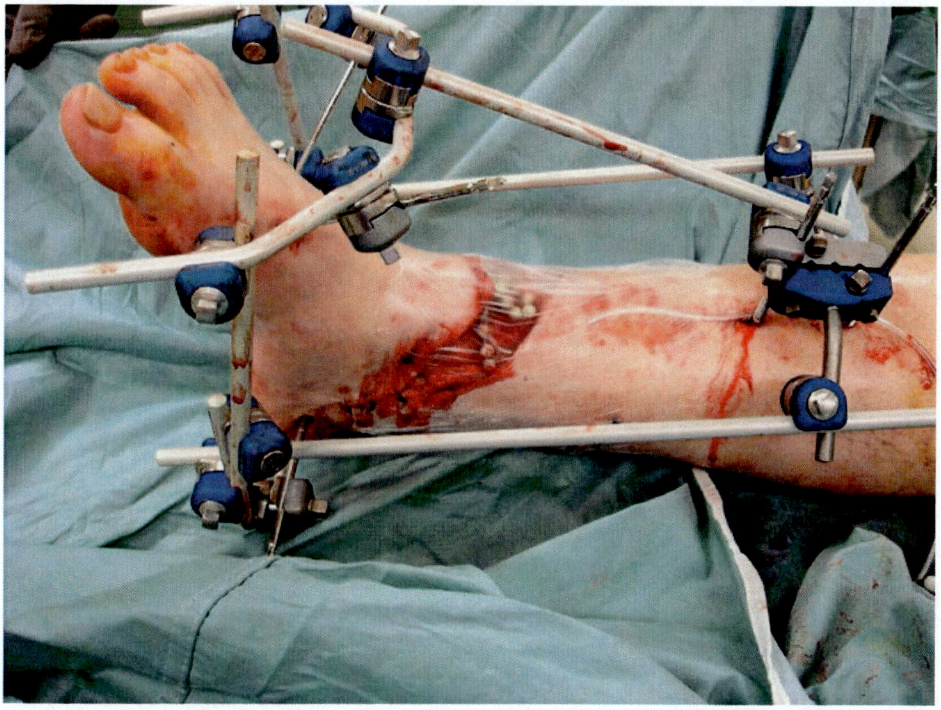

Fig. 2.5 Photograph of an across-the-ankle external fixator which includes the hindfoot as well as an antibiotic bead pouch

connect the hexagonal rings on the foot, three long rods to connect the tibial pin clamp to the foot rings, and bar-to-bar clamps. Options include a complete spanning of foot (hindfoot to forefoot) with proximal tibial pin clamp versus hindfoot pins (without forefoot pins) with tibial pin clamp (Fig. 2.5). Pitfalls include iatrogenic injury to the posterior neurovascular bundle, inadequate purchase in the calcaneus pin, iatrogenic anterior subluxation of the tibio-talar joint, and iatrogenic injury to digital vessels.

2.3.6 External Fixators Across the Ankle Sparing the Hindfoot

This montage is particularly useful for applications where the hindfoot needs to be spanned. Specific indications include mangled heel injuries or open calcaneus fractures or combined ankle and hindfoot articular injuries. Components include double-pin clamp with posts, one partial hexagonal ring, three long connecting rods, and bar-to-pin clamps. Options include first and fourth or fifth metatarsal half-pins plus tibial pin clamp versus first and fourth metatarsal half-pins plus tibial pin clamp (Fig. 2.6). Pitfalls include injury to digital neurovascular bundles and iatrogenic anterior subluxation of the tibio-talar joint.

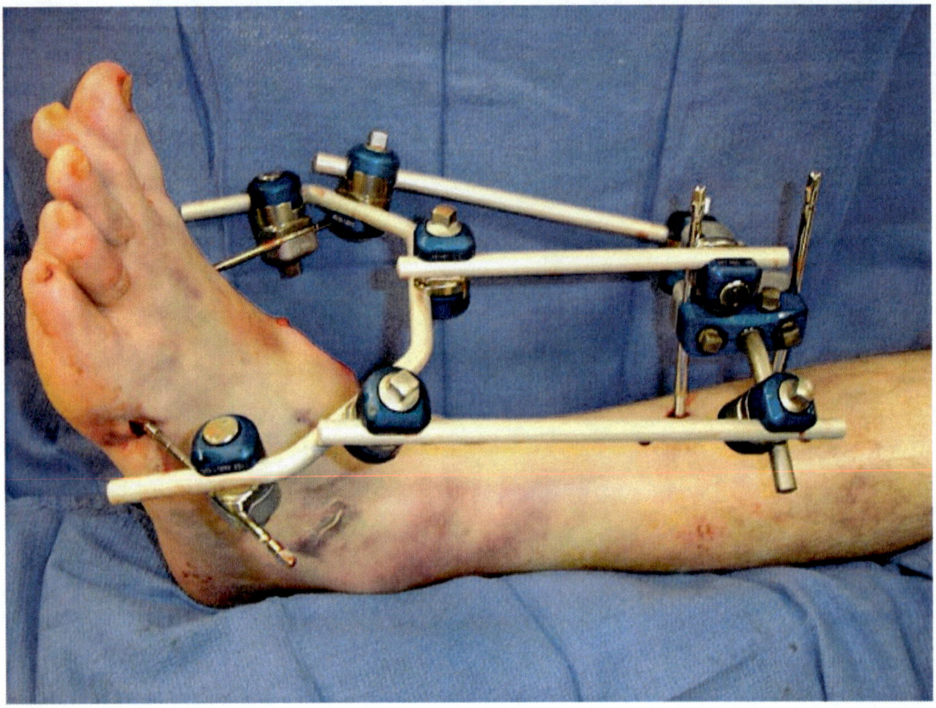

Fig. 2.6 Photograph of an across-the-ankle heel-sparing external fixator

2.4 Adjunctive Measures

2.4.1 Antibiotic Bead Pouches

Antibiotic bead pouches are useful for grossly contaminated open fracture wounds that will need additional staged debridements, as well as wounds that after debridement cannot be closed primarily. An antibiotic bead pouch consists of a porous plastic film placed over the soft tissue defect to establish a "closed" bead-wound-fracture environment containing high levels of antibiotics at the fracture site. Seligson et al. reported that antibiotic bead pouches lower infection rates after open fractures [8]. In a series of 227 open fractures in 204 patients with the antibiotic bead pouch technique, there was a 0% infection rate in grade I open fractures, 1.2% infection rate in grade II open fractures, and 8.6% infection rate in grade III open fractures [8].

One or more chains of antibiotic bead chains are placed in the wound. If more than one chain is used, the bead chains are connected to each other by twisting them together. A suction drain is brought out through normal intact skin and is used to collect overflow only and the suction is intentionally released. The soft tissue defect is covered with an occlusive wound dressing after ensuring that the surrounding skin is dry. Tincture of Benzoin or Mastisol is used to enhance the adhesiveness of the film to skin. The bead pouch dressing is changed in the operating room every

48–72 h. The advantages of the bead pouch are that the open wound is isolated from the hospital environment, high local concentrations of antibiotics are delivered locally in the wound, and systemic toxicity from antibiotics is avoided. One theoretical disadvantage is the development of resistant strains of bacteria; however, this has not been a clinical problem.

2.4.2 Negative Pressure Wound Therapy

Vacuum-assisted wound closure (VAC) is an application of negative pressure wound therapy which has increasingly been used for treating open fracture wounds. VACs were previously termed topical negative pressure (TNP), subatmospheric pressure (SPD), vacuum sealing technique (VST), negative pressure wound therapy (NPWT), and sealed surface wound suction (SSS) [9]. The VAC appears to increase the rate of granulation tissue formation compared with saline dressing-treated wounds [10]. The VAC may also reduce bacterial counts in wounds. In bacterial clearance studies, conducted by infecting wounds with *Staphylococcus aureus* and *Staphylococcal epidermidis*, bacterial levels remained below 10^5 organisms/g of tissue for all treated wounds while bacterial levels in control wounds remained above 10^5 organisms/g of tissue until day 11 [10, 11]. The VAC may also decrease the need for future free flaps or rotational flaps. The components of the VAC system include an electrically powered programmable pump capable of generating a negative suction with a controlled pressure usually ranging from 25 to 200 mmHg with the option of continuous or intermittent suction. This unit is connected to a system of disposable sterile sponge kits complete with tubing and plastic adhesive drape commercially available in three sizes: small, medium, and large. One end of the tubing originates from the dressing with a noncollapsible, side-ported evacuation tube. The other end is connected to a canister to collect the wound exudates. The essential part of the setup is the special pressure distributing dressing made up of open cell polyurethane foam which is positioned in the wound cavity or over the flap. The pore size is carefully designed to maximize tissue growth and is generally 400–600 μm [10]. A semipermeable occlusive adhesive dressing seals the wound from external environment. Portable vacuum-assisted wound closure systems, which are battery operated, are available for ambulatory and highly mobile patients.

The VAC has to be applied after the wound has been debrided. The foam dressing should be cut geometrically to fit the wound with care taken to place the foam material into the deepest portion of the wound. The sponge should be loose and expanded, not tightly packed. A plastic adhesive drape is then placed over the sponge, overlapping the wound margins by 5 cm or more to obtain an airtight seal. The plastic drape can be easily placed under or wrapped around external fixation devices to maintain the pressure seal. The tubing should be elevated off the skin surface and "flagged" by the adhesive drape to avoid undue tubing pressure to skin or bony prominences. After vacuum pressure is applied and an airtight seal is achieved, the sponge will collapse and apply equal subatmospheric suction pressure to the sides and base of the wound. An open wound is converted to a controlled, closed wound [12].

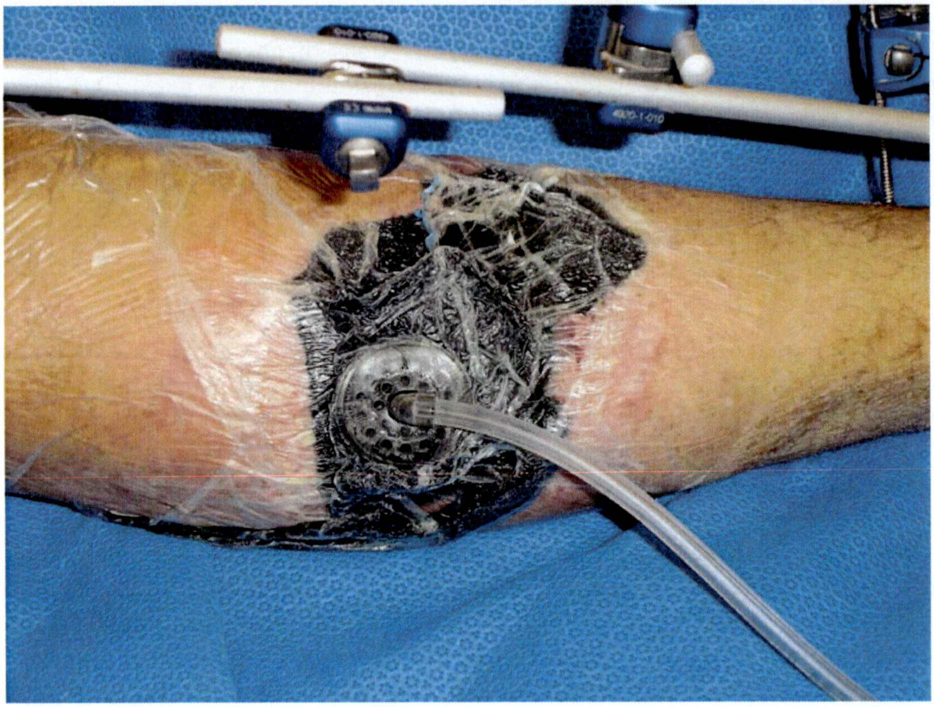

Fig. 2.7 Close-up photograph of a vacuum-assisted wound closure dressing

A sterile plastic occlusive dressing is used to cover the sponge (Fig. 2.7). The wound is not considered sterile, and a clean controlled approach to sponge change is entirely satisfactory. Vacuum-assisted closure sponges optimally should be changed every 48 h. Patients usually require pain medicine for sponge changes. Children and some adults may require sedation or anesthesia during changes. However, most dressing changes can be managed without difficulty at the bedside by specialized nursing staff. Patients with the VAC device can be managed outside of the hospital on an outpatient basis. Many patients who have been treated with antibiotic bead pouches or VACS have external fixation of long duration. External fixation of more than 3 weeks' duration can increase the chances of bacterial contamination of the intramedullary canal. Such cases often need removal of the external fixator combined with antibiotic nail insertion as a temporary bridge to sterilize the medullary canal in preparation for a staged nailing with a conventional, metal nail.

2.4.3 *Antibiotic Nails*

The antibiotic nail can be thought of as an intermediate step in a staged treatment of combined bony and soft tissue injuries of the lower extremity where definitive internal fixation is not safe because the soft tissue envelope is not intact. Antibiotic nail-

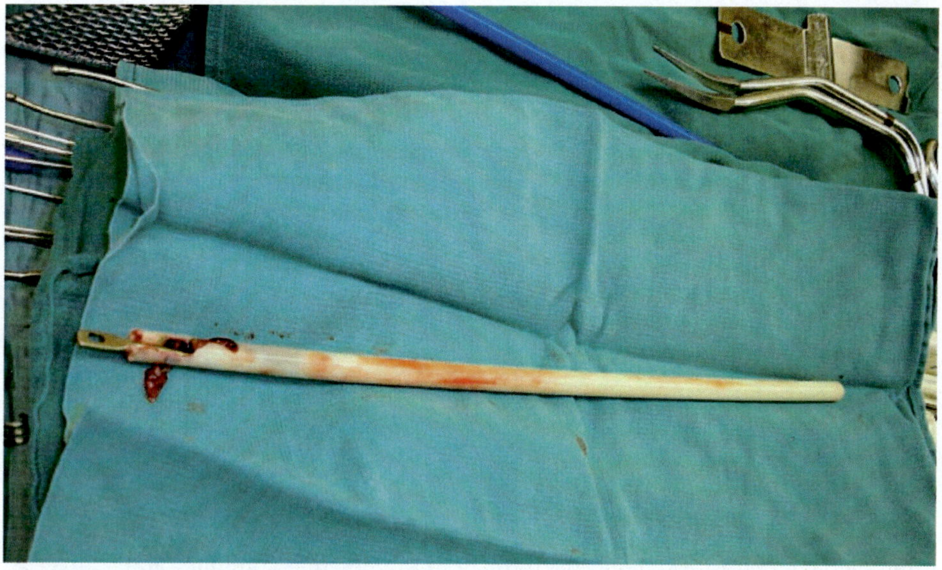

Fig. 2.8 Photograph of an explanted antibiotic nail

ing ought to be considered if external fixator has been prolonged (more than 3 weeks) even in the absence of a documented pin tract infection, or in the case of external fixation with a pin tract infection when intramedullary nail is desirable. Antibiotic-impregnated cement is capable of eluting high concentrations of antibiotics even 36 weeks after implantation [13]. The advantages of using an antibiotic nail include the opportunity to wait for definitive bone battery culture results from the intramedullary canal, time for the noninfected pin tracts to heal, temporary bony stability, and eluted high local antibiotic concentrations.

The technique of antibiotic nailing has been well described [14, 15]. After the external fixator is removed, the pin tracks are curetted and irrigated. The limb is then prepped and draped, and a standard nailing entry site is made with the knee flexed on a triangle. The medullary cavity is entered with a Küntscher awl and a ball-tipped guide wire is passed across the fracture site and confirmed by fluoroscopy. The medullary cavity is progressively reamed and the reamings are sent for culture. The antibiotic nail is usually prepared on the back table using an appropriate length 3.5 or 4 mm diameter Ender nail (Howmedica, Mahwah, NJ), antibiotic of choice (Gentamicin, Tobramycin, Vancomycin), two packs of 40 gm bone cement, vacuum cement mixer, cement gun, and a 40 French chest tube. Antibiotic nails made using a 40 French chest tube are of 10 mm diameter. Care is taken to ensure that the Ender nail extends over the full length of the cement or else fragmentation of cement tip can occur upon antibiotic nail removal. It is also important that the cement does not cover the proximal end of the Ender nail where the eyelet is located (Fig. 2.8). The nail is inserted by hand pressure or using a bone tamp on the end of the Ender nail using gentle taps. The antibiotic nail is usually not inserted as deeply as standard intramedullary nails in order to facilitate later extraction.

Table 2.1 Various montage types

Injury pattern	Montage
Fracture shaft femur	Femoral external fixator
Supracondylar femur	Anterolateral knee spanning fixator
Fracture patella	Knee-spanning fixator
Fracture tibial plateau	Knee-spanning fixator
Knee dislocation	Knee-spanning fixator
Floating knee	Knee-spanning fixator
Fracture tibial shaft	Tibial external fixator
Fracture tibial pilon	Ankle-spanning fixator
Ankle dislocation	Ankle-spanning fixator
Open calcaneus fracture	Ankle-spanning fixator (without hindfoot pins)

2.5 Conclusion

Limb damage control is an approach for limb salvage that combines and addresses complex soft tissue and bony lower extremity injuries. Although the mangled lower extremities are perhaps the best indication for a full limb damage control approach, a limited focus of limb damage control in the form of temporary external fixation is useful for complex periarticular injuries around the distal femur and both ends of the tibia. This approach emphasizes temporary external fixation coupled with wound coverage with antibiotic bead pouches or vacuum-assisted closure. Various options for limb damage control external fixation montages exist for these injuries (Table 2.1). Adjunctive measures such as antibiotic beads, VAC, and antibiotic nails are useful. Limb damage control as a limb salvage technique is supported by the LEAP study data. Prospective studies of limb damage control may be the key to answering unanswered questions about the timing of surgery and functional outcome. A limb damage control approach requires a multidisciplinary team, a global limb assessment, and orthopedic surgeons taking the lead in decision making [2].

References

1. Nanchahal J, Nayagam S, Khan U, Moran C, Barrett S, Sanderson F, et al. Standards for the management of open fractures of the lower limb: a short guide [pamphlet]. London: British Association of Plastic Reconstructive and Aesthetic Surgeons and British Orthopaedic Association; 2009.
2. Wolinsky PR, Webb LX, Harvey EJ, Tejwani NC. The mangled limb: salvage versus amputation. In: Egol KA, Tornetta III P, editors. Instructional course lectures, vol. 60. Rosemont: American Academy of Orthopaedic Surgeons; 2011. p. 27–34.
3. Hansen Jr ST. Overview of the severely traumatized lower limb: reconstruction versus amputation. Clin Orthop Relat Res. 1989;243:17–9.
4. Cannada LK, Jones AL. Demographic, social and economic variables that affect lower extremity injury outcomes. Injury Int J Care Injured. 2006;37:1109–16.

5. Mackenzie EJ, Boss MJ, Pollak AN, et al. Long-term persistence of disability following severe lower-limb trauma: results of a seven-year follow-up. J Bone Joint Surg Am. 2005;87(8):1801–9.
6. Harwood PJ, Giannoudis PV, Probst C, Krettek C, Pape HC. The risk of local infective complications after damage control procedures for femoral shaft fracture. J Orthop Trauma. 2006;50(3):181–9.
7. Roberts CS, Dodds JC, Perry K, Beck D, Seligson D, Voor MJ. Letter to the editor. J Orthop Trauma. 2004;18(1):57.
8. Henry SL, Ostermann PAW, Seligson D. The antibiotic bead pouch technique the management of severe compound fractures. Clin Orthop Relat Res. 1993;295:54–62.
9. Banwell PE, Teopl L. Topical negative pressure (TNP: the evolution of a novel wound therapy. J Wound Care. 2003;12(1):28–30.
10. Morykwas MJ, Argenta LC, Shelton-Brown EI, McGuirt W. Vacuum-assisted closure: a new method for wound control and treatment: animal studies and basic foundation. Ann Plast Surg. 1997;38:553.
11. Weed T, Ratliff C, Drake DB. Quantifying bacterial bioburden during negative pressure wound therapy: does the wound VAC enhance bacterial clearance? Ann Plast Surg. 2004;52(3):276–80.
12. DeFranzo AJ, Argenta LC, Marks MW, et al. The use of vacuum assisted closure therapy for the treatment of lower extremity wounds with exposed bone. Plast Reconstr Surg. 2001;108(5):1184–91.
13. Nelson CL, Hickmon SG, Harrison BH. Elution characteristics of gentamicin – PMMA beads after implantation in humans. Orthopedics. 1994;17:415–6.
14. Madanagopal G, Seligson D, Roberts CS. The antibiotic cement nail for infection after tibial nailing. Orthopedics. 2004;27(7):709–12.
15. Paley D, Herzenberg JE. Intramedullary infections treated with antibiotic cement rods: preliminary results in nine cases. J Orthop Trauma. 2002;16(10):723–9.

Chapter 3
Practical Biomechanical Considerations about External Fixators

Cyril Mauffrey, Dennis Beck, and Laura Ruhala

3.1 Introduction

External fixators can be categorized into three basic types: unilateral, circular, and hybrid. In general, a unilateral (or monolateral) frame is a bar attached to bone with simple groups of large-diameter pins (Fig. 3.1). These frames are analogous to plates fastened to bone with screws. The other style of frame originated in traction wires. Traction bows hold traction wires. Connect traction bows with bars, and the construct becomes a ring frame. This concept evolved into circular fixators that consist of groups of tensioned transfixion wires attached to rings around the bone; threaded bars connect these rings (Fig. 3.2). Hybrid devices combine the benefits of the strength of circular fixators with the ease of application of unilateral ones (Fig. 3.3). The clinically relevant biomechanics of external fixators include their components' individual material properties, geometry of construction, size of the fixateur pins, and spacing of components. The biomechanical concepts of external fixation are different for each of the basic fixator types.

The goal of most external fixation for trauma is to restore stability to fractured bones. With external fixators, any range of mechanical stability can be achieved. Stability is clinically assessed through the reduction of deformity and the reduction of fracture site motion. Stability can be achieved through fixateur stiffness, geometry, and material properties.

C. Mauffrey (✉)
Department of Orthopaedics, University of Louisville Hospital,
530 South Jackson Street, Louisville, KY 40202, USA
e-mail: cmauffrey@yahoo.com

D. Beck
Orthopaedics Associates, Evansville, IN, USA

L. Ruhala
Department of Engineering, University of Sothern Indiana, Evansville, IN, USA

D. Seligson et al. (eds.), *External Fixation in Orthopedic Traumatology*,
DOI 10.1007/978-1-4471-2197-8_3,

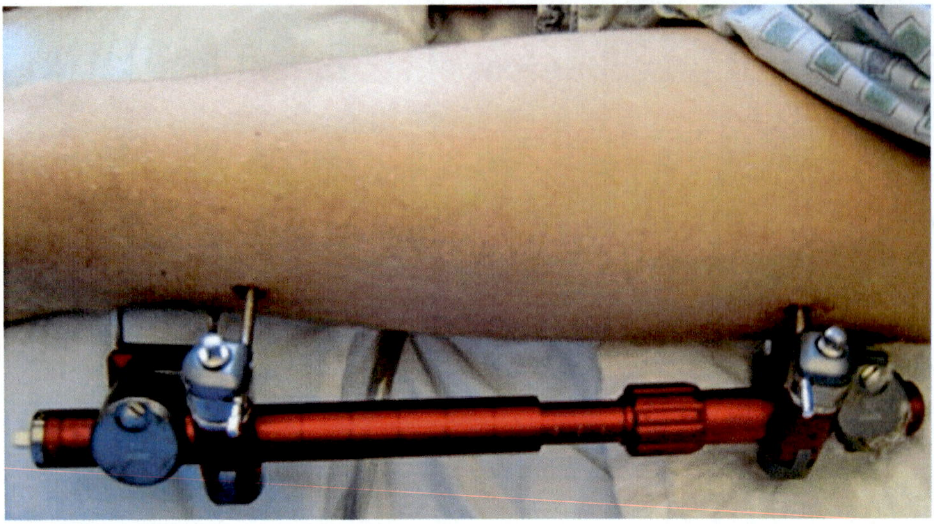

Fig. 3.1 Unilateral (or monolateral) frame is a bar attached to bone with simple groups of large-diameter pins

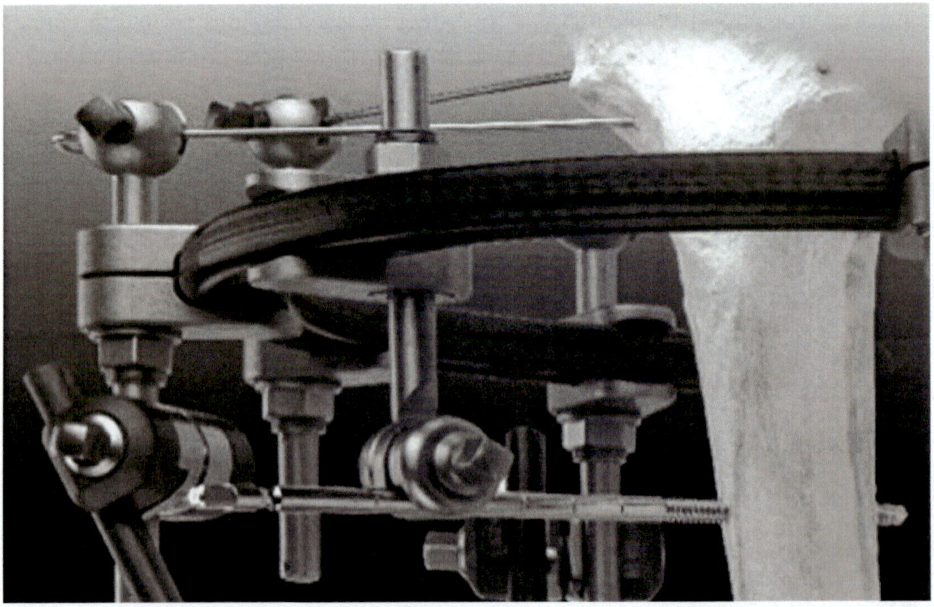

Fig. 3.2 Circular frame Illizarov type

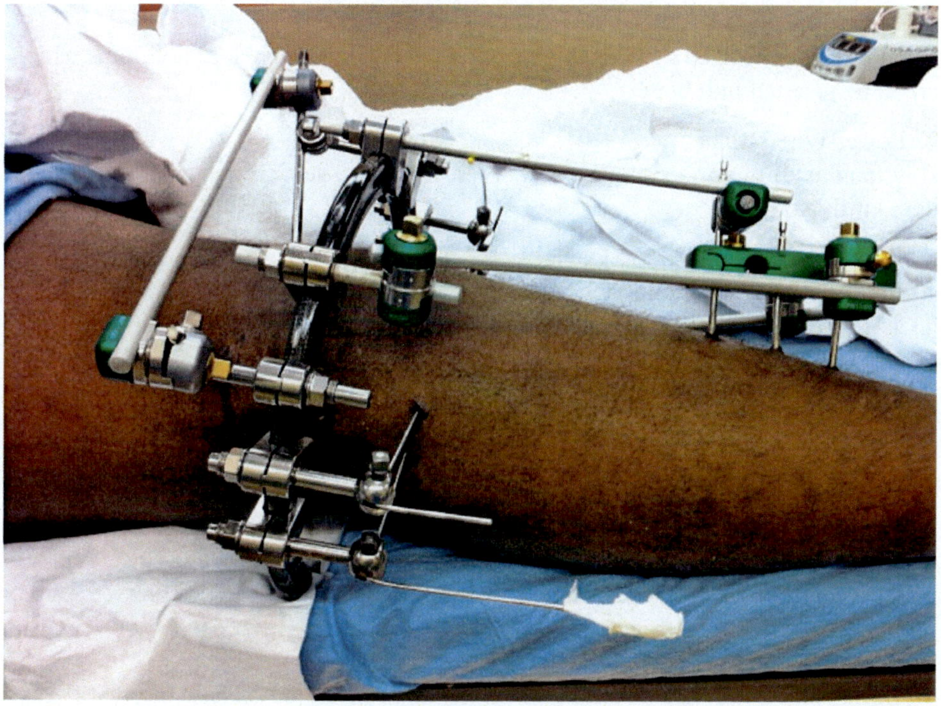

Fig. 3.3 Hybrid external fixation for a tibial plateau fracture

1. Pins
Stainless steel or titanium, partially or wholly threaded, rods inserted into a stable area of the bone. External fixateur pins can have surface treatments for specific biologic effects. For example, hydroxyapatite-coated pins adhere tightly to bone [1].

2. Wires
Wires are usually 1.5–2.5 mm. They are driven across bone and fastened to a ring in a circular external fixateur. An "olive wire" has a stop so it can be driven across but not passed entirely through the bone.

3. Clamps
Mechanical devices used to connect parts of a fixateur constructs, or the fixateur construct to the pins in the bone. Pin-holding clamps can hold pins at various angles. The connection between the clamp and an external fixateur rod can be adjustable.

4. Connecting Bars/Modular Connecting Device
Any material molded into usually a rod with none or any number of joints to allow for placement of frames in a variety of geometric configurations.

5. Manual Pin Driver
Any handheld, nonmotorized device used to insert pins into the bone – a handheld *wimble* increases the torque of external fixateur pin insertion.

6. Power Pin Driver
A handheld, motorized device which can be attached to a chuck to hold pins which are to be inserted into bone.

7. Power Wire Driver
Any handheld, motorized device to allow for rapid insertion of a thin wire (as in circular fixators).

8. Joint-Specific Connecting Device
A prefabricated connecting device designed to bridge a specific joint usually with an axis of rotation that closely matches the rotation of the joint involved.

3.2 Unilateral Fixators

Unilateral fixators are generally comprised of a single bar or contiguous piece of material attached to the bone through large-diameter (≥3mm) pins inserted into intact areas of the bone. These simple fixators can be used for temporary traction, limb lengthening, bone transport, or joint immobilization. Figure 3.1 shows a basic unilateral fixator with all individual parts labeled.

Unilateral fixators are generally less stiff than ring frames. The motion at a fracture site takes place with load. The bone ends travel a distance and return to their resting position when the load is removed. This hysteresis cycle is considered "elastic" fixation. The excursion of bone ends is greatest for simple monoaxial frames. Unilateral fixator stiffness is determinedly four essential elements: (1) pin diameter, (2) pin spread and quantity, (3) connection of pins to connecting bars, and (4) distance of connecting bars from bone [2]. The stiffness of a uniaxial frame is proportional to pin diameter – the thicker the fixation pins, the stiffer the frame. A useful rule of thumb is two 5 mm half-pins are as stiff as three 4 mm half-pins. The choice of pin diameter is also dependent on the anatomic location of the fracture and bone quality. Larger pins, which are stiffer, are not well suited for small areas of cancellous bone where they can overcome the stiffness of the bone and "toggle" out [2]. Conversely, smaller pins are not well suited for large, thick areas of diaphyseal bone such as the femur. Pin stiffness is proportional to the third power of the pin radius. However, how the pin-bone junction behaves depends not only on pin material and diameter but also on bone quality, rate, and direction of load.

Pin spread is the distance of individual pins from the fracture site, connecting rods, and connectors. The general clinical rule for pin placement is to maximize the distance between pins on each size of the fracture site, with one pin as close as possible to the fracture and one distant. This construct minimizes the torsion moment on the fracture through reduction of the distance of the lever arm of rotation. The addition of a supplemental pin out of plane of the others can be an easy way significantly to increase stability. The number of pins is also directly proportional to the stiffness of the fixator. Two pins on either side of the fracture are required so that there is rotational stability. More pins will add more stability.

Fixation clamps that are brand-specific joints that hold external fixation half-pins together in groups. Generally pin clamps accept from one to multiple pins in various planes, but universally group these pins together to create a fixation point with bone. Most pin clamps attach to pins using fraction created by tightening a bolt or screw. Pin clamps are generally more stable with more pins with greater spread between pins and with pins in different planes.

The distance of the connecting bars to the bone also influences fixator stiffness. Situate the connecting bars as close to the bone as anatomically possible by location and soft tissue condition. Connecting bar stiffness is like pin stiffness – directly proportional to the third power of the radius of the bar [2].

A uniaxial frame built with more than one connecting bar is more stable particularly when the bars are not in the same plane. Connecting bars can also have joints so they can be contoured around joint surfaces and anatomic curves. Generally, the location of the connecting bar joints is not clinically relevant to the stability of the connecting bar once the joints are locked [3].

Half-frame fixators should provide for equivalent fixation on either side of a fracture. If one side has more anchorage than the other does, motion will loosen the pins on the side with less of a grip on the bone. For example, to get equal holding across the elbow, place two 5 mm half-pins in the distal humerus and three 4 mm half-pins in the proximal ulna.

3.3 Ring Fixators

Circular fixators are generally the stiffest constructs. These frames use thin wires (≤2.5 mm) transfixed through the bone to the other side and tensioned anywhere from 50 to 100 kg depending on brand, material type, and anatomic location. Circular fixator stiffness is based also on six essential elements: (1) diameter of the rings, (2) spread of the thin wires and angle of placement relative to each other, (3) plane of thin wire fixation, (4) tension of thin wires, (5) connecting devices from wires to rings, and (6) quantity of rings in the montage [4].

The diameter of the rings is analogous to the distance of the unilateral frame connecting bar from the bone. The closer the ring is to the bone, the more stable the construct [5]. Two to three fingerbreadths distance between any soft tissue surface and the bone is a clinically relevant distance for clearance between the ring and the limb.

Fine wires are inserted with power, using a wet sponge to stabilize the wire as it is advanced through the bone. Thin wires are attached to rings with wire fixation bolts. The wires are tensioned with a wire tensioning device. More tension on a thin wire usually creates more stability.

A ring frame has at least one ring proximal and one ring distal to the fracture. Begin frame construction by placing one ring proximal and one ring distal to the fracture perpendicular to the long axis of the bone. The ring on the more stable side of the fracture is the reference ring. The two rings are connected by three or four threaded bars parallel to the long axis of the bone. This frame montage is a simple traction device. Since the rings can rotate about a single wire, the frame is not stable. The next step is to place a second fine wire either at an angle to the first or in a different plane from the ring through a second ring on through posts fastened to the ring. The second wire prevents the reference ring from tipping and makes the frame stable. Finally additional wires, rings, or half-pins can be added to the basic traction frame to compute the fixation. Wires can serve special functions. For example, a wire passed just anterior to bone can be fastened to the ring, with wire holding bolts situated slightly posterior. Tensioning the wire will pull the bone posteriorly. Wires with short thick stops (olive wires) can be sued to pull bone toward the tensioner or to prevent the limb from shutting in the frame [6].

Close to the knee, an open back (5/8) ring is used to permit knee flexion. To cross the ankle, fine wires are held by a foot plate. The use of the various elements of a fine wire ring fixateur depends on their design and materials. For example, a conventional Ilizarov carbon fiber foot plate needs a half-ring placed distally to keep the arms of the foot plate from bending when a wire is tensioned across the forefoot. The Tenxor foot plate can be used without a distal half-ring.

Ring frames are most commonly used for tibial pilon and plateau fracture, for hindfoot fractures, and for forearm fractures. The mechanics of small wire frames has been well studied. When only wires are reused, they allow for compression – distraction at a fracture site with relatively little bending, shear, or tension. Addition of half-pins creates an asymmetric restraint on motion of the bone ends and introduces greater motion of the fracture particularly in bending and shear.

3.4 Hybrid Fixators

Hybrid frames combine the stability of circular frames with the ease of application of unilateral frames. These montages typically consist of a ring connected to a unilateral or multiple connecting rods through special ring to rod clamps (Fig. 3.3). These fixators are designed primarily for periarticular fractures of the tibia plateau and pilon, but can also be used for bridging fixation across the ankle and knee. Hybrid frame biomechanics are determined by four essential elements: (1) crossed thin wires, (2) ring to connecting bar coupling, (3) attachment of the pins to the bone, and (4) geometry of the hybrid construct. The connection of the ring to the unilateral bar is a brand-dependent, specific device designed for use in a hybrid frame [7].

Connecting bar stiffness, like pin stiffness, is directly proportional to the third power of the radius of the bar.

A uniaxial frame built with more than one connecting bar is more stable particularly when the bars are not in the same plane. Connecting bars can also have joints so they can be contoured around joint surfaces and anatomic curves. Generally, the location of the connecting bar joints is not clinically relevant to the stability of the connecting bar once the joints are locked.

Half-frame fixateurs should provide equivalent fixation on either side of a fracture to prevent motion from loosening the pins on the side with less of a grip on the bone. For example, to get equal holding across the elbow, place two 5 mm half-pins in the distal humerus and three 4 mm half-pins in the proximal ulna [8].

3.5 Conclusion

There is a revival of interest in external fixation for trauma. Temporary frames damage control strategies increase the use of fixators for both civilian and military injuries (Chap. 5). Clearly temporary frames should be appropriately priced. Frames facilitate transport, increase patient comfort, and decrease intensive care stay. Possible solutions are reuse, material modifications, and design changes. Since the use of temporary frames is short and adjustment is not really an advantage, it may be more economic to design them for single use than to recycle frame components. A new modular lightweight frame constructed with nonreusable couplings (they melt in the sterilizer) is priced at less than new conventional or reprocessed frames (Fig. 3.4) [8]. Today's frame is steel, titanium, or carbon fiber. An improvement is the plastic frames, which can be taken into the magnetic resonance scanner. MRI compatibility is of particular advantage for the multiply injured patient. Tomorrow's frames will contain connectors that are easier to disassemble. The requirements for fracture healing are different from the requirements from temporary stabilization. Today we use the same frame for both indicators, tomorrow there will be greater differentiation of frame functions. Some of the possibilities are already available. Frames can transmit load to fracture sites. Adjusting the spring element in the monotube varies load and excursion of the fracture ends. A ring fixateur with electric drives stimulates bone regeneration. "Smart frames" fitted with strain gauges monitor fracture healing. The understanding of cutting technology prompted the development of self-cutting external fixation pins. Choice of the optimum rake angle created a pin design so a large half-pin could be safely drilled into dense conical bone without first drilling a pilot hole. The mechanical behavior of the bone-pin interface and its load transfer characteristics hold the key to improvement in the clinical use of external fixation. Previous work has emphasized the unique characteristics of the pin-bone interface. This interface is a relationship between a nonliving material and biologic tissue capable of healing. The rate and magnitude of load are only two of the important variables. The addition of ceramic or polymer materials to the pilot hole in bone could assure the integrity of pin anchorage, and thus reduce pin track infection and improve load transfer to bone.

Fixateur montages could be lighter, more elastic, and contain memory elements that could resend the load history of the construct. Engineering holds the key to exciting advances in external fixation for the future.

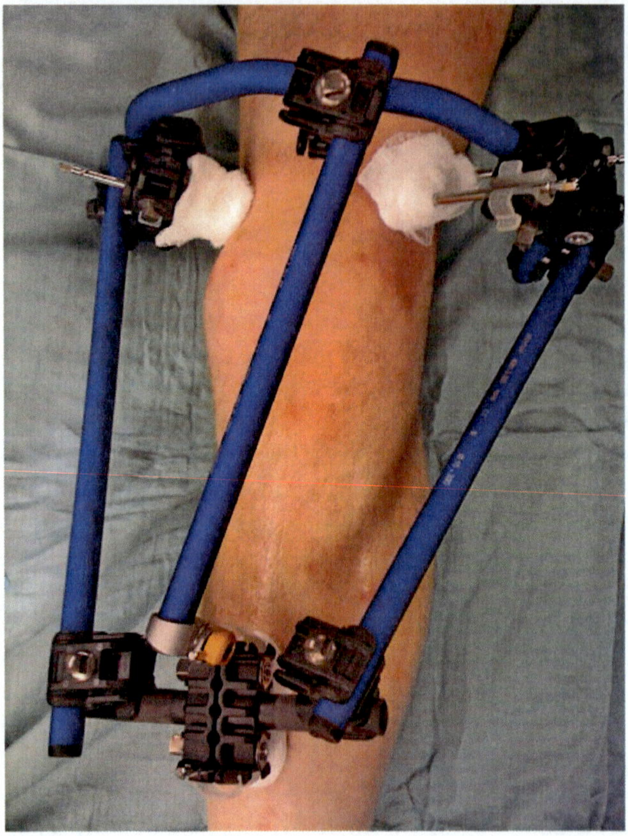

Fig. 3.4 Hoffmann Express external fixateur for a tibial plateau fracture

References

1. Schell H, Epari DR, Kassi JP, Bragulla H, Bail HJ, Duda GN. The course of bone healing is influenced by the initial shear fixation stability. J Orthop Res. 2005;23(5):1022–8.
2. Carmack DB, Kaylor KL, Yaszemski MJ. Structural stiffness and reducability of external fixators placed in malalignment and malrotation. J Orthop Trauma. 2001;15(4):247–53.
3. Ming JH, Zhou PH, Zhou JP. Biomechanical analysis of fracture fixation with external fixator in vivo. Chin J Traumatol. 2006;9(2):100–4.
4. Antoci V, Roberts CS, Antoci Jr V, Voor MJ. The effect of transfixion wire number and spacing between two levels of fixation on the stiffness of proximal tibial external fixation. J Orthop Trauma. 2005;19(3):180–6.
5. Metcalfe AJ, Saleh M, Yang L. Techniques for improving the stability in oblique fractures treated by circular fixation with particular reference to the sagittal plane. J Bone Joint Surg Br. 2005;87(6):868–72.
6. Rocchio TM, Younes MB, Bronson DG, Birch JG, Samchukov ML. Mechanical effect of posterior wire or half-pin configuration on stabilization utilizing a model of circular external fixation of the foot. Foot Ankle Int. 2004;25(3):136–43.
7. Ponsen KJ, van Dijke HGA, Joosse P, Snijders CJ. External fixators for pelvic fractures: comparison of the stiffness of current systems. Acta Orthop Scand. 2003;74(2):165–71.
8. Roberts CS, Dodds JC, Perry K, Beck D, Seligson D, Voor MJ. Hybrid external fixation of the proximal tibia: strategies to improve frame stability. J Orthop Trauma. 2003;17(6):415–20.
9. Seligson D, Douglas L. Experience with a large frame, disposable external fixateur. Orthopaedics. 2010;10:150–3.

Chapter 4
External Fixation in Economically Disadvantaged Areas

David Seligson, N.S. Laud, and Alfredo Aybar Montoya

4.1 Introduction

In 2001, 1.1 billion people had consumption levels below $1 a day and 2.7 billion lived on less than $2 a day [1]. For these populations, medical care is not readily available. High-speed trauma usually means death [2]. Patients with isolated extremity fractures, however, often survive [3]. They may be brought to hospital by makeshift transport. Ambulance services, emergency medical services, and field resuscitation equipment are not available [3, 4]. Even in highly industrialized countries, natural disasters like volcano eruptions and tsunamis can create mass casualties in a setting of hopelessly damaged infrastructure.

In hospital or hastily assembled temporary medical facilities, these survivors are admitted, occupy beds, and use resources. In this setting, judicious use of damage control strategies is a rational approach to maintaining life and limb.

A cost-effective use of minimal or native damage control external fixation devices is the basis for this approach. The patient can be treated ambulant with brief outpatient interventions. Results are acceptable and functional. The risks are low. In most of the world where expensive components of exotic materials, blood transfusion and

Chapter 4 was prepared in a time and a place before the widespread availability of megapixel phone cameras. The Chapter appropriately reflects solutions developed for the care of patients who for the most part were otherwise undersured and underserved. We present this material in this light.' Seligson, Mauffrey, Roberts, eds

D. Seligson
Department of Orthopaedics, University Hospital Louisville, Louisville, KY, USA
e-mail: seligson@louisville.edu

N.S. Laud
Department of Orthopaedics, Laud Clinic, 180, Hindu Colony,
Dadar (East), Mumbai, Maharastra, India

A.A. Montoya (✉)
Department of Orthopaedics, Av. San Felipe 142, Jesus Maria, Lima 14, Peru
e-mail: feday2000@hotmail.com

D. Seligson et al. (eds.), *External Fixation in Orthopedic Traumatology*,
DOI 10.1007/978-1-4471-2197-8_4, © Springer-Verlag London Limited 2012

costly antibiotics, and fluoroscopy units are all out of reach, the adaptation of external fixation concepts for the cure of the injured makes good sense [4].

In the past 50 years, there has been a dramatic evolution in the strategies for managing, for example, femur shaft fractures. What began as fracture treatment followed by cast bracing has become a "high tech" intervention.

One can remember patients kept in balanced traction until the fracture was "sticky" who were then cast-braced. Hospitalization lasted 2 months – unthinkable today. Today, in North America, length of stay has been shortened either by insurers or by state authorities.

In reality, the bed costs for an orthopedic patient with a limb fracture are not so great. Cost averaging across the spectrum of human disease has assigned the same value for a patient day in a traction bed as for a patient with metabolic failure. In today's first-world countries, it is likely that the patient with an uncomplicated femur shaft fracture will be home within a week if not sooner. Economic factors in so-called third world countries are entirely different.

4.2 How We Get Things Done When the Time Arrives

In the developed world, a highly organized system of Emergency Medical Services delivers the injured to the accident department [5]. Often patients with severe internal trauma and skeletal fractures survive because resuscitation begins within moments of injury. Either technicians are trained in intubations and intravenous fluid administration or casualty physicians are on ambulances or helicopters to provide initial care in the field [6–8].

This is in contrast to the situation in the less developed land. Here patients are brought to hospitals in ersatz transportation – in the bed of a truck, on the back of an animal, or in a cart – days or possibly weeks after injury [3, 9–11]. These patients are, in essence, the survivors of accidents and usually do not have life-threatening internal injuries – the patients with potentially lethal injuries died before they ever got to the hospital [12, 13].

In a study of infection after compound fracture, the hypothesis that limb injury infections were correlated with injury severity was investigated. The reasoning was that higher sepsis rates would be present in the multiply injured because of bacteria from pneumonia, indwelling catheters, and urinary infections. Not only was this correlation not found, but also patients with arm and leg fractures were a distinctly different group from the patients with chest, abdominal, and pelvic injury. When one thinks about it, apparently one either is hit to the body or one catches an arm or a leg.

In the undeveloped world, the casualty area consists of a few stretchers, some facility for plain x-ray, and splinting materials. In much of the world these are private hospitals, owned by doctors and staffed by their employees [3]. There is an abundance of kindness, expertise, and willingness to treat but there are no CT machines, no fluoroscopy, and little in the way of specialized appliances for fracture care. What is available will be used and reused and repaired because it cannot be replaced.

4.3 Cost Comparisons

Forty years ago, a US manufactured Küntscher nail cost $90 and a reusable external fixateur was several hundred dollars. Mobile image intensifiers were unavailable. A basic fracture table was used for hip nailing. To pin a hip, the position of the implant was controlled with biplanar portable x-rays. A good private orthopedist could fix a hip in under an hour. Most of this equipment is still unavailable for the treatment of most of the world's people.

Percutaneous medullary nailing was introduced in the US by Dr. Kay Clawson and the group in Seattle. Clawson imported to the US a fluoroscopy unit and fracture table from Germany. There began the saga of technological improvement with more complicated, costly devices which extend the indications for operative fracture care, shortened hospitalizations, and improved results for complex fracture problems. Parenthetically, the surgeon's fee did not keep pace with implant costs.

Today's medullary nails with interlocking cost several thousand dollars and external fixateurs cost about $5,000 each. We are further in an information age where lectures, technical brochures, and journal articles are universally available at no cost over the Internet.

The price of implants produced in economically advantaged countries includes not only the added cost of advances in manufacturing and quality but also expenses imposed by regulatory agencies and by law. Certainly, intramedullary nails produced by gun-drilling as compared to historical devices which were folded from strips of steel are more expensive to make. MRI-compatible fixateurs and ex-fix pins with surface treatment are costly but improve performance and safety.

Today, introducing a new device requires a team of lawyers and engineers skilled in securing the requisite approval from the Food and Drug Administration so the product can be sold in the United States. Innovations are subject to a multiphase approval process which can cost millions for products which are considered new and/or have consequences for life support. Adverse outcomes of fracture treatment are a top cause of product liability or malpractice. Both the company and the physician can be charged and prosecuted for well-meaning attempts to improve fracture care.

There is then a tremendous gulf between the need of people throughout the world to have access to established treatment that will improve results, and the ability of large manufacturers to devote themselves to less advanced and perhaps less reliable but certainly less expensive solutions to common skeletal injury problems.

4.4 Practical Solutions

Damage Control Strategies in which simple external fixateurs are followed by or combined with internal fixation is particularly attractive for economically disadvantaged areas. The external fixateur can be inexpensive and can be applied easily and at low risk. Thoughtful administrative strategies could create centers where more expensive equipment such as a mobile c-arm would be located. The fixateur lends itself to patient transport to a place where an intense short stay intervention can be performed.

There are several practical solutions to providing low-cost external frames. One is the distribution of used appliances via voluntary efforts. Probably very little comes of these efforts. The frames may not arrive at places they can be understood and used. The parts are incomplete and local components do not fit the sets that are sent. Similarly companies could send their outdated models to Third World centers. It is not likely that sufficient material is available to make a significant contribution and manufacturers are interested in selling, not in undercutting potential markets. Since those networks who have means usually buy what they need from distributors, it would be against good commerce if similar devices were placed without charge at charity hospitals.

A more practical solution is the manufacture of simple appliances in the local area – devices that are affordable because they are made from inexpensive components and because they do not contain the added costs imposed by regulation and by the legal system of the developed world.

For example, a straightforward small-sized external fixateur for wrist fractures can be constructed using basic turnbuckles. The frame is placed with transfixing Kirschner wires. This montage provides distraction at the fracture site and is adjustable. The risks are low and the benefits considerable.

In another strategy, simple metal elements are connected to pins using flexible tubes. The tubes are hardened with inexpensive plastic material. A variety of these devices can be constructed. There is a lack of adjustability of articulated couples but, nonetheless, these devices are suited to a wide variety of fracture problems. The montages can be combined with classic internal fixation as definitive treatment for many important clinical problems.

4.5 Practical Cases

4.5.1 The UMEX (Fig. 4.1)

In the first example, the author N.S. Laud has designed and used a simple inexpensive external fixateur for the acral skeleton. The device, the Universal Mini-Modular External Fixateur (UMEX), is locally manufactured in India and consists of three sizes of basic units which lock knurled rods to K-wires by jamming the rod against the K-wire. The stability of the connection has been verified by mechanical testing. The connection rods, basic units, and K-wires are fabricated in stainless steel.

4.5.1.1 Case 1

This 50-year-old orthopedic surgeon sustained a comminuted distal radius fracture in a road traffic accident. The AP (Fig. 4.2a) and lateral (Fig. 4.2b) x-rays show

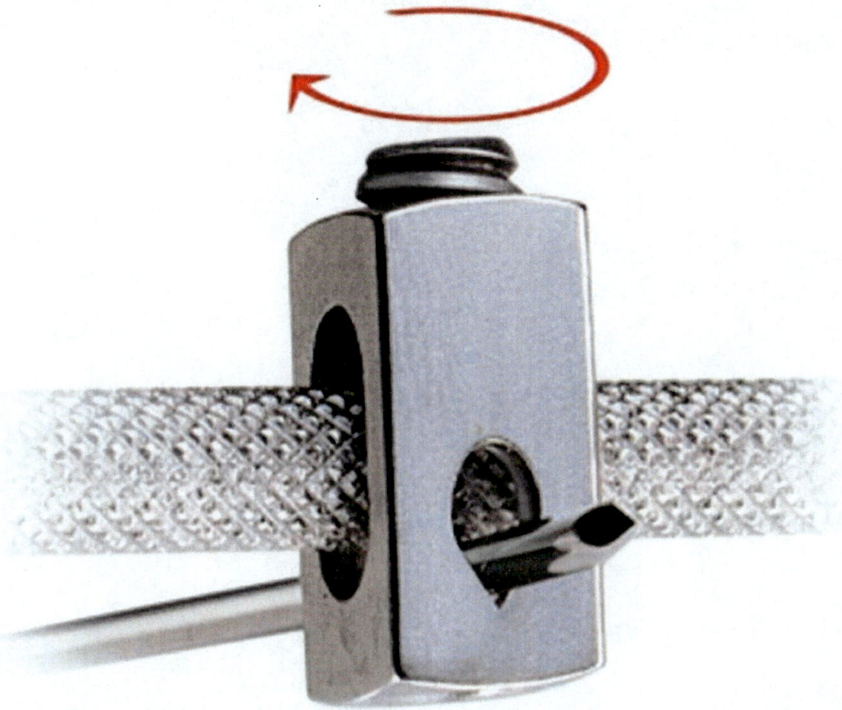

Fig. 4.1 Detail of the rod-pin-basic unit of the Universal Mini-Modular External Fixateur (UMEX)

shortening of the radius, loss of physiologic volar facing of the joint surface, and an ulnar "die punch" fragment. Reduction was achieved with K-wire fixation which was augmented with a UMEX frame (Fig. 4.2c and d). At 3 months, the x-ray shows maintenance of the reduction (Fig. 4.2e), and at 6 months the healing has been satisfactory as shown on comparison x-ray of both wrists (Fig. 4.2f). Function is good and the orthopedist can operate again (Fig. 4.2g). UMEX is a particularly inexpensive and flexible system. The modular components can be cleaned and reused.

4.5.1.2 Case 2

RP, a 45-year-old workman, was injured in a car accident. He sustained a highly comminuted proximal tibia fracture (Schatzker type VI). On plain x-ray (Fig. 4.3a–c), the bicondylar aspect of the fractures is evident. The 3-DCT (Fig. 4.3d, e) shows the severity of the comminution. At surgery, the large fracture fragments were assembled with percutaneous screws and the forces across the knee were neutralized with the UMEX frame (Fig. 4.3f–i). At 6 months after injury, there is good alignment of the leg, satisfactory joint surface reduction, and good knee function (Fig. 4.3k).

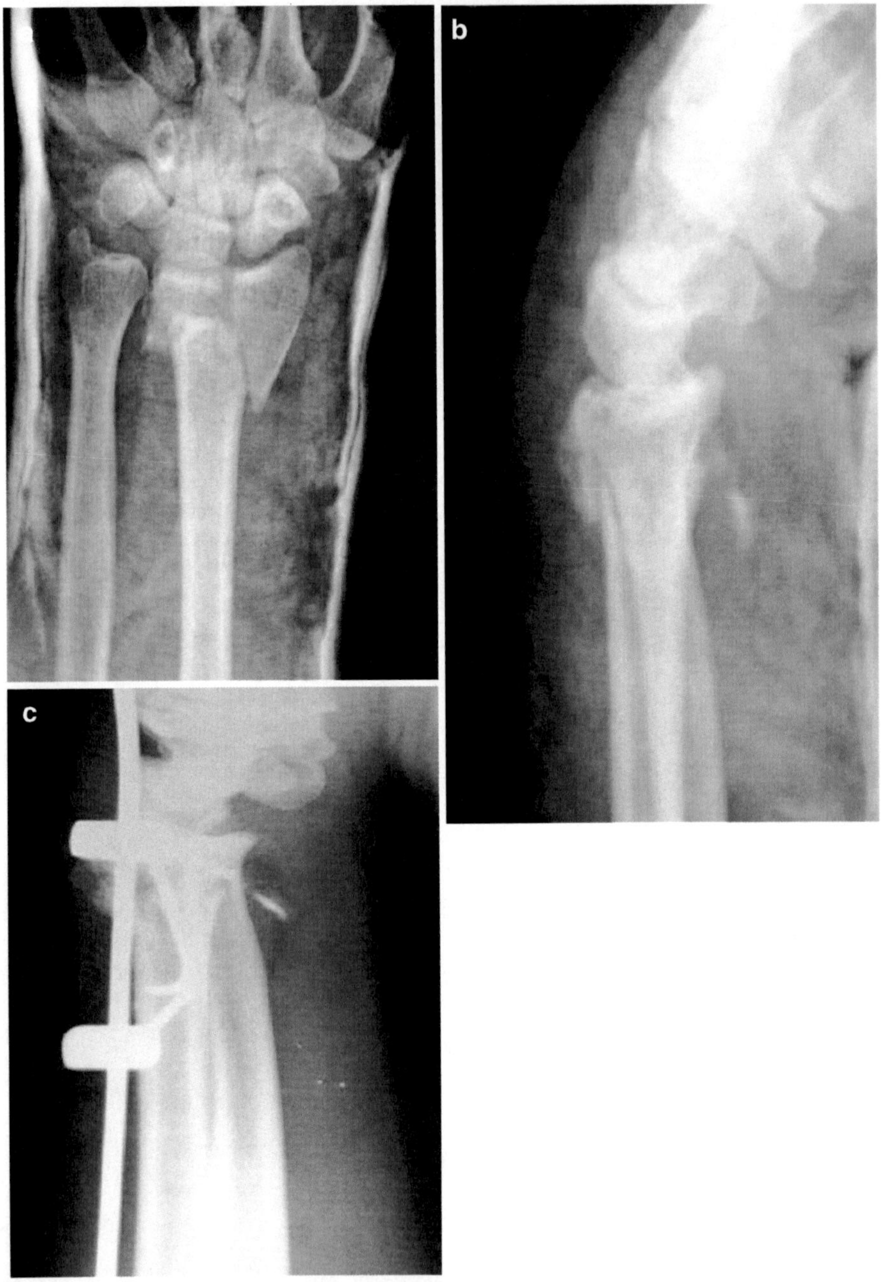

Fig. 4.2 (**a**) AP radiograph of an intra-articular distal radius fracture. (**b**) Lateral radiograph of an intra-articular distal radius fracture. (**c**) Lateral radiograph showing that reduction was achieved with K-wire fixation which was augmented with a UMEX frame. (**d**) AP radiograph showing that reduction was achieved with K-wire fixation which was augmented with a UMEX frame. (**e**) Maintenance of reduction at 6 weeks. (**f**) AP radiograph at 6 months showing healing of the fracture. (**g**) Lateral radiograph at 6 months showing healing of the fracture

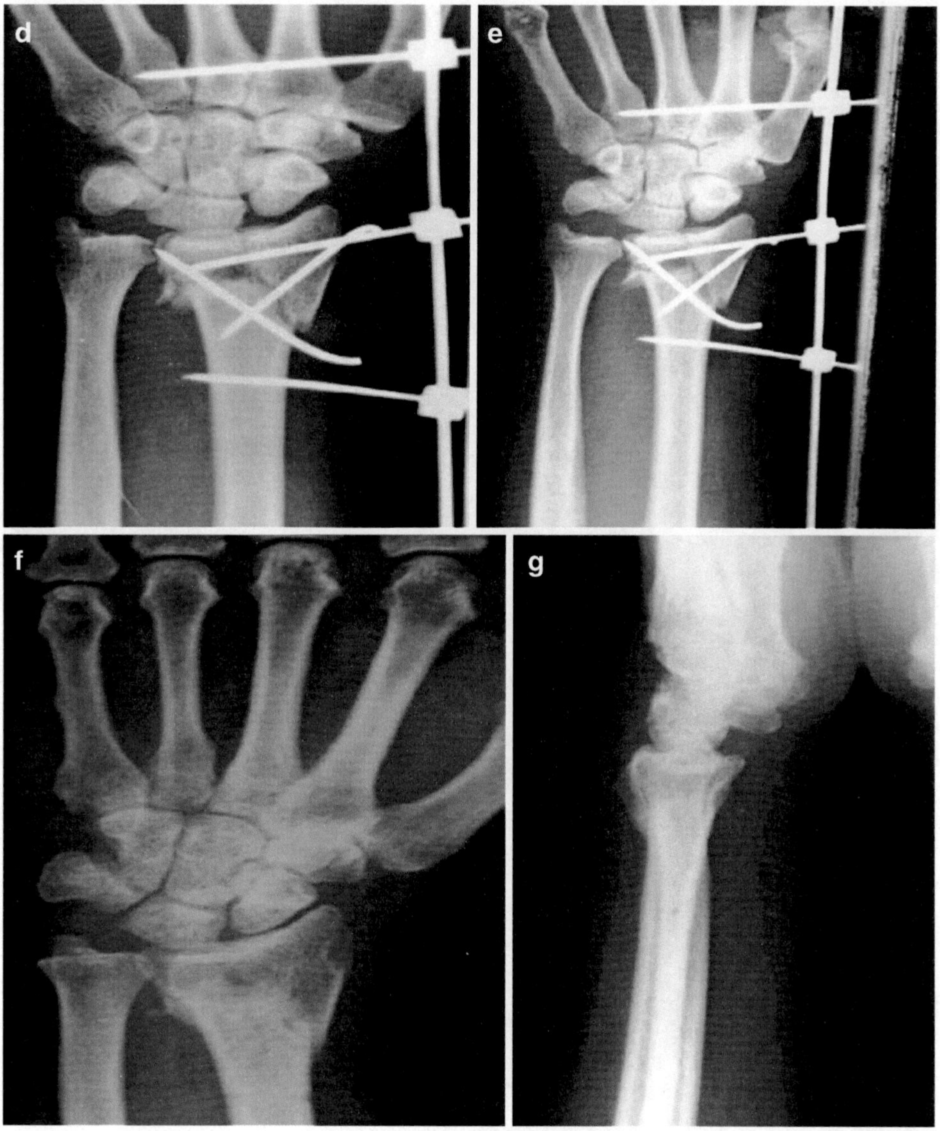

Fig. 4.2 (continued)

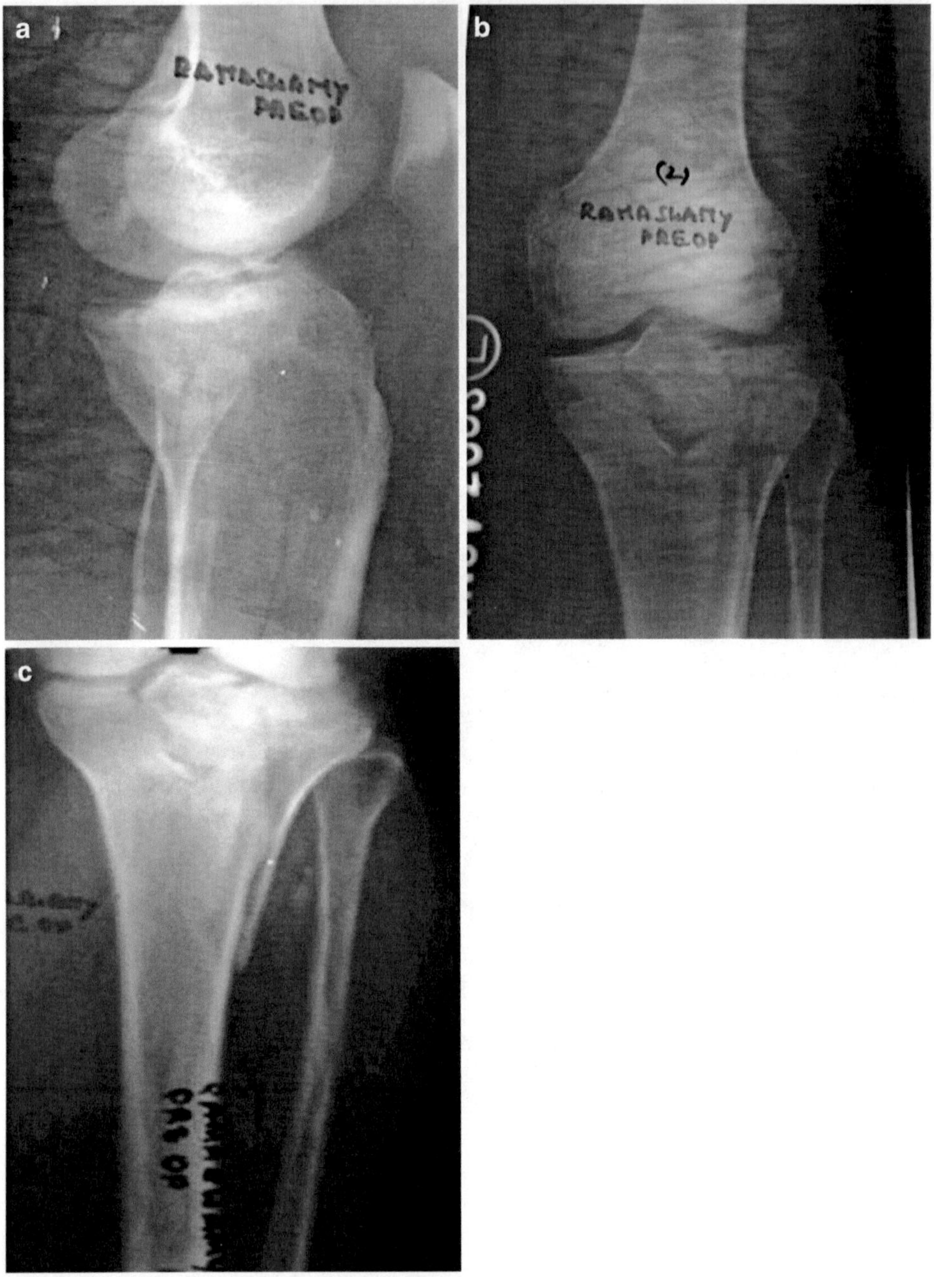

Fig. 4.3 (**a**) Lateral radiograph of a tibial plateau fracture. (**b**) AP radiograph of a tibial plateau fracture. (**c**) AP radiograph of a tibial plateau fracture. (**d**, **e**) 3D reconstruction views of a tibial plateau fracture. (**f–j**) The large fracture fragments were assembled with percutaneous screws and the forces across the knee were neutralized with the UMEX frame. (**k**) Patient with UMEX frame

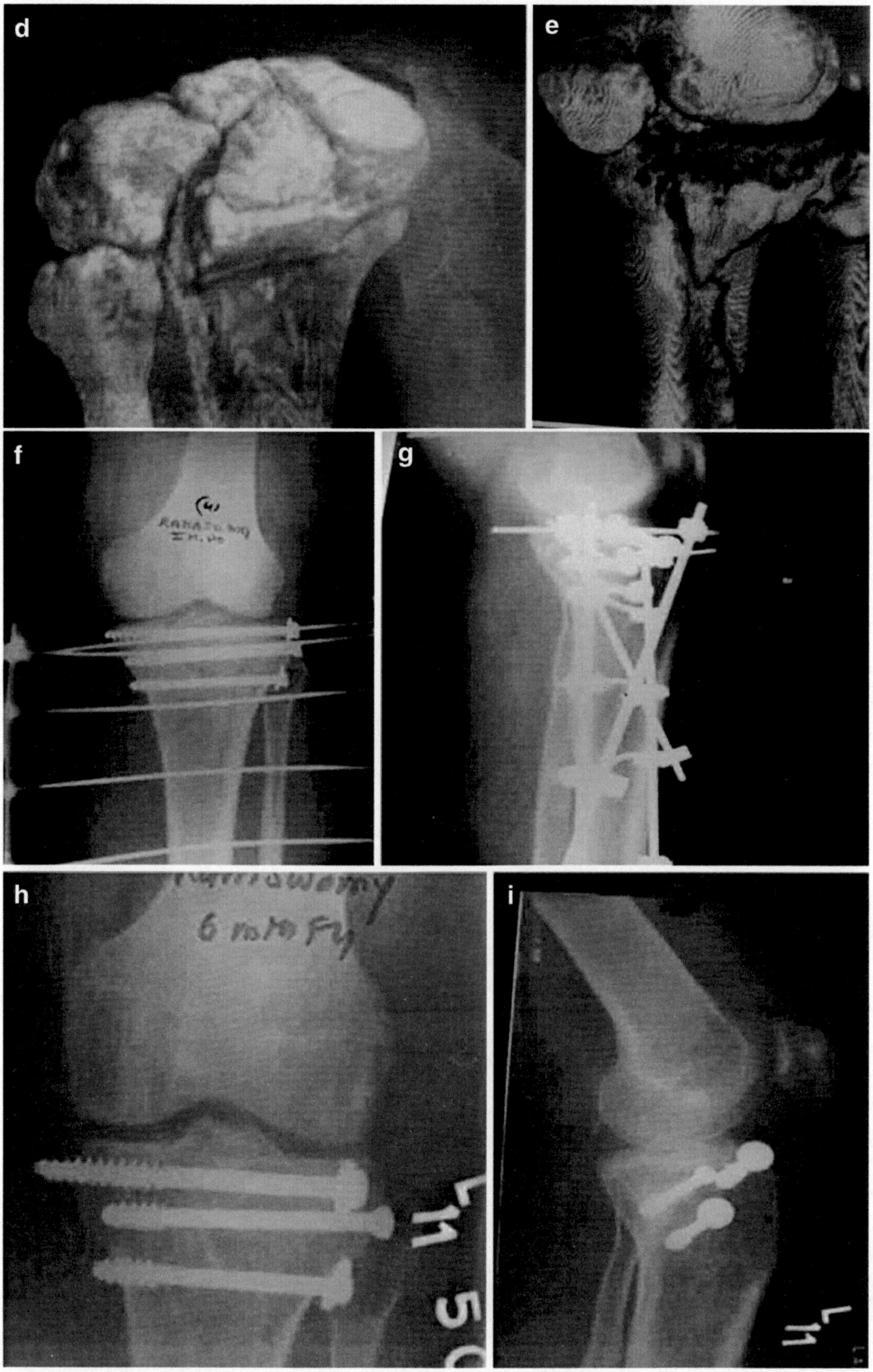

Fig. 4.3 (continued)

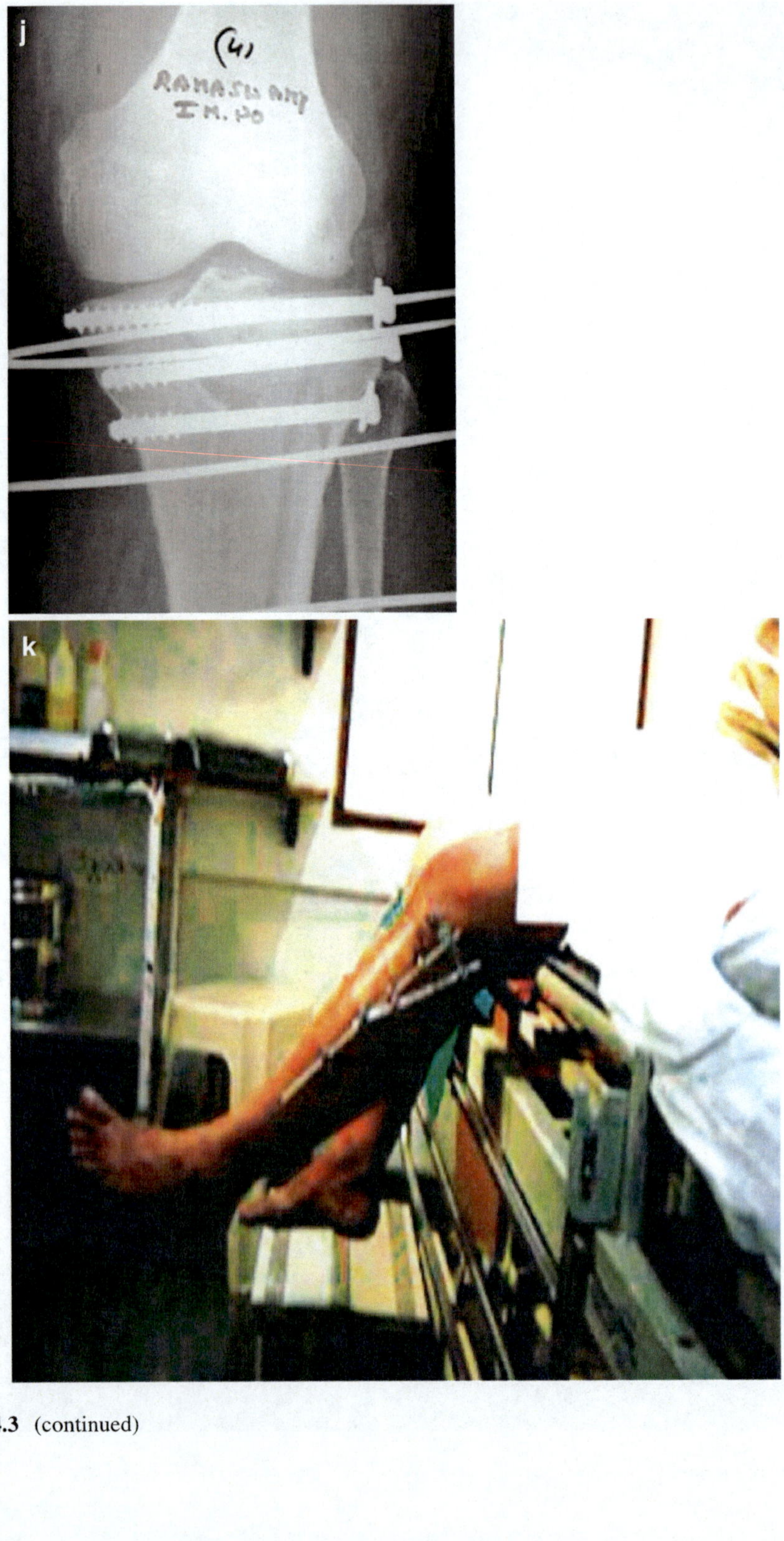

Fig. 4.3 (continued)

4.5.2 Disposable External Fixateur

Our second example is a full-frame, locally manufactured fixateur from Peru. The system is called the Fixateur External Disposable (Fijación Externa Descartable – FED). The device is usually assembled as a full frame – that is, with transfixing pins and a connecting bar on each side of the limb. However, half-frame application is also possible. The system has two sets of hardware: (1) tracto-compressor instrument and (2) the disposable set (aluminum bars and acrylic cement).

The first step is to place the transfixing pins, then to assemble the tracto-compressor instrument on the pins. The hardware FED has multiple positions and adjustable connecting rods. The pins are held in the hardware FED with locking collets. Next, the fracture is reduced by manipulating the pin and the hardware. Finally, a soft aluminum bar is fitted around the fixateur pins, and the pins are set in dental acrylic. The tracto-compressor instrument can then be reused and reused. The pins and acrylic-aluminum connectors are discarded when the frame is removed by cutting the pins off between the bars and limb.

The hardware FED (tracto-compressor instrument), mode bilateral, helps to reduce and maintain, transitorily, the fracture with its plates (Fig. 4.4a). Later, this is replaced by the discarded components (aluminum bars and acrylic cement).

The help instrument is placed and the fracture reduced (Fig. 4.4b). Next, the aluminum rods and dental acrylic are placed around the pins (Fig. 4.4c). Finally, the tracto-compressor instrument is removed and the assembly is complete (Fig. 4.4d, e).

4.5.2.1 Case 1

This 28-year old was injured in a traffic accident. His treatment began 1 month after injury. An amputation had been recommended. Figure 4.5a shows clinical appearance of the leg and (Fig. 4.5b) x-ray shows segmented fracture with bone loss and comminution. After repeat debridement and external fixation with FED, the gap was 13 cm (Fig. 4.5c). Corticotomy and lengthening were performed (Fig. 4.5d). After plastic skin coverage (Fig. 4.5e) and consolidation of the bone (Fig. 4.5f), the result was good (Fig. 4.5g). The author, Dr. Alfredo Aybar, has used this home-grown system with success both for acute fracture care and for reconstruction for more than a decade.

4.6 Conclusion

External fixation was introduced into North American practice in the late 1970s. At that time, the trauma movement was at its height. In the post-Vietnam War era medical education, the treatment of shock and airway management brought patients to trauma centers who had previously not survived. Immediate and comprehensive fracture treatment improved survival.

The importance of the upright position to pulmonary function was appreciated. The treatment of simple fractures with simple frames was neglected. The use of

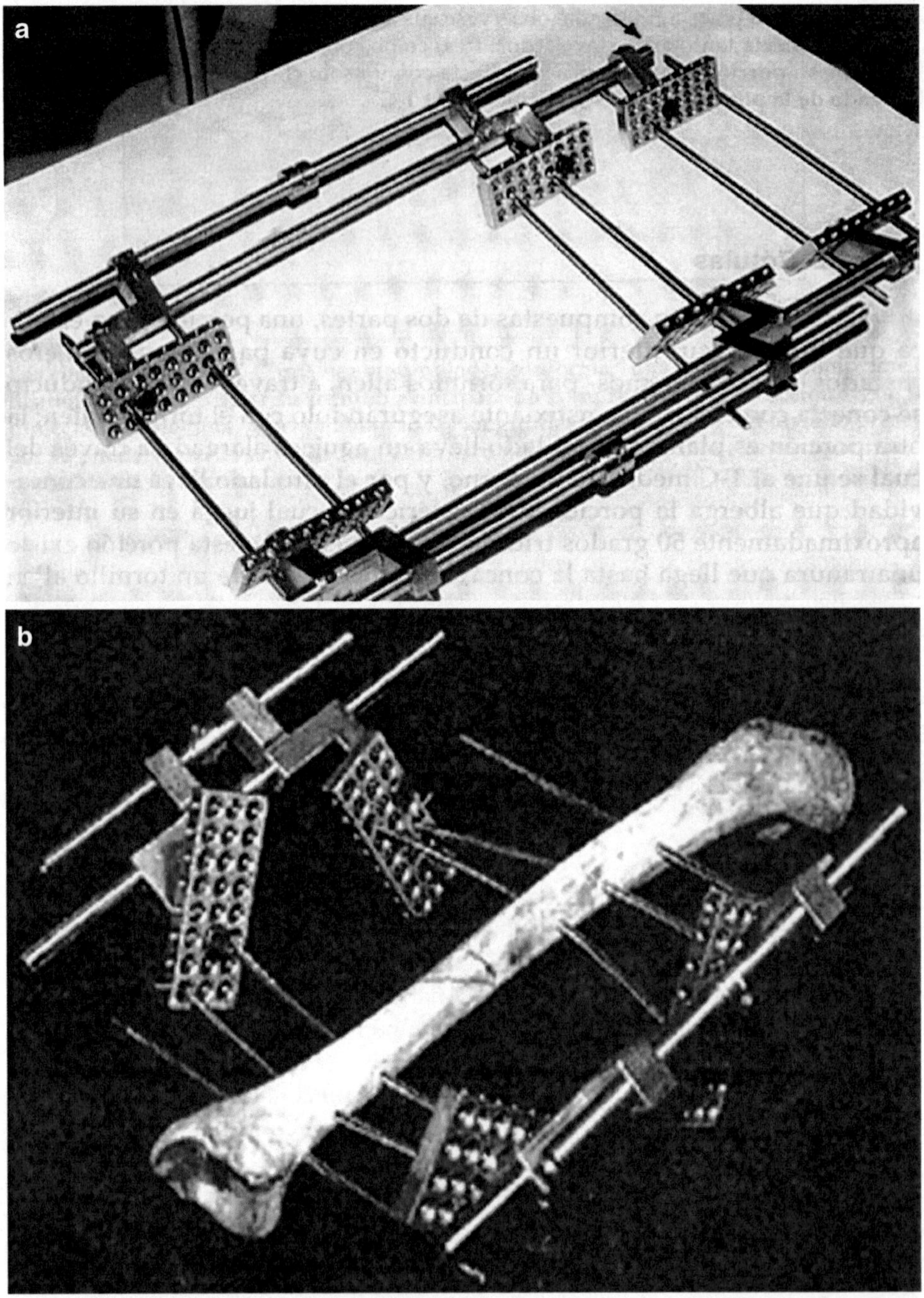

Fig. 4.4 (**a**) The hardware FED (tracto-compressor instrument), mode bilateral, helps to reduce and maintain, transitorily, the fracture with its plates. (**b**) The help instrument is placed and the fracture reduced. (**c**) The aluminum rods and dental acrylic are placed around the pins. (**d**) The tracto-compressor instrument is removed and the assembly is complete. (**e**) clinical photograph of limb without tracto-compressor instrument

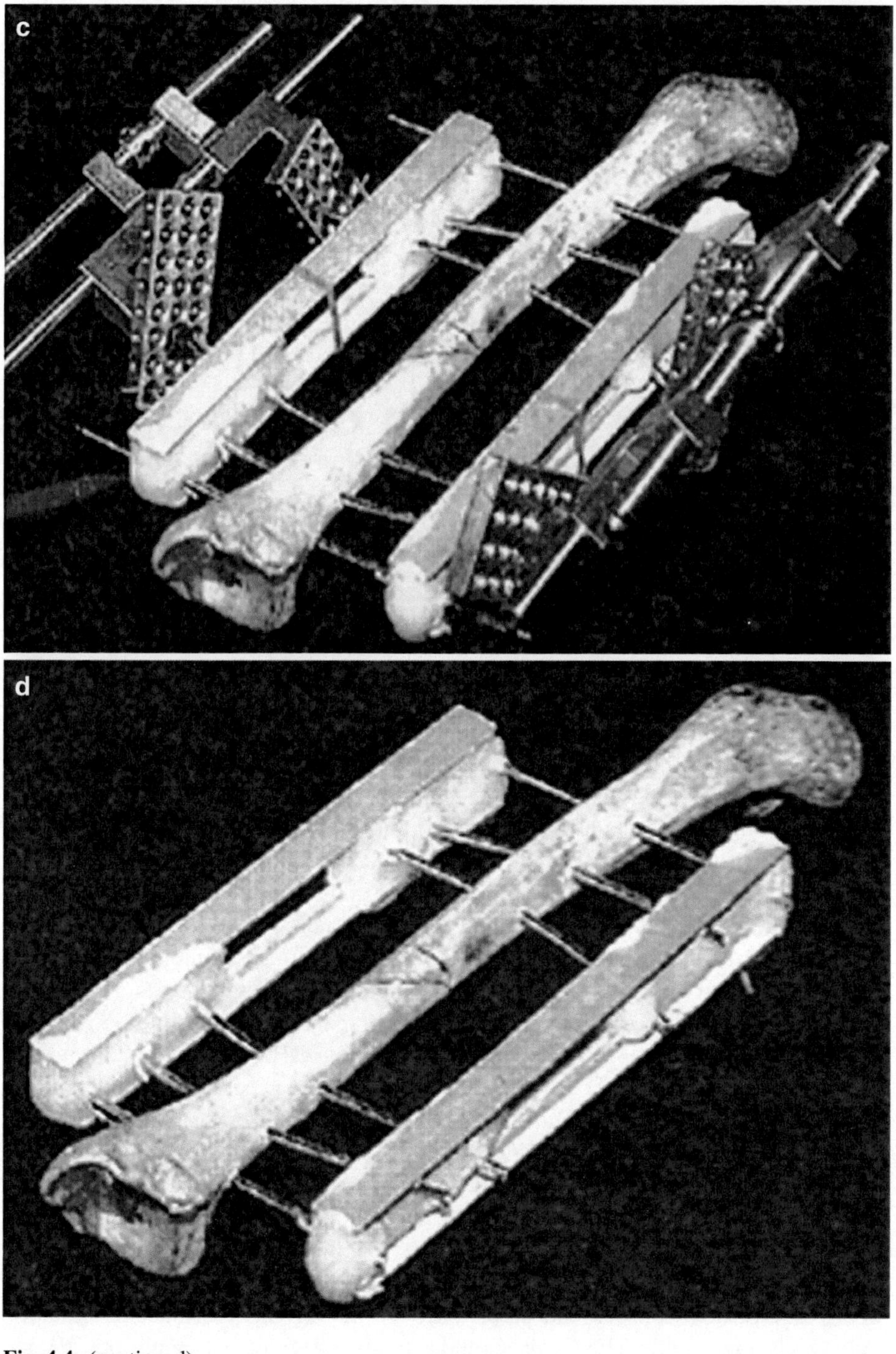

Fig. 4.4 (continued)

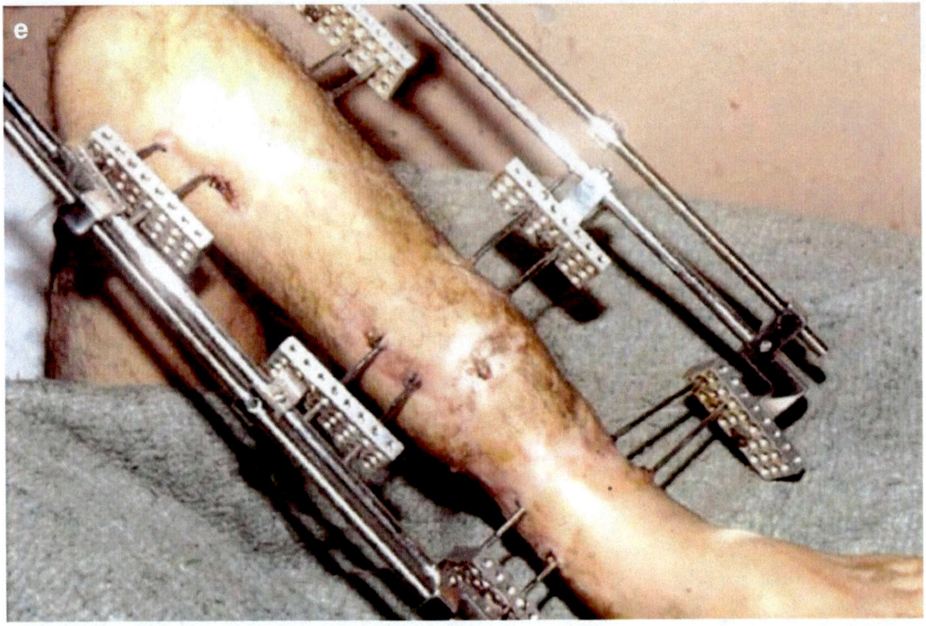

Fig. 4.4 (continued)

Hoffmann's elegant osteostaxis frames for initial and comprehensive care of fractures was limited. The exceptions were few but important – compound tibia, pelvic ring, and distal radius. Fixateurs were used mostly for complex posttraumatic reconstruction – for osteomyelitis, lengthenings, or axis correction.

Today, in developed countries, we are coming full circle and using frames in a "damage control" strategy. Though more costly, our equipment has not become more sophisticated. Medical costs have escalated and so has the price of equipment. The goal should be to apply the strategy and the concept in the developing world without the price tag. It is possible, as has been shown, to do a whole lot with very little. The approach should be to encourage simple methods with basic constructions made locally. The problem of mass casualty also requires a solution involving external fixation. The logistics as was demonstrated in Haiti, needs to be thought out. Even the best teams of skilled orthopedists cannot successfully stabilize fractures without power for light and running clean water for sterility. The injured are more mobile, more comfortable with externally stabilized fractures, but there is the obligation to "do no harm." Definite care can be horribly compromised by imposing infection on already damaged limbs by the injudicious use of external frames.

The feasibility of regionalized care allows for low-cost solutions based on the economy of scale and centralization. Much real information about the optimum timing of treatment phases and algorithms for management of specific fracture problems is unavailable. How soon should a compound fracture be debrided? What is the best time to convert a frame to a nail or a plate? Is conversion to a cast or a brace possible? Does "early motion" or early weight bearing really improve results? Doubtless as these factors are studied and evidence rather than opinion comes to direct treatment, many shibboleths will fall, and we will all be better for it.

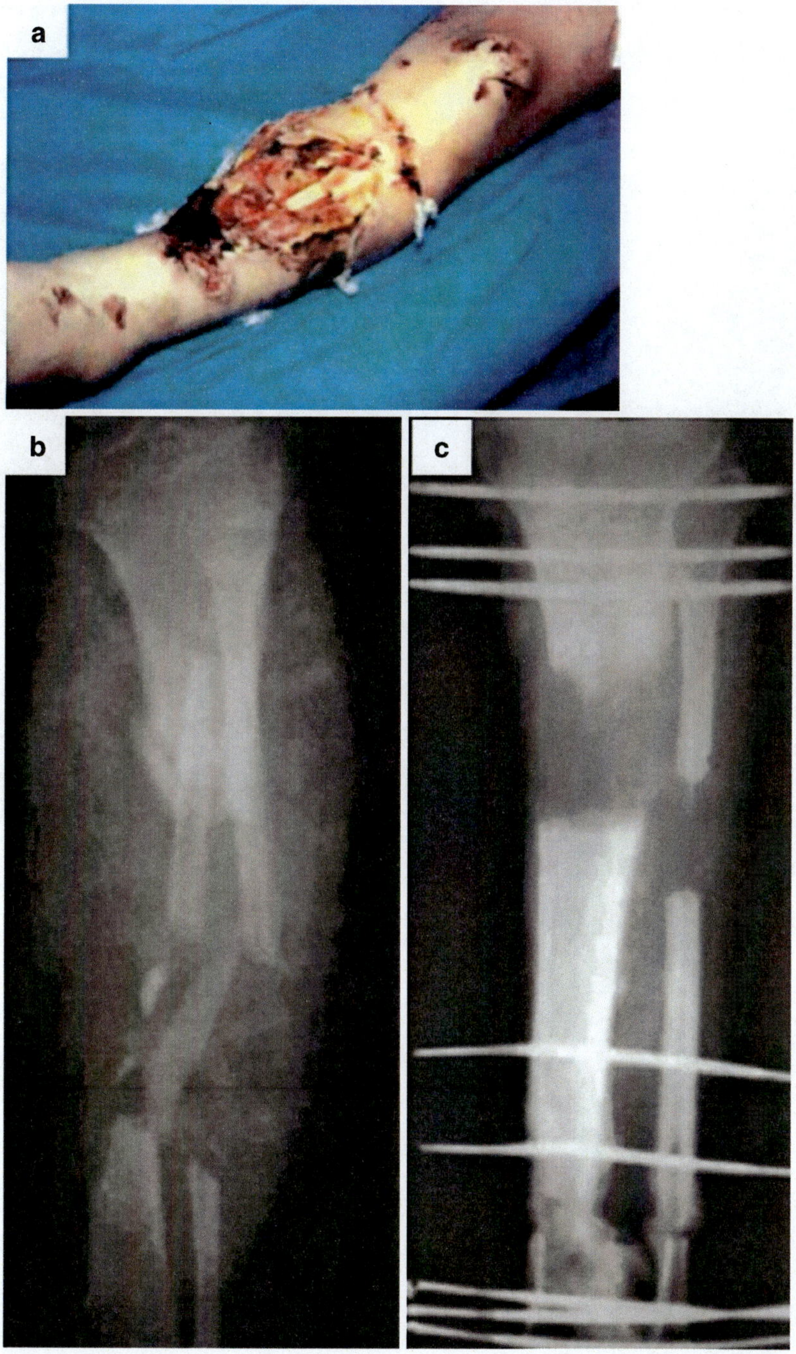

Fig. 4.5 (**a**) Clinical appearance of a leg with open contaminated fracture of the tibia and fibula. (**b**) X-ray showing segmented fracture with bone loss and comminution. (**c**) After repeat debridement and external fixation with FED, the gap was 13 cm. (**d**) After corticotomy and lengthening were performed. (**e**) After plastic skin coverage. (**f**) Consolidation of the bone at 6 months. (**g**) Consolidation of the bone at 1 year

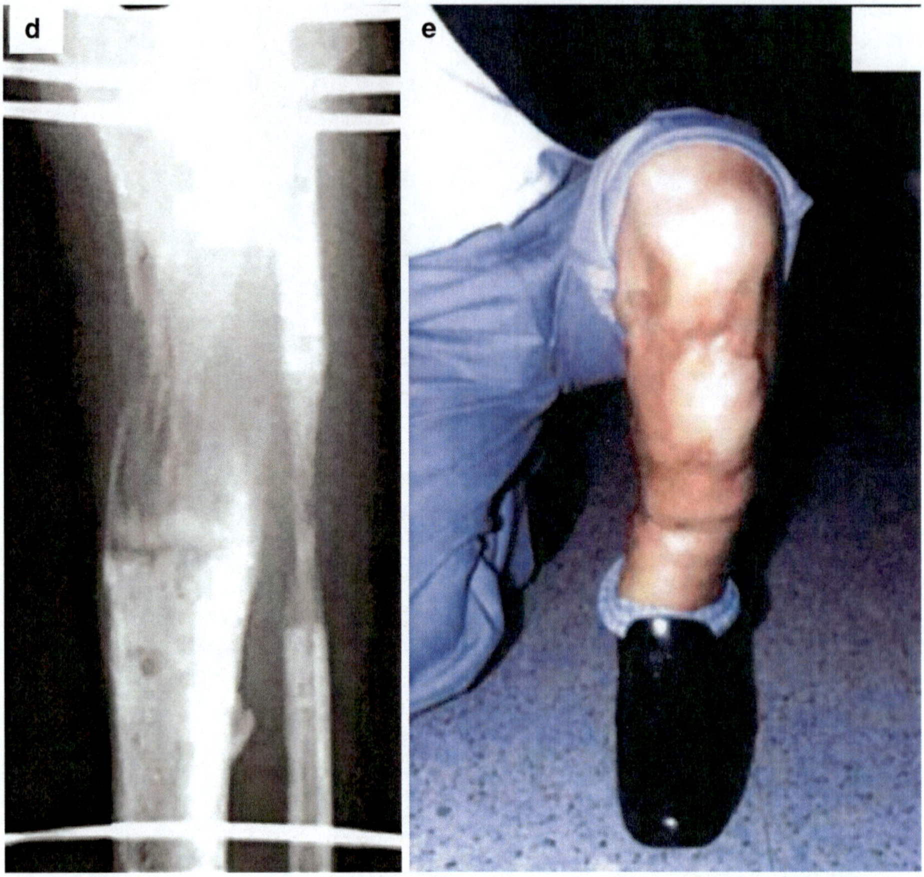

Fig. 4.5 (continued)

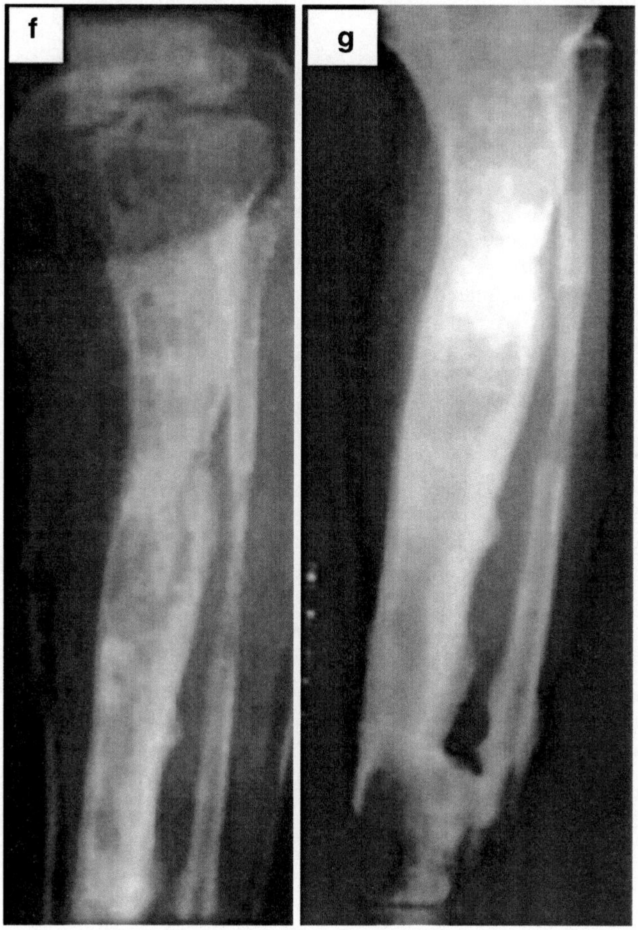

Fig. 4.5 (continued)

References

1. The World Bank, 2007, Understanding Poverty. Web.worldbank.org. 2005-04-19. http://web.worldbank.org/WBSITE/EXTERNAL/TOPICS/EXTPOVERTY/0,,contentMDK:20153855~menuPK:373757~pagePK:148956~piPK:216618~theSitePK:336992,00.html. Retrieved 24 Oct 2010.
2. Goosen J, Bowley DM, Degiannis E, Plani F. Trauma care systems in South Africa. Injury Int J Care Injured. 2003;34:704–8.
3. Joshipura MK, Shah HS, Patel PR, Divatia PA, Desai PM. Trauma care systems in India. Injury Int J Care Injured. 2003;34:686–92.
4. Mock C, Arreola-Risa C, Quansah R. Strengthening care for injured persons in less developed countries: a case study of Ghana and Mexico. Inj Control Saf Promot. 2003;10(1–2):45–51.
5. MacFarlane C, van Loggerenberg C, Kloeck W. International EMS systems: South Africa-past, present, and future. Resuscitation. 2005;64(2):145–8.
6. Gupta R, Sudhakar R. Major trauma transfer in Western Australia. ANZ J Surg. 2003;7:372–5.
7. Queipo de Llano E, Mantero Ruiz A, Sanchez Vicioso P, Bosca Crespo A, Carpintero Avellaneda JL, de la Torre Prado MV. Trauma care systems in Spain. Injury Int J Care Injured. 2003;34(9):709–19.
8. Duke T. Transport of seriously ill children: a neglected global issue. Intensive Care Med. 2003;9:1414–6.
9. Thomson N. Emergency medical services in Zimbabwe. Resuscitation. 2005;65:15–9.
10. Oestern HJ. Management of polytrauma patients in an international comparison. Der Unfallchirurg. 1999;102(2):80–91.
11. Rogers FB, Shackford SR, Osier TM, Vane DW, Davis JH. Rural trauma: the challenge for the next decade. J Trauma. 1999;47(4):802.
12. Suthorn Bavonratanavech. Trauma care systems in Thailand. Injury Int J Care Injured. 2003;34:720–1.

Chapter 5
External Fixation in the War Zone

Paul J. Dougherty and Kimberly M. Kesling

5.1 Introduction

The major form of initial long bone fracture stabilization to care for US or allied soldiers in battlefield hospitals is presently external fixation [1]. The use of external fixation by the military is similar to current usage in civilian trauma centers as a means to temporarily stabilize a limb [2–4]. What is different is the fact that the wounded soldier is transported to a site of definitive care after initial stabilization at a battlefield hospital. Once in a stable environment, the receiving surgeon can continue with external fixation or change to another treatment method [1, 5–7].

Caring for civilian casualties of war has also seen the use of external fixation. Though civilian casualties sustain the same types of injuries as soldiers in conflict regions, their treatment is often more complicated because of limited resources and the uncertainty of follow-up care [8–10].

Use of external fixation to treat fractures of those injured in conflict is not new, having been used since the nineteenth century with varying degrees of success. Until recently, external fixation use was for definitive treatment of the fracture, rather than to initially stabilize the fracture until the patient is transported to a more stable environment.

This chapter is meant to provide information about external fixator use in an area of conflict whether the surgeon is treating wounded civilians or soldiers.

P.J. Dougherty (✉)
Department of orthopaedics, University of Michigan, Ann Arbor, MI, USA
e-mail: pauldoug@med.umich.edu1

K.M. Kesling
Department of orthopaedics, Clinical Services, Darnall Army Medical Center, Ft Hood, TX, USA

D. Seligson et al. (eds.), *External Fixation in Orthopedic Traumatology*,
DOI 10.1007/978-1-4471-2197-8_5, © Springer-Verlag London Limited 2012

5.2 History

A system of external fixation had been developed during the 1930s by Stader, Hoffmann, and Anderson that allowed for the treatment of a variety of fracture patterns. Use of external fixation for military casualties, however, has been limited until recently but was described by Hoffmann himself back in 1942 [11, 12].

Shaar et al. reported on the use of the Stader device for treating tibia and fibula fractures in both military casualties and accidents. They reported on 21 patients who were cared for at Philadelphia Naval Hospital early in the war. The authors felt this was an ideal treatment for more comminuted fractures or segmental fractures, and also felt that it decreased the time to union. The authors were trained in the use of the device and they were able to follow all of their patients [13].

Bradford and Wilson reported on use of external fixation for the treatment of war casualties at the American Hospital in Britain early in World War II. The authors felt external fixation was indicated for patients who had infected fractures, and fracture patients who are in shock. The surgeons were well trained in the use of external fixation, and were using the devices for patients who in the opinion of the authors would not be treated as well with skeletal traction or casting alone [14].

During World War II, initial enthusiasm for the device decreased as complications (sepsis) became known. Use of external fixators at the time required a certain level of skill and training. Because of the large number of surgeons who were brought on active duty during the conflict, most had no experience with the device. As a consequence, poor results were obtained. Because of this, external fixation was withdrawn for general use as a means of treating fractures. Indications for use of external fixation were considered to be long bone fractures with comminution or segmental defects and also those with persistent malalignment when treated with skeletal traction. Patients with burns in conjunction with fractures were also an indication for the care of these patients [15–17].

Because of the experience in World War II, there was limited use for treating battle fractures during both the Korean and Vietnam Wars by US surgeons [6, 7].

During the 1973 Yom Kippur War and 1982 War, Israeli battle casualties were treated with external fixation for definitive care in certain cases [18–21]. Reis et al. [19] reported on 110 limbs of 99 patients from both conflicts that were treated with external fixation. The intent of the authors was to use the fixator for definitive care. Patients with severe soft tissue injuries or with extensive comminution or bone loss were candidates for the use of external fixation. Thirty-two of the patients needed to be changed to another method of treatment primarily because of pin site sepsis.

The above examples use external fixation as the primary means to treat a fracture, leaving the frame on the patient's limb until healing is complete. More recently, external fixation has been used temporarily as a bridge to span a period of time for patients who are severely injured and cannot tolerate more extensive surgery or for those who have a severe limb injury and a more extensive procedure would compromise the limb. Temporary external fixation has been used for the tibia, femur, ankle, and knee in this manner with reported good success [2–5].

As discussed below, temporary external fixation is a good option in caring for soldiers who are wounded overseas and need to be transported home. It allows for standardized treatment of patients with a minimal physiological insult leaving the maximum options open for surgeons at the site of definitive care.

5.3 Requirements for a Military External Fixation System

During the 1980s, several attempts were made to obtain a standardized external fixator system for the military in order to be prepared to treat casualties. Prior to the Gulf War, requirements for a fixator were made by Department of Defense doctors who desired a peel packaged, self-contained unit that had all of the tools included to allow for the application of a frame without power and in an austere environment. Additionally, any fixator system should be of a common enough design so the frame could be removed or modified by tools used with the nonmilitary frames of the same manufacturer. The military fixator would also have to withstand field sterilization without a loss of biomechanical properties and also have equivalent biomechanical strength as the commercially available product of the same manufacturer [22].

The Howmedica (Rutheford, NJ) Ultra-X was purchased by the Department of Defense during the Gulf War. Though easy to apply, the biomechanical strength was less than that of the comparable Hoffmann external fixator. After the Gulf War, this system was withdrawn from use by the Department of Defense [22].

In the late 1990s, similar requirements were made for an external fixator to be purchased by the Department of Defense. Additional requirements were the capability to build up or build down a construct as the patient's condition progressed, a frame that could be applied to a limb with a minimum number of pins (usually four total), need only hand tools for application, not require predrilling for pin insertion, and have the ability to reduce a fracture after the application of the frame. The last requirement is important as the external fixator may be applied without radiographic support and later, when the patient is in a stable environment, needs to have the fracture reduced [22, 23].

On the basis of the new requirements, the Hoffmann II external fixator was available to the military in two forms: a simple peel pack that contained four pins, one bar, and two clamps for a single application and an autoclavable tub that contained enough equipment for the application of several frames [1, 23].

It is unclear just what the minimum biomechanical requirements for an external fixator system should be [22–29]. Patients with lower extremity fractures are not required to bear weight on the limb and are transported via litter in the evacuation system. Though less demanding than weightbearing, the patient with a lower extremity fracture may be capable of non-weightbearing on crutches. Minimizing fracture site motion while being transported to a site of definitive care is important to prevent pain and retain reduction. Because of limited x-ray capability, any system should allow for fracture reduction even after application.

5.4 Care of Nonmilitary Patients

Military surgeons are often asked to care for nonmilitary patients in regions of conflict or natural disaster as part of humanitarian assistance measures. Caring for nonmilitary patients is often difficult because in strife-torn areas, the patients are often homeless, the host country does not have any medical care system, and military missions are often for a limited period of time, allowing for limited follow-up [1, 8–10].

Nongovernmental organizations provide care to nonmilitary patients in regions of conflict or natural disaster.

There are limited reports of external fixator use in caring for refugee patients. Hammer et al. [9] reported limited follow-up of 96 fractures treated with the "Hammer external fixator system." This external fixator is a peel pack single-use device with adjustable multipin clamps connected by a single bar. The authors reported no short-term complications of deep infection or pin site sepsis. However, their follow-up was limited in both time and number of patients.

Rowley compared patients who were treated with plaster casting or traction to those who had an external fixator placed at ICRC hospitals in Northern Kenya and Afghanistan. He reported on 64 tibia fractures (24 by casting and 40 by external fixation) and 86 open femur fractures (51 skeletal traction and 36 external fixation) sustained tibia and fibula fractures. The author reported that there was no decreased hospital stay of femur fractures treated with external fixation and that alignment with both groups was about the same. For patients with tibia fractures, hospitalization was 62 days for the external fixator group, as opposed to 32 for the casting group. There were also fewer complications with the group treated with casting. The author concluded that use of external fixation was more likely to have a complication and require further, more extensive care beyond the capability of the hospital. Because he was caring for refugees, the patients stayed longer in the hospital than one would expect in a stable country where there is a medical system in place [8].

Has et al. reported on the use of external fixation for temporary and definitive treatment of 192/760 patients who had open fractures during the "war against Croatia" in the early 1990s. Thirty-nine percent of all patients admitted to the authors institution ($n = 1,658$) were nonmilitary and the rest of the admissions were "Croatian national guard and Croatian police." The rate of osteomyelitis in these patients was 13/147 (8.8%) and 7/68 (10.3%) for upper limbs. Eight of the patients who had lower limb injury and thirteen of those with upper limb injury had a delay in healing and were treated with internal fixation and bone grafting. Of those, 5/8 of the upper limb and 4/13 for the lower limb developed osteomyelitis.

Caution must be used in treating patients with external fixation if the treating surgeon cannot be assured of the patients' follow-up care. Application of a device without reasonable assurance as to safe follow-up care and removal of the fixator should not be undertaken in a combat zone if these conditions cannot be met.

5.5 Current US Military Doctrine

The present conflicts in Afghanistan and Iraq Operation Enduring Freedom/ Operation Iraqi Freedom (or OEF/OIF) have provided experience in the care of both service members as well as nonmilitary casualties. For service members, fracture care is rendered from the point of injury through various medical treatment facilities to a site of definitive care in the United States. The simultaneous goals of treating the fracture and allowing for safe transportation differ from the routine care provided to trauma patients at a major trauma center in the United States.

Service members who are wounded on the battlefield provide first aid to themselves or receive first aid from another soldier or a medic as soon as possible. First aid includes stopping hemorrhage, dressing the wound, and splinting. Additional care may be the insertion of an intervenous line and fluids, IV antibiotics, and pain control. The wounded soldier with a fracture due to battle wounds is then moved either directly to a site of initial surgical care or to an intermediate facility (battalion aid station or medical company) [5].

Initial surgical care for service members in Iraq or Afghanistan is performed as soon as possible in order to minimize the morbidity and mortality of a given wound. For open fractures, this allows treatment to prevent infection and for fracture stabilization. A patient will then undergo evacuation to a site of definitive care as soon as feasible. The wounded service member usually goes to Lanstuhl, Germany, and from then on to the United States for definitive care. Treatment in Germany consists of further fracture reduction, wound care (either in the operating room or at bedside), and in certain cases further fracture treatment. Surgeons caring for patients in both Afghanistan and Iraq are mindful of the fact that they are preparing the patients to undergo evacuation, which may mean that a patient is en route for several days, with possibly less attendant care. Because of this, elaborate surgical procedures that require close postoperative monitoring are avoided during the initial surgery [1, 5–7].

External fixation and casting are the two means available for care of wounded soldiers at the first surgical echelon of care. Using slab splints has been shown to be unacceptable for use in patients who will undergo transportation during both the Vietnam War and OEF/OIF [30]. External fixation is presently the most common method of stabilizing lower extremity fractures of the femur, tibia, knee, and ankle. Standardized constructs, which respect "at risk" anatomical structures for fixators, are to be placed on limbs in a consistent manner. This also facilitates consistent training of surgeons who prior to deployment may have little experience with fixator use. The austere nature of battlefield hospitals also means there may be no radiographic capability available when applying an external fixator to a limb [1, 5–7].

External fixator use today is a temporary measure used to stabilize a fracture until the patient can be moved to a site of definitive care. Once at a site of definitive care within the continental United States, the fixator may be changed to another device, such as an intramedullary nail, or the fixator may be continued as the method of treatment. The decision for definitive stabilization should be made within 2–3 weeks to avoid increasing the risk of sepsis [5, 31]. If more than 3 weeks had elapsed or if the patient arrives with pin sepsis, other types of stabilization may still be used. The patient may have to undergo a staged procedure, however. The goals for patient care in Combat Zone facilities are to prepare the patient for transportation and allow the maximum number of options to be available for the receiving surgeon [1–7].

5.6 Application Techniques

As mentioned before, the fixator system currently used by the Department of Defense is the Hoffmann II (Stryker, Rutherford, NJ). The guidelines used in this chapter are applicable to other systems as well. The examples given here are based on the NATO Emergency War Surgery Handbook (Fourth US revision) [1]. The purpose of this section is to show how to apply simple standard frames for patient care to allow for safe transportation of the wounded soldier. As radiographic capabilities may be limited, these examples also may be applied without the use of x-ray or C-arm. Some fixator constructs, such as around the elbow, should not be applied without having radiographic support. Any surgeon applying external fixation should be familiar with the system, its limitations, and the anatomy of the limb for which the fixator is used as treatment.

Concern has been raised about using the single-bar, four-pin construct for stabilization of a long bone fracture [32]. Clasper and Philips reported revising 13 of 15 external fixators because of complications, of which frame instability was present in 10. The authors used both Centrafix (Forward Medical Technology, Oxford, UK) and Hoffman II (Stryker Howmedica Osteonics, Rutherford, NJ) external fixator systems, and found the single-bar constructs insufficient for long bone stabilization.

5.6.1 Treatment of the Soft Tissues

Fractures caused by explosive munitions or small arms (pistols, rifles, and machine guns) are open, contaminated wounds different than that routinely seen at a civilian trauma center [30]. With each new conflict, surgeons often relearn the principals of soft tissue wound care due to these injuries [33, 34]. The term "débridement" comes from the French verb "débrider" which means to release or unbridle. A surgeon of Napoleon's army, Larrey, described this technique of war wound care to be primarily an incision to allow for exposure of the wound, "to relieve tissue tension and establish free wound drainage." Presently it is more often used to describe excision of nonviable tissue as a means of preventing infection [34–36]. Both aspects described, the longitudinal incision of the wound to open up and expose the wound and to relieve tension, as well as removal of nonviable tissue, are important tenets of wound surgery to prevent infection and potentially allow for later closure [35, 36].

Skin is incised longitudinally along the axis of the limb centered over the wound. At the wound itself, only obviously dead tissue should be removed. Incisions should be planned to avoid any skin bridges that may occur. The fascia should be incised to allow for both exposure and to relieve the tension of the tissue. Once skeletal muscle is exposed, it should be evaluated for areas of dead tissue. The "four Cs," color, contractility, circulation (bleeding), and consistency, are often used to determine the viability of skeletal muscle. Scully et al. [36] evaluated 60 biopsy samples during the Korean War of tissue removed from war wounds 3–8 h from surgery and found good correlation between contractility, bleeding, and consistency and determining viability. The wounds should be irrigated to remove contaminated material from the wound. At the end of the procedure, the wound should be left open and covered with a dressing. Wounds should not be packed or plugged to allow for drainage.

5.6.2 *Humerus*

Open diaphyseal humerus fractures due to war wounds are, in general, initially stabilized with splinting or a Velpeau dressing after initial surgery. External fixation may also be used but should only be done by an orthopedic surgeon who is experienced in this technique because of potential nerve or vascular injuries. Relative indications for applying an external fixator to an arm include polytrauma patients, a patient with a chest or neck injury, bilateral injuries, or wounds that require more frequent inspection. Keller [37] reviewed 37 soldier and nonmilitary patients with gunshot fractures who were treated at his Red Cross Hospital in Lopiding, Sudan. He treated seven of these patients with external fixation of which he found a higher rate of delayed union when compared to using a functional brace or traction. Because of this, he did not recommend this treatment for gunshot wounds of the humerus.

For a patient with a diaphyseal humerus fracture, the external fixator is applied after the soft tissue wounds have been surgically treated. In addition to the 5 mm half-pins that are commonly available, 4 mm half-pins may be used. A surgeon and assistant are needed to facilitate both the application and reduction of the limb. Just as with any fracture patient, prior to surgery a careful nerve and vascular exam should be done. If a patient is obtunded, this should also be noted.

The limb should be prepped as widely as possible to include the neck. This allows for extension of the surgical incisions, if necessary, when performing irrigation and debridement of the soft tissues.

After treatment of the soft tissues, the external fixator is applied. For temporary frames, two half-pins proximally and two half-pins distally are generally used (Fig. 5.1). Insertion of proximal pins should be from an anterior to lateral plane. The first pin should be inserted at least 2 cm from the fracture and out of the zone of injury. A 1.5 cm stab incision should be made, with blunt dissection and spreading with a clamp of the soft tissues down to bone after the incision is made. The pin should be inserted through a soft tissue protector. Using a multipin clamp as a guide, a second proximal pin is inserted more proximally along the limb away from the fracture site.

Distally, pins should be inserted from a posterior to anterior direction. Using a multipin clamp should be done as far distally on the humerus as possible, just above the olecranon fossa. This is the safest area for pin insertion. By extending the elbow, the surgeon should be able to insert the first pin 2 cm above the olecranon fossa as described above. Using the multipin clamp as a guide, a second pin should be inserted outside of the zone of injury. Careful spreading of the soft tissues and use

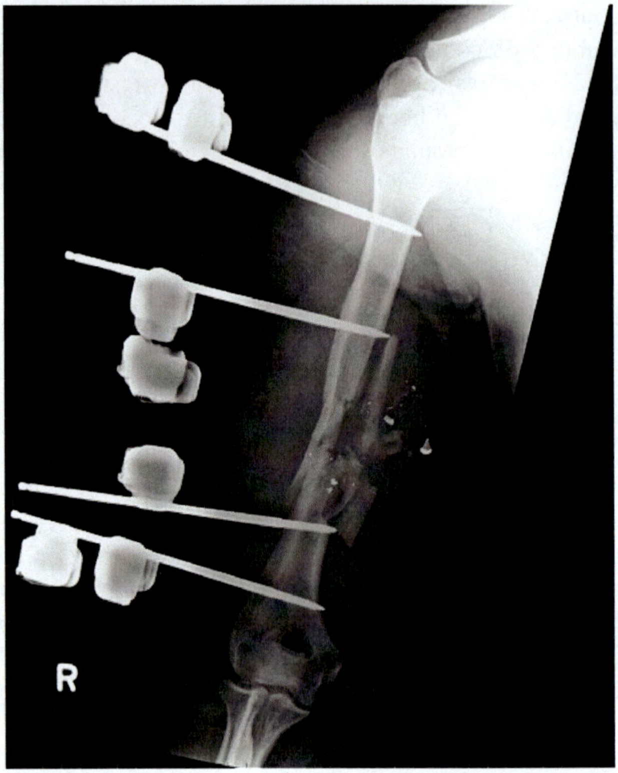

Fig. 5.1 Humerus external fixator

of a soft tissue sleeve should be done to prevent nerve injury. The soft tissues should be released enough to allow for elbow flexion and extension. The two multipin clamps are then connected via elbows and two bars after reduction of the fracture.

Because of binding of the triceps tendon distally, the frame described should be only used as a temporary external fixator, and not as the final method of treatment for patients.

5.6.3 *Tibia*

A surgeon and assistant are required for applying a frame to a tibia. The limb is initially prepped and draped above the knee for an isolated tibia fracture. The tibia is palpated along the anterior medial border of the limb. The first pin should be located on the proximal or distal main fragment outside of the zone of injury and a minimum of 2 cm from the fracture site. A 1.5 cm incision is made over the medial border, centering the incision on the posterior 1/3 and middle 1/3 of the tibia (Fig. 5.2). A single 5 mm half-pin is then inserted perpendicular to the medial face of the tibia (Fig. 5.3). The surgeon should feel two cortices during the insertion of the pin to obtain bicortical purchase (Figs. 5.4 and 5.5).

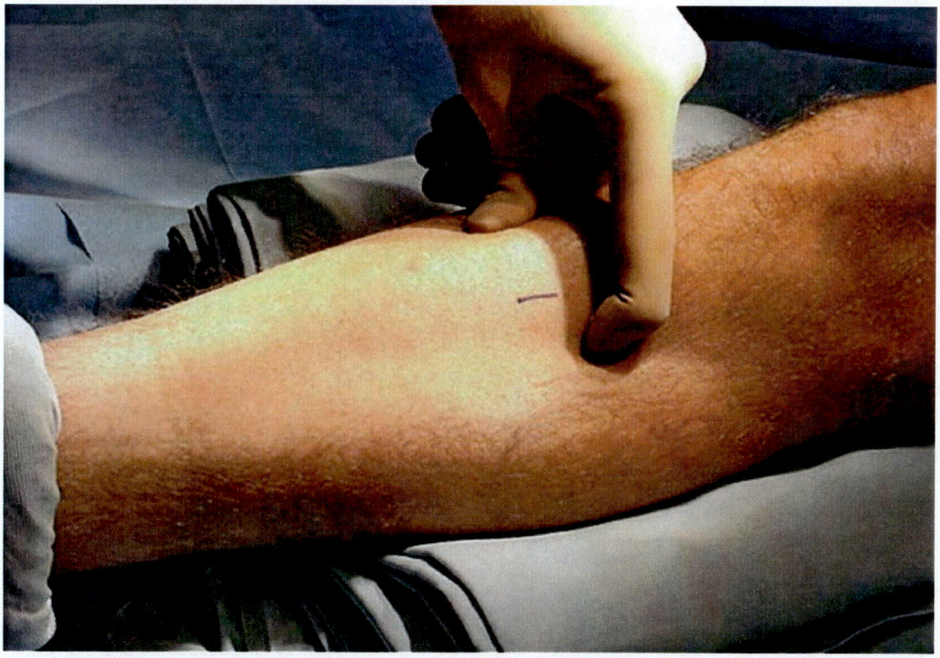

Fig. 5.2 Skin incision for 5 mm half-pin placement on the anterior medial border of the leg

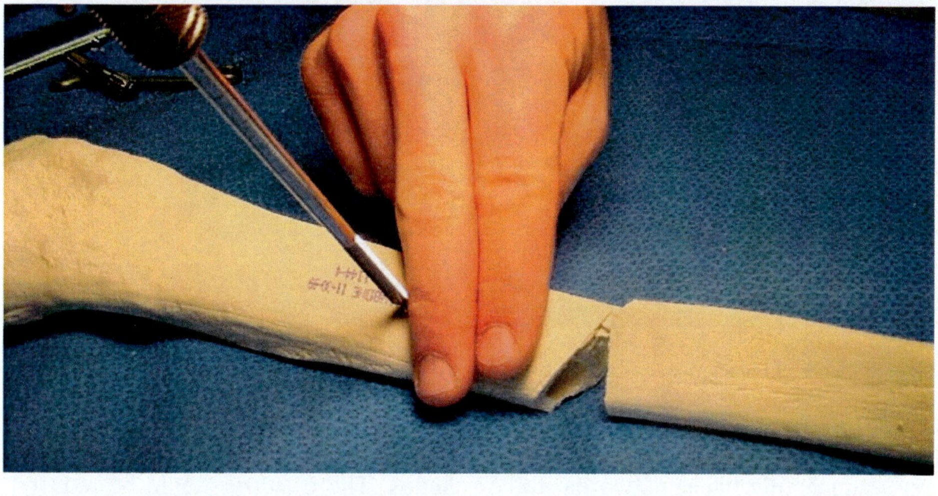

Fig. 5.3 Insertion by hand of 5 mm half-pin

Using a multipin clamp as a guide, a second pin is inserted to the tibia on the side away from the fracture site (Figs. 5.6 and 5.7). The maximum distance possible between pins should be used to obtain the best stability. Once inserted, the clamp should be tightened to the two pins. The process should be repeated on the other main fracture fragment of the tibia with two 5 mm half-pins and a multipin clamp (Fig. 5.8). The two clamps are then connected with a bar that spans the fracture site

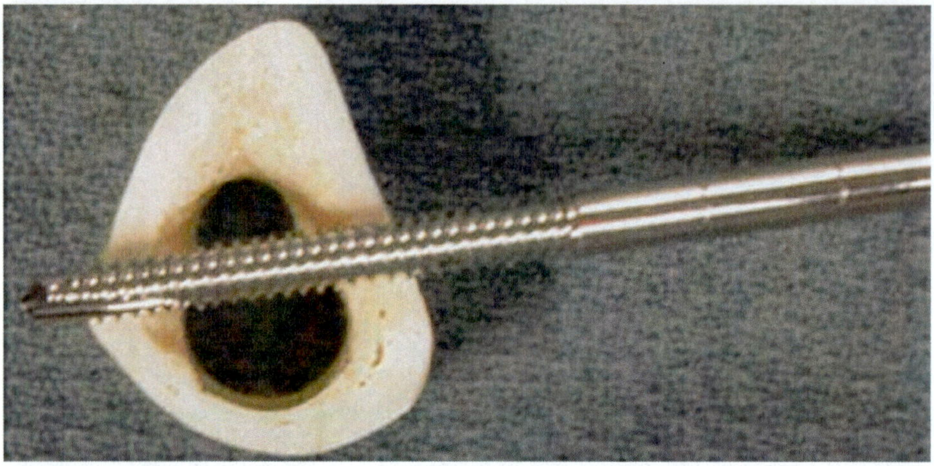

Fig. 5.4 Correct bicortical pin placement

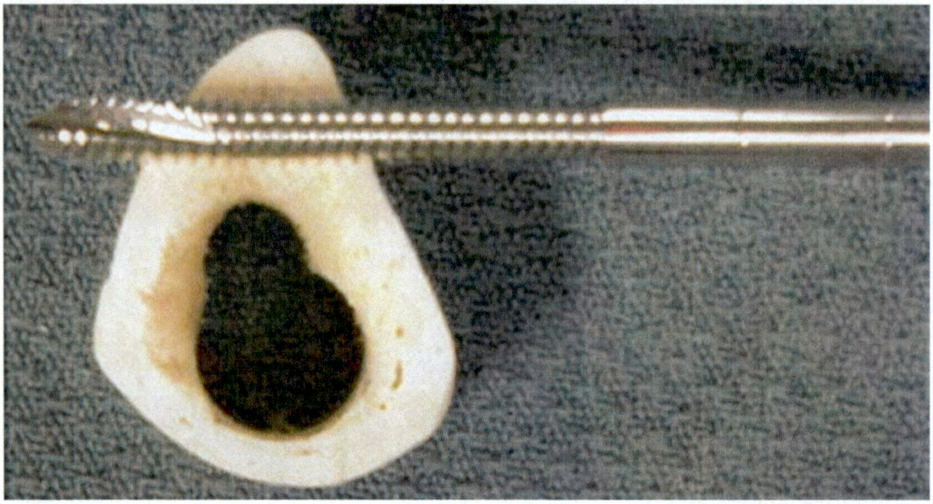

Fig. 5.5 Incorrect placement

via a connecting bar and two bar-to-bar clamps. The fracture should be reduced prior to final tightening of the frame (Fig. 5.9).

Though only one bar is included with the peel pack, experience during the present conflict has shown that two bars are generally needed for battlefield fractures. This may necessitate opening a second peel pack. Otherwise, a second bar can be obtained from the set if that system is used (Fig. 5.10).

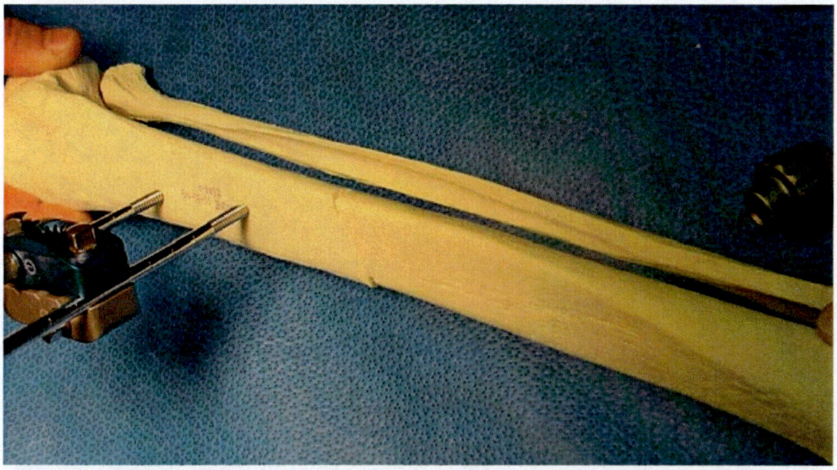

Fig. 5.6 Insertion of second half-pin using multipin clamp as a guide

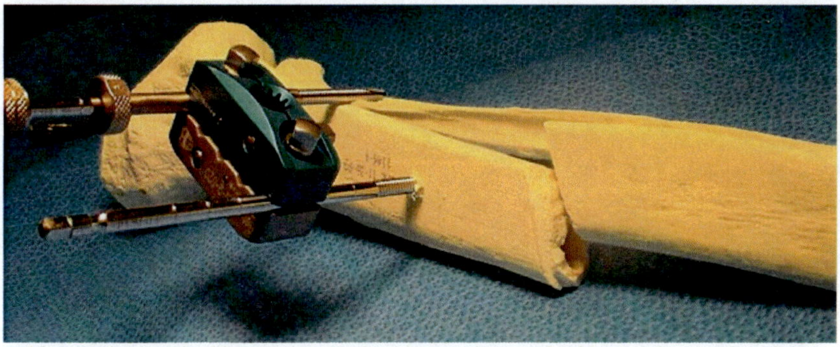

Fig. 5.7 Tactile feedback is important to avoid missing the bone

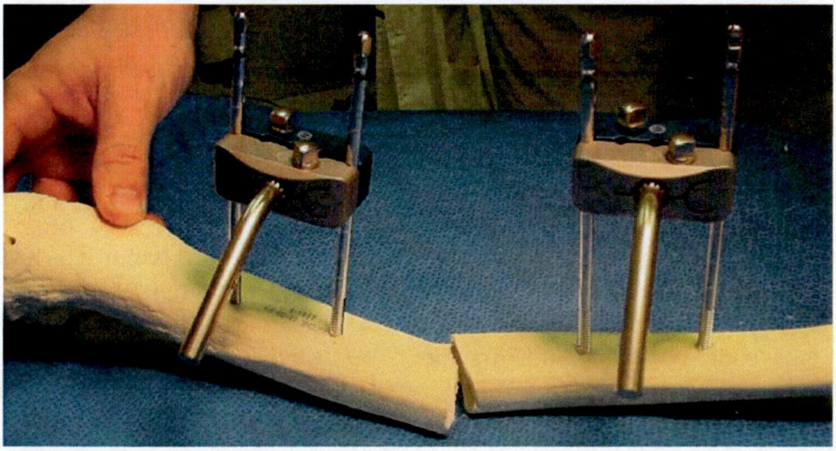

Fig. 5.8 Repeat the same steps distal to the fracture site

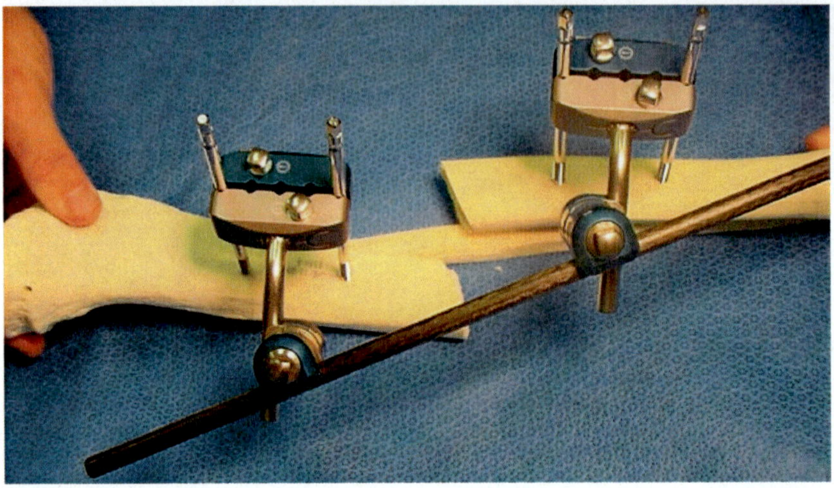

Fig. 5.9 Attach bar to pin clamps and connect the clamps with a 8 mm rod

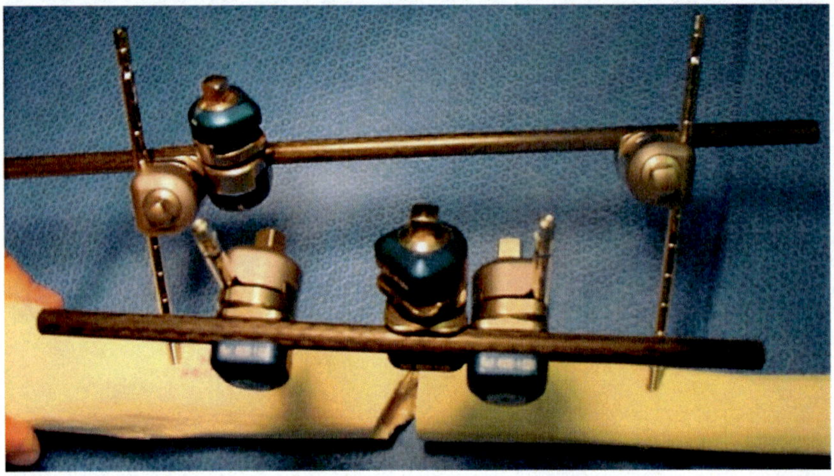

Fig. 5.10 A second bar should be attached to provide optimal stability

5.6.4 Femur

A surgeon and assistant are required for applying a frame to the femur. The patient should have the entire thigh and hip prepped out to apply the frame. Open wounds should be thoroughly cleaned, with obvious dead tissue and foreign debris removed from the wound. For a diaphyseal fracture, a sterile bump is placed under the mid-thigh (Fig. 5.11). A 1.5 longitudinal incision is made over either the proximal or distal femur fragment. Blunt dissection is used to spread the tissue down to bone. A single 5 mm pin is then inserted into the bone. Care must be made to ensure that the pin is centered on the bone and a good bicortical purchase is obtained. Good tactile feedback is essential to ensure this occurs in the absence of radiographic support.

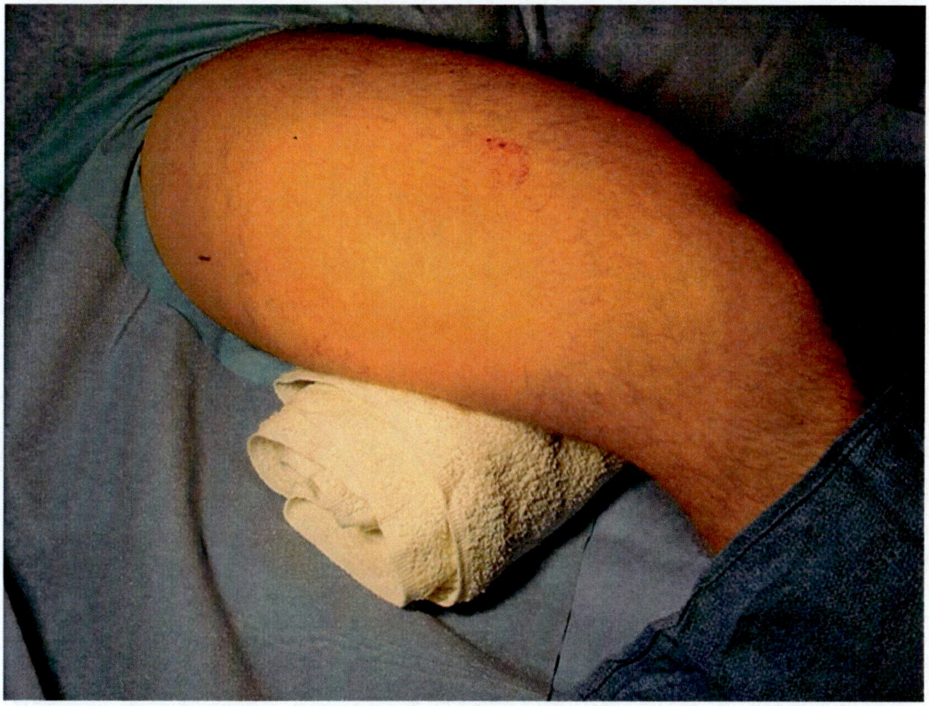

Fig. 5.11 A bump should be placed under the thigh to aid reduction

Once the first pin is inserted, a second pin is placed in the other main fracture fragment (either proximal or distal). Two single pin/bar clamps are then connected to the pins, and a bar connects the clamps together. Traction should be placed on the limb prior to tightening the bar to the pin and clamp. Reduction may be checked through the open wound if present. A second set of pins are then inserted on each major fragment, 2 cm proximal or distal to the previously inserted ones. This second set should also be parallel to the longitudinal axis of the femur and should be offset by 45° in an axial plane to enhance the stability of the construct. The two parallel bars are then connected by a *third* bar to enhance the stability of the frame. Prior to final tightening, the reduction should be assessed. Care should be taken to insert the pins outside of the zone of injury at least 2 cm from the fracture site. This may be difficult to determine without radiographic support with a comminuted fracture.

5.6.5 Knee Spanning

Knee injuries that have a proximal tibia or distal femur fracture may be stabilized in Combat Zone hospitals with a spanning external fixator. Careful monitoring of the vascular status should be done because of their prevalence in knee injuries.

The limb should be prepared from the hip to the foot. A minimum of a surgeon and assistant are needed to complete this surgery. Open wounds should be cleaned and irrigated with removal of obvious foreign material. Bone fragments should be

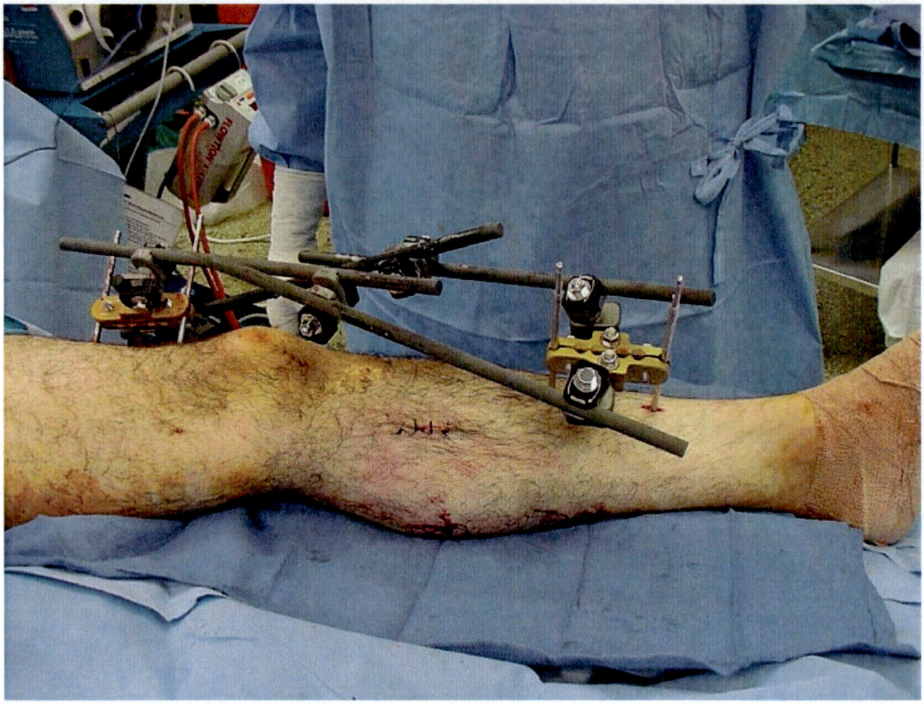

Fig. 5.12 Use of independent pin placement for temporary femoral external fixator use

preserved if at all possible. Wounds near the knee joint should be explored to look for penetration into the joint. If questionable, a formal arthrotomy should be done to explore the joint. Failure to remove debris or contamination from a knee joint could result in sepsis that may manifest itself when the patient is undergoing medical evacuation with minimal medical support.

After initial irrigation and removal of dead tissue and foreign material, the external fixator may be applied. Proximal to the fracture site by at least 2 cm, a 1 cm stab incision should be made over the anterior lateral aspect of the thigh. Blunt dissection is then done to access the bone. Feeling the curvature of the bone, a 5 mm half-pin is then inserted into the bone by hand. Using a multipin clamp as a guide, the process is then repeated with a second pin more proximal to the first. A third pin may be inserted through the multipin clamp to enhance stability.

Distal to the knee on the anterior medial surface of the leg, a 1 cm stab incision is made at least 2 cm distal to the fracture or along the proximal 1/3 of the tibia if there is no fracture. A single 5 mm half-pin is then inserted proximally, and then using a multipin clamp as a guide the steps are repeated and a second pin is inserted on the multipin clamp distally.

The two multipin clamps are then connected with two 8 mm bars. The multipin clamp elbows are connected to the bars with bar-to-bar clamps. The two bars are then connected with a third bar to provide the best stability. A minimum of two bars must be used to span the knee. The knee should be in slight flexion (about 5°) when the frame is tightened. A "bump" made of hand towels may facilitate the reduction. The bars should sit far enough away from the skin to allow for dressing changes (Fig. 5.12).

5.7 Conclusion

Use of a temporary external fixator to stabilize a long bone fracture is one of the primary means available for the initial treatment of wounded US or allied soldiers. One of the landmark papers for the use of external fixator in the warzone dates back from 1942 and is still remarkably modern [38]. A surgeon who is caring for soldiers or wounded nonmilitary should be proficient in the use of external fixation in an austere environment. This chapter is meant to provide guidelines on the safe application of standardized external fixator constructs during mass casualty situations under austere circumstances.

References

1. Dougherty PJ. Chapter 23: Extremity fractures. In: Lounsbury DE, editor. Emergency War Surgery. Third United States Revision. Washington, DC: US Government Printing Office; 2004.
2. Antich-Androver P, Marti-Garin D, Murias-Alvarez J, Puente-Alonso C. External fixation and secondary intramedullary nailing of open tibial fractures. J Bone Joint Surg. 1997;79B:433–7.
3. Blachut PA, Meek RN, O'Brien PJ. External fixation and delayed intramedullary nailing of open fractures of the tibial shaft. J Bone Joint Surg. 1990;72A:729–35.
4. Nowotarski PJ, Turen CH, Brumback RJ, Scarboro JM. Conversion of external fixation to intramedullary nailing for fractures of the shaft to the femur in multiply injured patients. J Bone Joint Surg. 2000;82A:781–8.
5. Bhandari M, Zlowodzki M, Tornetta 3rd P, Schmidt A, Templeman DC. Intramedullary nailing following external fixation in femoral and tibial shaft fractures. J Orthop Trauma. 2005; 19(2):140–4.
6. Burkhalter W. Penetrating Wounds of the Thigh with Associated Femur Fracture. In: Burkhalter WE, Burkhalter WE, editors. Surgery in Vietnam Orthopaedic Surgery. Washington, DC: Office of the Surgeon General and Center for Military History; 1994. p. 21–37.
7. Burkhalter W. Penetrating wounds of the leg, with associated fractures of the tibia. In: Burkhalter WE, editor. Surgery in Vietnam. Orthopaedic Surgery. Washington, DC: Office of the Surgeon General and Center for Military History; 1994. p. 39–51.
8. Rowley DI. The management of war wounds involving bone. Jour Bone Joint Surg. 1996;78B: 706–9.
9. Hammer RRR, Rooser B, Lidman D, Smeds S. Simplified external fixation for primary management of severe musculoskeletal injuries under war and peace time conditions. J Ortho Trauma. 1996;10:545–54.
10. Has B, Jovanovic S, Wertheimer B, Mikolasevic I, Grdic P. External fixation as a primary and definitive treatment of open limb fractures. Injury. 1995;26:245–8.
11. Anderson R. An automatic method of treatment for fractures of the tibia and fibula. Surg Gyn Ob. 1934;58:639–46.
12. Lewis KM, Breidenbach L, Stader O. The Stader reduction splint. Ann Surg. 1942;116:623–36.
13. Shaar CM, Kreuz FP, Jones DT. Factures of the tibia and fibula. Treatment with the Stader reduction and fixation splint. Surg Clin. 1943;23:599–630.
14. Bradford C, Wilson PD. Mechanical skeletal fixation in war surgery. Surg Gyn Obst. 1942;75: 468–76.
15. Laning RH, Small WD, Flower CF. Management of fractures in the United States Navy. Surg Clin. 1941;21:1703–22.
16. Hampton, O. Chapter VII: External fixation. In: Surgery in World War II. Orthopaedic surgery in the Mediterranean theater of operations. Washington, DC: Office of the Surgeon General, US Government Printing Office; 1957. p. 203–10.
17. Mazet R. Use and abuse of anatomical splint. J Bone Joint Surg. 1943;25:839–58.

18. Reis ND, Zinman C, Besser MIB, Shifrin LZ, Rosen H. A philosophy of limb salvage in war: use of the fixateur externe. Mil Surg. 1991;156:505–20.
19. Zinman C, Reis ND. External fixation in wartime limb surgery. Isr J Med Sci. 1984;20:308–10.
20. Simchen E, Sacks T. Infection in war wounds: experience during the 1973 October War in Israel. Ann Surg. 1975;182:754–61.
21. Simchen E, Raz R, Stein H, Danon Y. Risk factors for infection in fracture war wounds (1973 and 1982 wars, Israel). Mil Med. 1991;156:520–7.
22. Bosse MJ, Holmes C, Vossoughi J, Alter D. Comparison of the Howmedica and Synthes Military External Fixation Frames. J Ortho Trauma. 1994;8:119–26.
23. Dougherty PJ, Vickaryous B, Conley E, Hickerson K. A comparison of two military temporary femoral external fixators. Clin Ortho. 2003;412:176–83.
24. Sladicka SJ, Duffin SR, Erpelding JM. A biomechanical strength comparison of external fixators. J Trauma. 1998;44(6):965–9.
25. Carmack DB, Kaylor KL, Yaszemski MJ. Structural stiffness and reducibility of external fixators placed in malalignment and malrotation. J Ortho Trauma. 2001;15:247–53.
26. Finlay JB, Moroz TK, Rorabeck CH, Davey JR, Bourne RB. Stability of ten configurations of the Hoffmann external-fixation frame. J Bone Joint Surg. 1987;69A:734–44.
27. Moroz TK, Finlay JB, Rorabeck CH, Bourne RB. External skeletal fixation: choosing a system based on biomechanical stability. J Ortho Trauma. 1988;2:284–96.
28. Broekhuizen AH, Boxma H, van der Meulen PA, Snijders CJ. Performance of external fixation devices in femoral fractures; the ultimate challenge? A laboratory study with plastic rods. Injury. 1990;21:145–51.
29. Sarmiento A, McKellop HA, Llinas A, Park SH, Lu B, Stetson W, et al. Effect of loading and fracture motions on diaphyseal tibial fractures. J Ortho Res. 1996;14:80–4.
30. Camuso MR. Far-forward fracture stabilization: external fixation versus splinting. J Amer Acad Ortho Surg. 2006;14:s118–23.
31. Dougherty PJ, Silverton CD, Yeni Y, Tashman SL, Weir R. Conversion from temporary external fixation to definitive fixation: shaft fractures. J Am Acad Ortho Surg. 2006;14:s124–7.
32. Clasper JC, Phillips SL. Earl failure of external fixation in the management of war injuries. J R Army Med Corps. 2005;151:81–6.
33. Debakey ME. Military surgery in World War II, A backward glance and a forward look. NEJM. 1947;236:341–9.
34. Fackler ML. Misinterpretations concerning Larrey's methods of wound treatment. Surg Gyn Obs. 1989;168:280–2.
35. Lounsbury D, editor. Chapter 22: Soft tissue injuries. In: Emergency war surgery handbook, Third United States Revision. Washington, DC: US Government Printing Office; 2004. www.bordeninstitute.army.mil. Accessed 27 Mar 2005.
36. Scully RE, Artz CP, Sako Y. An evaluation of the surgeon's criteria for determining the viability of muscle during debridement. Arch Surg. 1956;73(6):1031–5.
37. Keller A. The management of gunshot fractures of the humerus. Injury. 1995;26:93–6.
38. Hoffmann R. Closed osteosynthesis with special reference to war surgery. Acta Orthop Scand. 1942;86:235–66.

Chapter 6
External Fixation of the Pelvis in Damage Control Orthopedics

Madhusudhan Yakkanti and Craig S. Roberts

6.1 Introduction

Damage control orthopedics for pelvic fractures involves early identification of the potentially lethal injury which can cause exsanguination [1], and prompt decision making to determine which fracture patterns require pelvic external fixation.

6.2 History

Hoffmann's diagrams show fixators for pelvic fractures. Pennal and Sutherland applied the concept of external fixation to stabilize pelvic injuries in the 1950s using the Roger-Anderson fixator [2]. Twenty years later, Slatis and Karaharju popularized the use of external fixation in pelvic ring injuries by applying Hoffmann's anterior frame [3, 4].

The use of the external fixator for pelvic ring injuries is viewed as part of patient resuscitation [5]. Recent trends in pelvic external fixation use temporary applications of external fixation with early conversion to anterior and posterior internal fixation. The need for an external fixation device that can be rapidly applied to stabilize the posterior pelvis led to the development of the pelvic C-clamp [6, 7] (Mathys Ltd., Bettlach, Switzerland) and the pelvic stabilizer (Ace Medical, Los Angeles, CA).

M. Yakkanti (✉)
Department of Orthopaedic Surgery, University Hospital Louisville,
Louisville, KY, USA
e-mail: madhuyakkanti@gmail.com

C.S. Roberts
Department of Orthopaedic Surgery, University Hospital Louisville,
Louisville, KY, USA
e-mail: craig.roberts@louisville.edu

D. Seligson et al. (eds.), *External Fixation in Orthopedic Traumatology*,
DOI 10.1007/978-1-4471-2197-8_6, © Springer-Verlag London Limited 2012

6.3 Anatomic Considerations

The anatomy of the iliac crest can make intraosseous pin placement between the narrow iliac tables technically challenging. There are probably no serious consequences if an iliac crest pin passes either in or out of the iliac tables. The subcrestal pin placement is an alternative which may avoid complications [8]. The anterior pillar of the iliac crest contains the densest portion of bone, thereby providing the most desirable placement for fixation of external fixator half-pins. In the supine position, an intact pelvis is oriented such that the symphysis pubis, the anterior superior iliac spines, and the anterior pillar lie in a plane nearly parallel to the floor [9]. The plane of the angle of the opening of the true pelvis is at a 45° angle to the horizontal plane. The medial-lateral angulation of the iliac crest is also at a 45° angle in the intact pelvis [10]. Due to the curvature of the iliac crest, pins cannot be placed in a straight line. The overhanging outer lip of the iliac crest requires that pin insertion start on its inner third [9]. Placement of pins in the anterior inferior iliac spine, with its potential anatomic hazards especially in the presence of altered anatomy due to injury, is usually done under fluoroscopic control. In an anatomic study of placement of half-pins in the supra-acetabular region, Haidukewych et al. reported that the extent of the superior reflection of the hip capsule above the joint was an average of 16 mm (range, 11–20 mm) [11]. The lateral cutaneous nerve was found to be at risk for injury during pin insertion, and was as close as 2–10 mm from the pins which had been placed under fluoroscopy [11]. In addition, anatomic studies have revealed that the lateral femoral cutaneous nerve has an extremely variable course which increases its vulnerability to injury [12, 13].

The frontal cross sections of the pelvis on computerized topography (CT) demonstrate different orientations of the plane of the lateral cortex of the iliac wing proximal and distal to the pelvic brim. The change of orientation forms a consistent "groove" on the outer bony surface of ilium. This specific region represents the lateral aspect of the sacroiliac (SI) joint, and is the recommended site for the placement of the pins of a pelvic C-clamp. This site is also used as an entry point for transiliosacral screw fixation of sacroiliac joint dislocations and sacral fractures. To access this anatomic landmark, a skin incision of approximately 1.5–2.0 cm in length is made and blunt dissection of the fibers of the abductor muscles accomplished by palpation with a blunt instrument [14].

6.4 Biomechanics

A biomechanical study of pressure volume characteristics of intact and disrupted pelvic retroperitoneum suggested that low-pressure venous hemorrhage may be tamponaded by an external fixator; however, the pressure generated will not be sufficient to stop arterial bleeding [15]. In order for the fixator to be effective, a large volume of fluid must be lost into the pelvis which underscores the dictum of the requirement to replace a large volume of colloid or blood in pelvic ring injuries.

Bottlang et al. reported that application of circumferential compression to the pelvic soft tissue envelope with a pelvic strap was an efficient means of achieving controlled reduction of external rotation-type pelvic fractures [16]. Biomechanical studies have revealed that the pelvic C-clamp decreases motion at the disrupted sacroiliac joint, while anterior frames decrease motion to a greater degree at the disrupted rami [17]. A mechanical study in synthetic bone achieved sacroiliac compression using a femoral distractor as an anterior pelvic compressor with supra-acetabular pins [18]. An external frame applied anteriorly, even with a double-cluster arrangement, cannot restore enough stability to an unstable type C-3 injury to permit weightbearing before fracture union is achieved [19]. Patients with an open-book (B-l) or lateral compression (B-2) injury may mobilize without risking major re-displacement. These studies support the addition of internal fixation to both the anterior and posterior aspects of the pelvis to restore stability to a partially stable (type-B) injury, and to promote adequate consolidation of an unstable (type-C) injury. This has led to a greater emphasis on definitive open reduction and internal fixation (ORIF) of anterior symphyseal disruption and posterior sacroiliac injuries [19]. Archdeacon et al. reported that an orthogonal pelvic external fixator pin construct produced a significantly stiffer construct for in-plane loading (flexion/extension moment) compared with either parallel pin construct; however, a parallel supra-acetabular pin construct was stiffer for out-of-plane loading [20].

Finite element studies [21] have shown that the stability of open book fractures with external fixation accomplished with pins placed either high (iliac crest) or low (supra-acetabular) was similar; however, stability was greatly increased when both pin positions were used. External fixation did not effectively stabilize rotationally and vertically unstable fractures. Adequate stabilization was achieved only by using internal fixation [22]. The relative pullout strength of half-pins placed high in the superior iliac crest above the anterior superior iliac spine, and between the anterior superior and anterior inferior iliac spines, has been shown to be equivalent [23].

6.5 Indications

The indications for pelvic external fixation include resuscitation of patients with hemodynamic instability from pelvic bleeding, a temporary frame in a borderline patient prior to open reduction and internal fixation with a SI screw, a definitive frame in anterior-posterior compression (APC-I) injuries, a "comfort" frame in stable lateral compression injuries which are painful and limiting mobilization of the patient, and open pelvic fractures.

The primary indication for the application of the pelvic external fixator is the hemodynamically unstable patient with a blood pressure which cannot be maintained at or greater than 90 mmHg in spite of adequate resuscitative measures. The term hemodynamic instability is based on the classification by Bone, which indicates an estimated overall blood loss of more than 2,000 mL (class III and IV) [24]. The tamponade effect produced by an external fixator is usually sufficient to control venous bleeding. Persistent hypotension, despite of the application of an external fixator and blood replacement, indicates possible arterial bleeding for which angiography and embolization should be considered. Anterior pelvic frames contribute to hemostasis by decreasing pelvic volume, allowing tamponade, and decreasing the bony motion of the pelvis which allows clotting.

Bleeding in association with pelvic fractures may originate from arterial, venous, or bony (fractured cancellous bone surfaces) sources. Arterial bleeding occurs in approximately 10% of cases and can be torrential, originating from iliac vessels and their branches (particularly the internal iliac artery and its branches) [25]. The incidence of arterial injury as a source of bleeding was reported in one study to be as high as 78% when a group of patients with unstable fractures of the pelvis was evaluated angiographically for uncontrolled hypotension [26]. Venous bleeding typically originates from the rich pre-sacral venous plexus, which is low in pressure but troublesome if adequate resuscitative measures are not begun early. The retroperitoneum can accommodate up to 4 L of blood before the pressure can overcome the intravascular venous pressure and produce a physiologic tamponade. This hemorrhage can easily turn into life-threatening exsanguination if associated with extensive retroperitoneal muscle disruption, or an open pelvic fracture [15].

The pelvic external fixator is the treatment of choice for complex pelvic trauma. This entity represents a pelvic fracture combined with a concomitant soft-tissue lesion in the pelvic region with injury to the urogenital system, hollow visceral injuries, neurovascular injuries, and significant damage to the integument. These complex trauma cases represent only approximately 10% of all pelvic fractures, but have a mortality rate as high as 33% [27]. Traumatic hemipelvectomy has been described as an indication for pelvic external fixation [28].

The external fixator is effective as a definitive care device in stable and partially stable fractures (B-l open book, B-2 lateral compression) [29]. Treatment of type B lateral compression injuries of the pelvic ring with anterior distraction external fixation is a highly effective yet relatively simple and minimally invasive treatment method. Surgical time and blood loss are minimal and the patients can be effectively and rapidly mobilized [30]. The role of external fixation alone in the definitive treatment of unstable fractures (type C) has not been satisfactory and requires supplementation with either open reduction and internal fixation or supracondylar pin traction depending on the general condition of the patient [31]. External fixation of the pelvis is particularly useful for type C fractures in which there are multiple rami fractures anteriorly in order to avoid a potentially dangerous anterior approach.

Pelvic external fixation has also been used for disruption of the anterior pelvic ring with bony avulsion of the symphysis pubis during a spontaneous delivery [32]. Unstable insufficiency fractures associated with rheumatoid arthritis have been treated with this device [33]. Pelvic external fixation may also have a role in the treatment of pelvic fracture nonunions and treatment of chronic SI joint instability postpartum, although plating of a symptomatic postpartum diastasis of the symphysis is more common. Temporary pelvic external fixation can be of value as a reduction instrument during image-guided percutaneous fixation of acetabular fractures under fluoroscopic navigation. Iliac wing fractures are usually a contraindication to pelvic external fixation.

The external fixation concept has also been used as a table-skeletal fixation as an adjunct to pelvic ring reduction [34]. The external fixator in this technique rigidly stabilizes the intact hemipelvis to the operating room table. The fractured and displaced fragments can then be manipulated around the securely fixed uninjured pelvis. This allows the application of more directions and greater magnitude of force for reduction maneuvers.

6.6 Diagnosis and Classification

Understanding the conditions of the accident and the mechanism of injury can aid in the diagnosis of specific injury patterns. Pelvic fracture patients in the emergency room are initially categorized as either hemodynamically stable or hemodynamically unstable (shock). Careful physical examination of the patient with suspected pelvic injury is critical and must include observation for pelvic contusions, patterned abrasions, abdominal distension, and bleeding from the urethral meatus, rectum, or vagina. Pelvic instability should be carefully assessed in both anterior-posterior and medial-lateral directions. The presence of a pelvic binder can obscure direct visualization of wounds, deformity, and the degree of fracture displacement and instability.

Radiographic evaluation should include anterior-posterior, inlet, and outlet views of the pelvis. The AP view will show injury to the pubic rami, symphysis pubis, and sacroiliac joint including some sacral fractures and vertical displacement of the hemipelvis. The inlet view with the radiograph beam angled at 60° toward the patient's feet allows visualization of the pelvic brim, sacroiliac joints, pubic rami, ala and body of the sacrum, and anterior-posterior displacement of a hemipelvis. The outlet view taken with the beam angled at 45° toward the patient's head visualizes the sacrum and any vertical displacement of a hemipelvis or fracture.

Modern CT scanning is a powerful diagnostic tool which provides additional information regarding injuries that involve the posterior pelvis (especially the sacrum) and acetabulum. Radiographic signs of pelvic ring instability include sacroiliac displacement of 5 mm in any plane, a posterior fracture gap rather than impaction, and an avulsion of the fifth lumbar transverse process, lateral border of sacrum, or ischial spine.

Pennal and Sutherland described a classification system of pelvic injuries based on the magnitude and direction of three possible injury forces: anterior posterior compression (APC), lateral compression (LC), and vertical shear (VS) [35–37]. The classification system of Tile divides pelvic ring injuries into three types and is extremely useful for decision making [38]. Type A fractures are stable injuries that do not involve the ring and are treated nonoperatively. Type B fractures are the result of rotational forces applied to the pelvis, and are due to anteroposterior compression or lateral compression. These fractures are rotationally unstable, but vertically stable. Type C injuries are unstable both rotationally and vertically and occur from shear forces.

The Young and Burgess classification system includes an understanding of the mechanism of injury and injury severity. This system detects posterior ring injury

Table 6.1 Advantages and disadvantages of each type of pelvic external fixators

Type of fixator	Advantages	Disadvantages
Superior iliac crest pin external fixator	Easy to apply	Only controls anterior pelvis
Low pin/supra-acetabular external fixator	Useful with iliac wing fractures	Proximity to hip joint
C-clamp/pelvic stabilizer anterior placement	Controls posterior pelvis	Proximity to hip joint
C-clamp/pelvic stabilizer posterior placement	Controls posterior pelvis	Proximity to sciatic notch

and predicts local and distant associated injuries, resuscitation needs, and expected mortality rates. APC types II and III, lateral compression type III, vertical shear (VS), and combined mechanical injuries are indicative of major ligament disruption. APC III injuries require the most blood replacement.

6.7 Technique: Pelvic Slings, Binders, and Sheets

The use of a bed sheet, pelvic sling, pelvic binder, or belt for emergency stabilization of pelvic fractures is widely accepted as adequate compression is achieved without compromising access to the patient [16, 39]. These external methods are the simplest, least invasive, and inexpensive techniques of external fixation of the pelvis. Most of these approaches use radiolucent devices which should not be removed before adequate arrangements have been made to proceed with immediate fixation to prevent the patient from going into shock [40, 41]. Disadvantages include skin pressure problems, and loss of access to the lower abdomen.

6.8 Types of External Fixators

There are various types of external fixation devices, including the pelvic C-clamp (Mathys Ltd., Bettlach, Switzerland), pelvic stabilizer (Ace Medical, Los Angeles, CA), and anterior external fixators. There are advantages and disadvantages of each type of fixator (Table 6.1). Fixators can be temporary or definitive, used to achieve reduction or hold reduction, for compression or distraction or as comfort frames.

6.8.1 Pelvic C-Clamp

The pelvic C-clamp has two pins for fixation on the posterior ilium in the region of the SI joints [6] (Fig. 6.1). The compression and stability at the posterior aspect of the

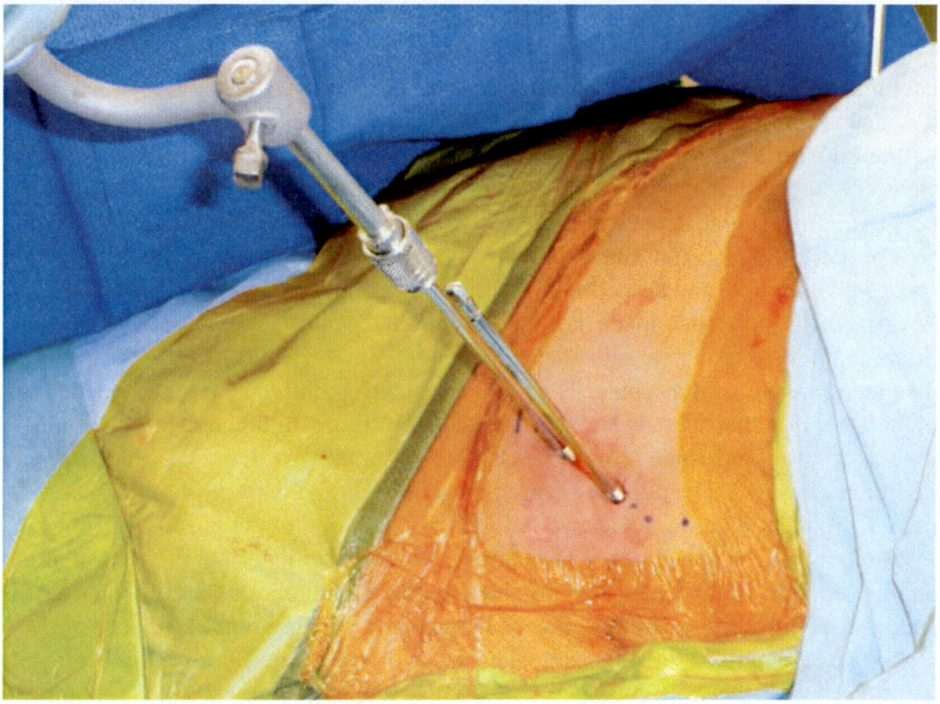

Fig. 6.1 Photograph of a pelvic C-clamp

ring at the point where the greatest bleeding occurs is adequate and effective as a tamponade. The application of the C-clamp has a definitive role in the management of polytraumatized patients with unstable pelvic ring injuries [7]. A study which compared AO and ACE pelvic clamps for unstable injuries showed satisfactory primary compression and stability was achieved with both clamps [42]. However, it was more difficult to achieve good rotational stability with the ACE clamp.

The pelvic stabilizer described by Buckle et al. is similar to the pelvic C-clamp and has two semicircular arms [43]. However, this stabilizer was taken off from the market in the United States due to limited demand and is no longer commercially available.

Anterior and posterior pin placement locations have been described for the pelvic C-clamp and pelvic stabilizer. The anterior pins are placed 4–5 cm inferior to the iliac crest on the dense column of bone just above the acetabulum. This is located midway along a line drawn between the tip of the greater trochanter and a spot on the iliac crest three finger breadths posterior to the anterior superior iliac spine. Posterior pins are placed 4–5 cm anterior to the posterior iliac spine on the dense iliac bone opposite the sacroiliac joint. Reynolds et al. in a cadaver study verified the anterior versus posterior pin placement of pelvic C-clamp in relationship to anatomical structures. Anterior pin placement is further from all anatomical structures with the exception of the hip joint capsule. The posterior pins are closer to the sciatic nerve, sciatic notch, and superior gluteal neurovascular bundle. Clinical decision making for C-clamp placement should be individualized on a case-by-case basis [44].

An alternative location for pin placement, the so-called "trochanteric C-clamp," was recently reported by Archdeacon and Hitatzka [45]. Pins are inserted into the lateral aspect of the greater trochanter instead of the ilium. Reported advantages of this technique include rapid application with provisional reduction of the pelvis without the need for immediate radiographs or fluoroscopy, unobstructed access to the pelvis and abdomen, and decreased risk of iatrogenic injury by pins placed adjacent to neurovascular structures [45].

The patient is placed in the supine position and the skin over the pelvic region is prepped with iodine and draped. The displacement of the pelvis is reduced manually. A 1.5–2.0 cm incision is made at the point where the superior extension of the axis of the femur crosses a perpendicular line that extends from just slightly posterior to the anterior superior iliac spine. The outer surface of innominate bone is reached by blunt dissection that spreads the fibers of the glutens maximus and medius. By moving the tip of the instrument on the surface of bone, the groove on the outer surface of ilium is exposed. The pins are secured by gentle hammer blows. The clamp is connected and the reduction reassessed before final clamping of the pins is performed.

The advantages of the pelvic C-clamp and pelvic stabilizer are that they can be quickly applied in emergency room and provide excellent access to the abdomen and upper thigh for procedures such as laparotomy and angiography. The pin sites are located away from most incision sites that would require access to conventional definitive ORIF that would be performed later, thus avoiding possible contamination due to pin tract infections. These devices may be used to hold innominate bones in a reduced position during definitive internal or external fixation. Further, they are preferred in the pediatric population because the fixation points do not violate areas of cartilage or physeal growth [46].

A disadvantage of these clamps is the inability to achieve reduction of the vertically displaced component. The pelvic ring must be reduced by manual or skeletal traction before the application of the device. In addition, if left for more than a few days, the fixation is likely to become loose. Therefore, the fixator must be assessed for integrity of stabilization, and additional compression may be achieved as required by turning the compression knobs. The pelvic C-clamp and pelvic stabilizer cannot be used in presence of iliac fractures or transiliac fracture dislocations. Complications such as injury to the gluteal nerves and vessels and secondary nerve injury as a result of over-compression in sacral fractures have been reported [27, 47]. Additional complications include pin penetration of the ilium and pin slippage into the greater sciatic notch with injury to the superior gluteal vessels or sciatic nerve. Contraindications for the pelvic C-clamp and pelvic stabilizer include stable pelvic ring disruptions with < 2.5 cm of anterior diastasis or 1 cm of vertical displacement, internal rotation deformities resulting from lateral compression, or major acetabular fractures. It is also possible to place a single pin in each iliac crest with local anesthesia in the emergency room or intensive care unit and connect these pins with a bar.

The classical method of anterior external fixation of the pelvis uses half-pins connected by vertical and horizontal bars with universal clamps. The half-pins may be placed in the high (anterior iliac crest), low (supra-acetabular), subcristal, or parasymphyseal position using either open or percutaneous techniques.

6.8.2 High Pin Placement (Superior Iliac Crest) (Hoffmann) for External Fixation

The high (or standard) pin placement is located in the superior iliac crest above the anterior superior iliac spine. The patient is placed in the supine position on a radiolucent table. The patient is anesthetized, prepped, and draped sterilely. The bladder is catheterized unless contraindicated. The surgical field extends from the costal margin to the pubic symphysis, and laterally must include the anterior half of the iliac crest.

Half-pins may be inserted either percutaneously (Figs. 6.2–6.6) through separate transverse stab incisions, or through an open incision. For open insertion, a 4–5 cm incision is made from the anterior superior iliac spine (ASIS) posteriorly along the mid-portion of the iliac crest. If there is marked displacement of the hemipelvis, it must be accounted for by moving the incision medially or laterally to compensate for changes in skin tension that occur after reduction [48]. If this is not done, there will be excessive skin tension and drainage at the pin sites. The skin incision is carried sharply down to fascia. The edges of the iliac crest are palpated. In some cases, it may be necessary to incise the fascial insertion on the iliac wing for better definition of the inner and outer walls of the iliac crest. The disadvantage of this step is the potential loss of the tamponade effect on the pelvic hematoma.

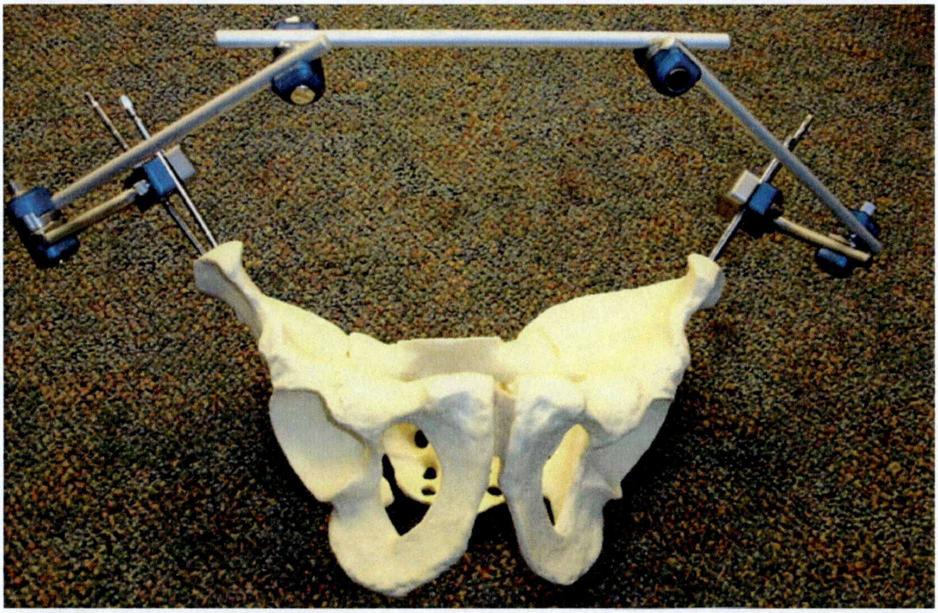

Fig. 6.2 Independent pin placement (high pin position) using a percutaneous insertion technique into the iliac crest

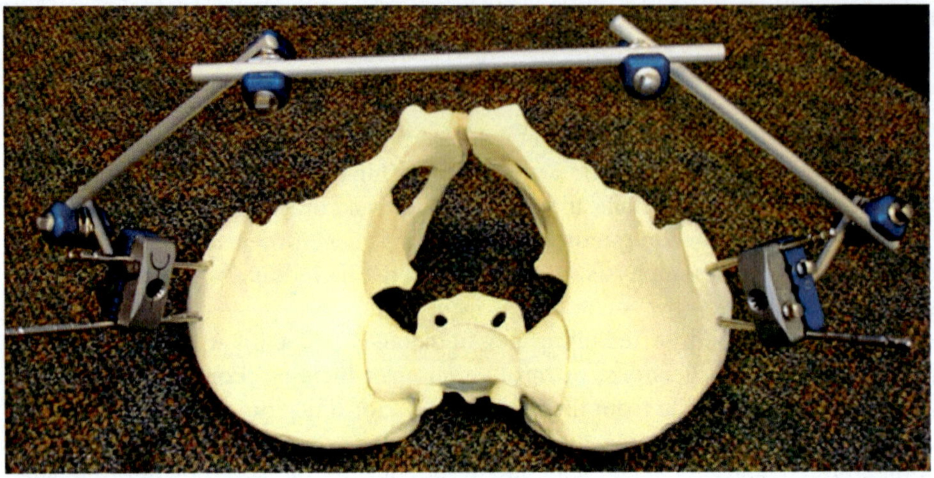

Fig. 6.3 Saw bones model of an external fixator with pins inserted into the high iliac crest location

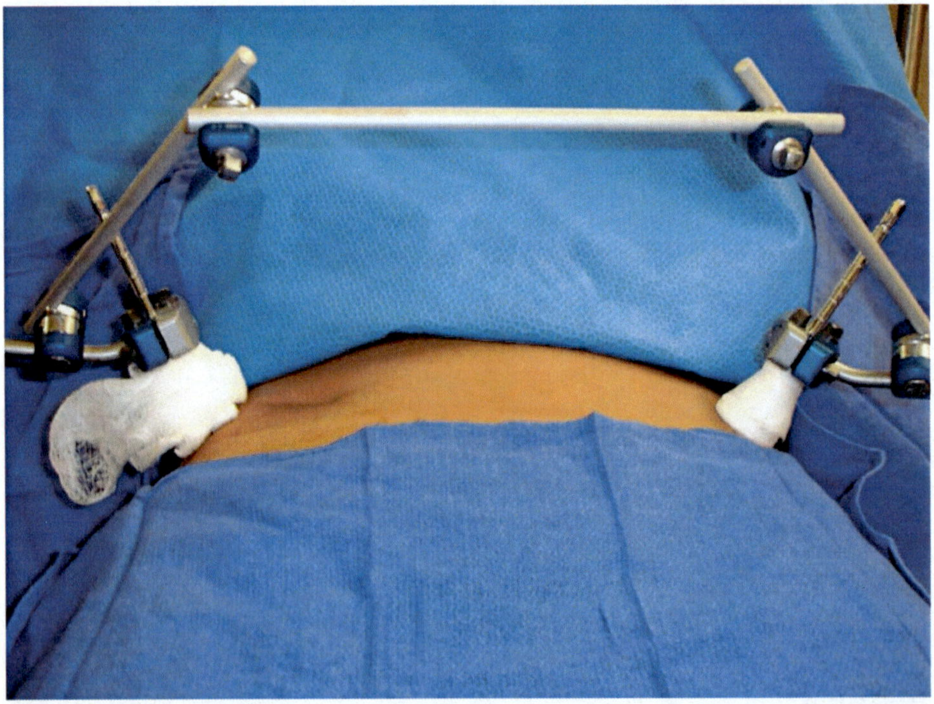

Fig. 6.4 Inlet view of saw bones model of an external fixator with pins inserted into the high iliac crest location

The first hole is placed 1 cm posterior to the ASIS. Subsequent holes are placed approximately 1–2 cm apart. Two pins are usually placed on each side. Self-drilling half-pins may be inserted manually without pre-drilling. Alternatively, half-pin holes may be predrilled for half-pins that are not self-drilling. A 5 mm pin is inserted to a depth

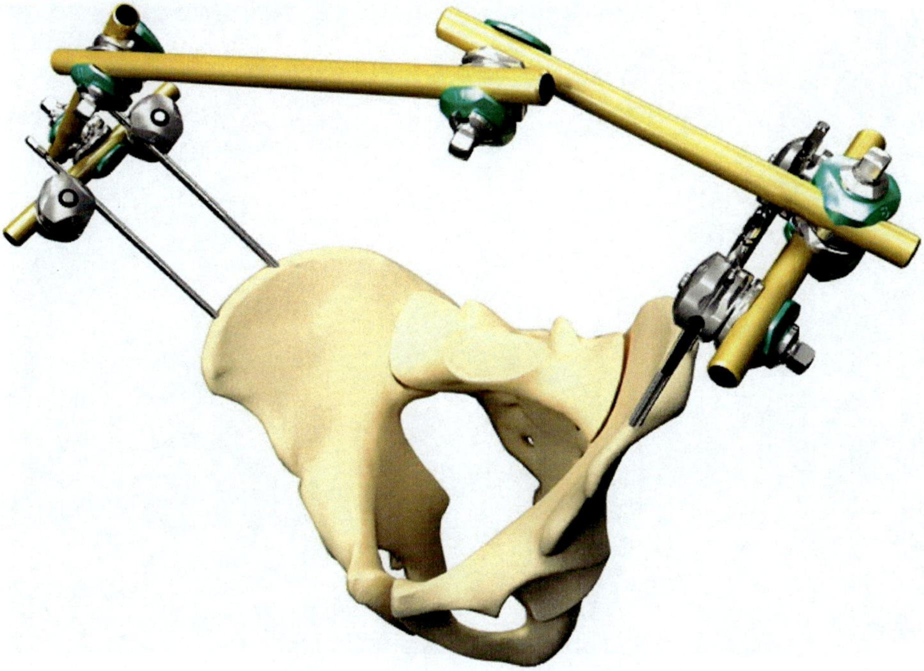

Fig. 6.5 Hoffmann III eternal fixation using two pins in the iliac crests

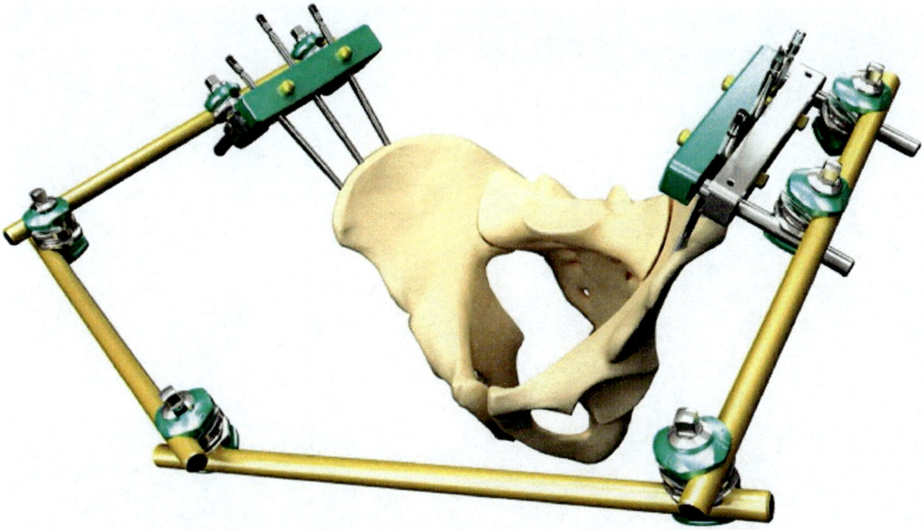

Fig. 6.6 Hoffmann III external fixator using numerous pins in the iliac crests

of approximately 5 cm, or until all the threads are buried in the iliac wing. Pin lengths of 180 mm are used for most patients; however, obese patients often require longer half-pins of >200 mm (Figs. 6.7–6.9). For open pin insertion, wound closure is performed in a standard manner. The percutaneous technique of half-pin insertion is similar to the

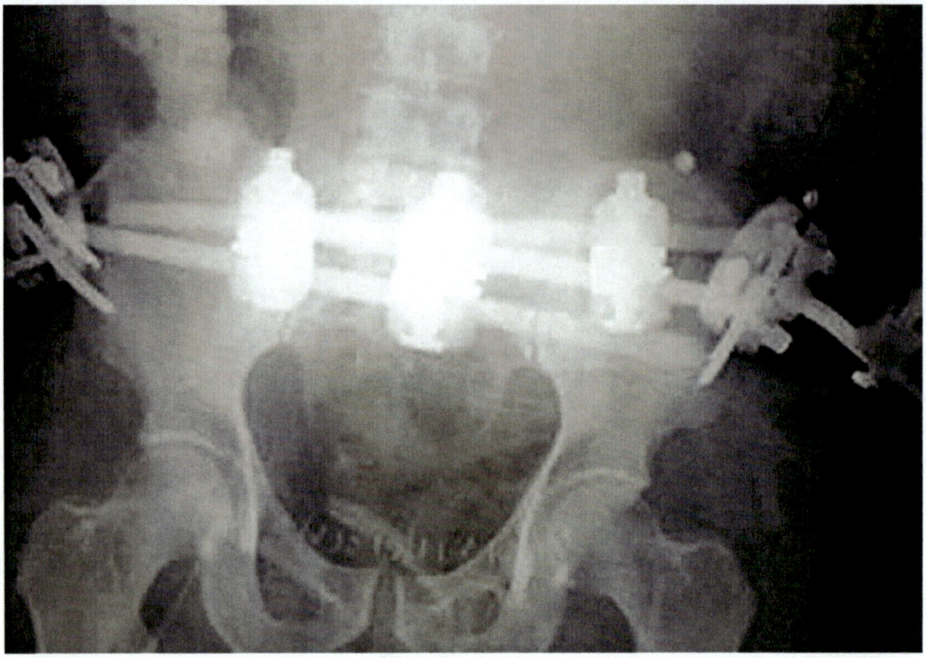

Fig. 6.7 Clinical photograph of an external fixator in place. External fixator bar configuration using a transverse bar

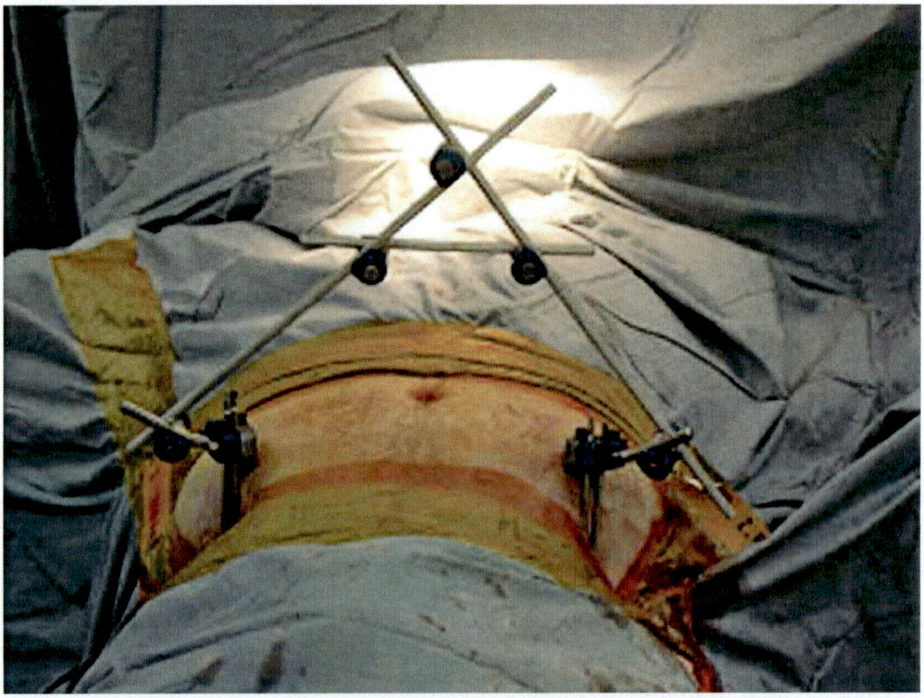

Fig. 6.8 AP pelvic radiograph of an external fixator. Of note is the presence of staples from a urologic procedure

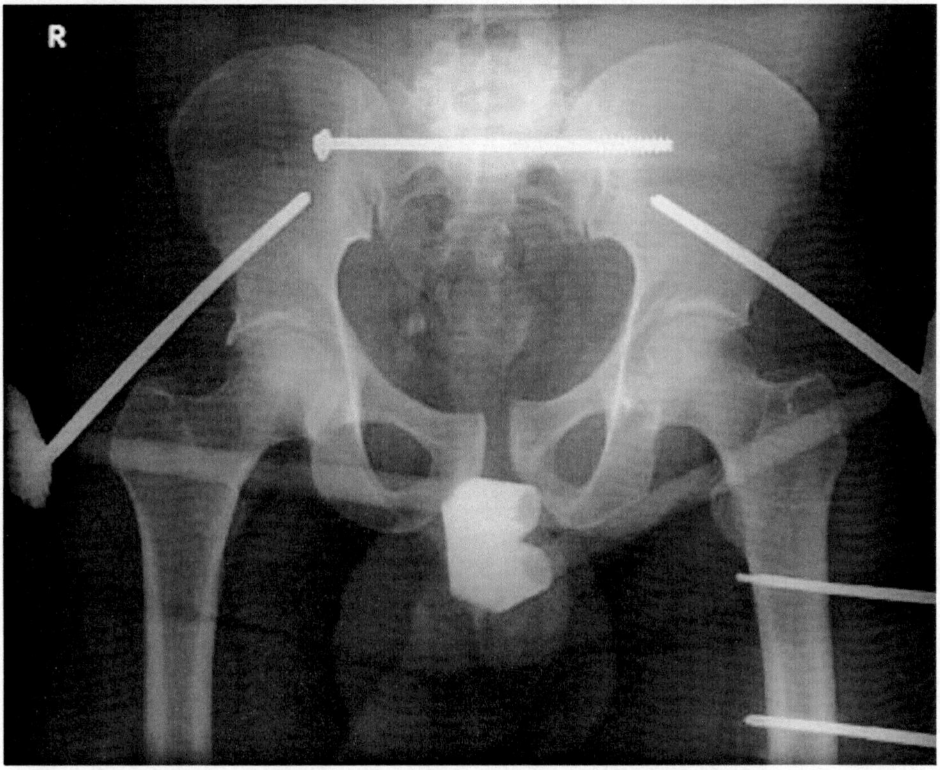

Fig. 6.9 Clinical photograph of an external fixator with an "A"-shaped bar configuration

open technique. It is worth remembering to start the half-pin insertion point closer to the inner border of the iliac crest. The inner table of the iliac crest can be palpated using K-wires prior to pin insertion. The disadvantages of the traditional pin placement on the anterior iliac crest are a compromised anterior approach to the SI joint, limited access to the abdominal wall, increased skin pressure from the fixator, and pin tract infection.

6.8.3 Low Pin Placement (Supra-Acetabular) for External Fixation

The lower pin position between the anterior spines is recommended when improved abdominal access is required. Half-pins can be placed in the dense supra-acetabular bone using fluoroscopic guidance. The patient is placed in the supine position on a radiolucent table. The surgical field extends from the umbilical line to the pubic symphysis, and laterally must include the anterior three-quarters of the iliac crest. The area of access for the application of the half-pins is proximally delimited by the anterior superior iliac spine and distally by the femoral arterial pulsation. Radiographically, the implant site for the half-pins is delimited distally by the roof and proximally by the

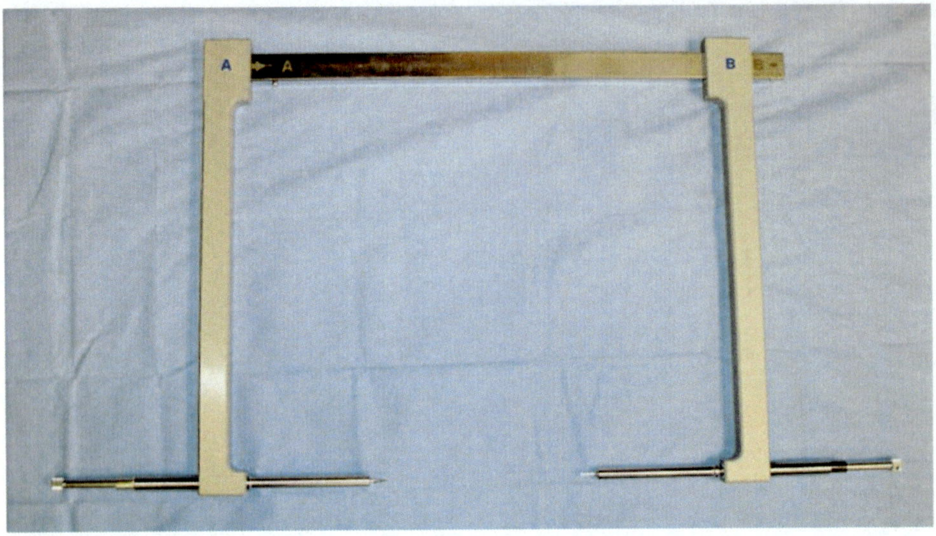

Fig. 6.10 AP pelvic radiograph of an external fixator with low anterior (supra-acetabular) pin placement. Also shown is external fixation of the femur and bilateral iliosacral fixation by a single screw

anterior superior iliac spine. Once the field has been defined, it is advisable to palpate and mark the femoral artery pulse and the anterior superior iliac spine. Five millimeter self-drilling half-pins (180–250 mm in length for obese patients and 150–180 mm in length for slim patients) are used [49]. The position of the reference point is verified under image intensification using a needle placed 7–8 mm proximal to the contour of the acetabular roof. Through a small incision, the first half-pin is applied distally above the acetabulum. The half-pin must be placed in a near vertical position, perpendicular to the long axis of the body. The pin is advanced inward at a 10° angle. A second half-pin may be placed proximal to the first half-pin at the same angle. Insertion of pins at least 2 cm above the hip is recommended to avoid penetration into the hip capsule (Fig. 6.10). There is no risk to the femoral nerve and artery, but the lateral cutaneous nerve of the thigh is at risk and caution is warranted [11, 50].

The open method requires a 3–5 cm incision which is initiated just below the anterior superior iliac spine and extended distally. The skin and subcutaneous plane is traversed, taking care to preserve the lateral femoral cutaneous nerve of the thigh if visualized. The anterior inferior iliac spine is palpated and the ridge of bone extending up from it is identified. The first pin is placed just above the anterior inferior iliac spine. Some authors have described a combination of low and high pin placements (iliac crest and supra-acetabular) creating an orthogonal construct between the two pins connecting both sides (Fig. 6.11).

A femoral distractor has been used as a compressor to achieve improved reduction of the posterior elements instead of the conventional connecting bar with the supra-acetabular pins [51].

The advantages of supra-acetabular pin placement are improved abdominal access, more favorable biomechanical positioning for closure of the pelvic disruption,

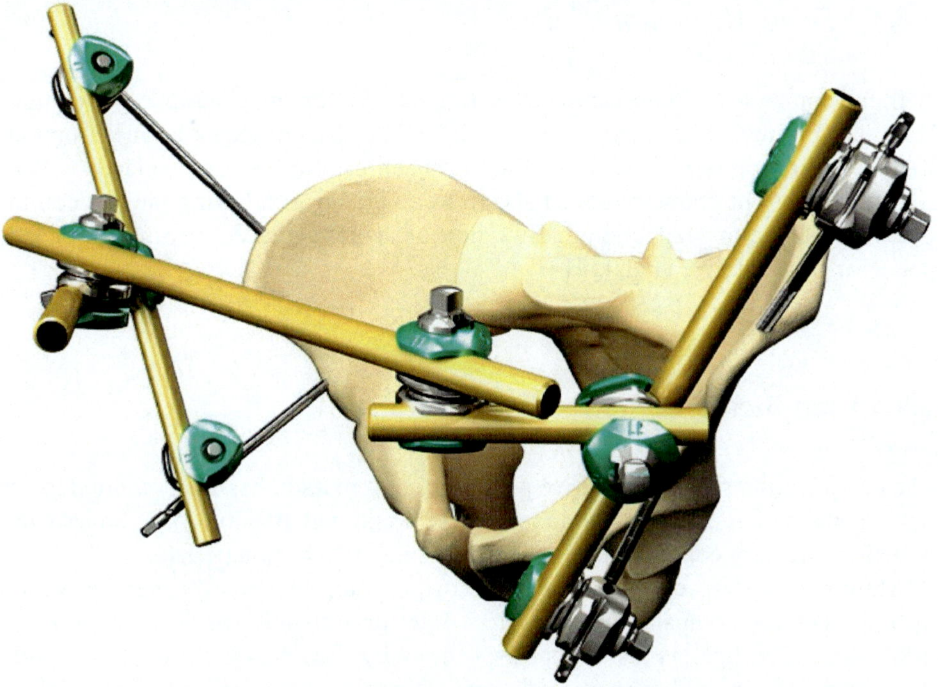

Fig. 6.11 Orthogonal positioning of iliac crest and supra-acetabular pins using the Hoffmann III external fixator

and the avoidance of violating the skin over the iliac crest that might be later used as part of an ilio-inguinal approach [31]. The disadvantages are limitation of hip flexion beyond 95°, risk of hip sepsis, hip joint penetration, need for fluoroscopy for pin insertion, and iatrogenic lateral femoral cutaneous nerve injury.

6.8.4 Subcristal Pelvic External Fixator

The pins are inserted from the anterior superior iliac spine (ASIS) in the subcortical bone of the iliac crest and parallel with the crest [52]. The advantages are easier pin placement, less skin irritation, less pin tract infection, and loosening and less interference with hip flexion, while allowing dressing, sitting, and walking.

6.8.5 Parasymphyseal Fixator Pins

The new concept of parasymphyseal pin fixation connected to an external fixator of the pelvic ring produces a considerable increase in stability for the treatment of type C pelvic injuries, as does an increase in pin diameter [53].

6.8.6 Pelvic Reduction Frame

A frame comprised of two carbon-fiber rings which are attached to the operating table and by means of external fixator pins to the patient (Starr Frame, Limited Liability Corporation, Richardson, TX) has been used to reduce displaced pelvic ring fractures. The frame has been shown to be effective, allowing the surgeon to obtain a satisfactory reduction and fixation of acute displaced disruptions of the pelvic ring by Lefaivre et al. [54].

6.9 Complications

The complication rate for definitive pelvic external fixation has been reported to be 62%, compared to 21% for temporary pelvic external fixation [55]. Superficial infections are very common, but osteomyelitis has also been reported [56].

Mason et al. [55] reported a 50% rate of pin tract infection for definite pelvic external fixation, compared to only a 13% rate for temporary pelvic external fixation. These investigators stated that the temporary use of external fixation of the pelvis was safe and effective, as definitive external fixation for prolonged periods was associated with a high rate of infection and aseptic pin loosening. The variables that may cause pin tract infection include diameter of the pins, thermal necrosis with self-tapping pins, the pin-bone interface, local pin care, soft tissue mantle between skin and bone, and duration of external fixation [57–60]. Skin tension around pins, believed to be a major factor by Hoffmann, is particularly applicable to pelvic external fixation and must be relieved by incision to prevent infection [57].

The use of hydroxyapatite coating to the threads of half-pins improves bone to pin osseous integration and interface strength. The improved stability appears to decrease the likelihood of infection. However, the application of this coating does make removal of half-pins more difficult [61, 62].

The lateral femoral cutaneous nerve of the thigh may be injured due to its anatomic variability. Penetration of pins at the back of the iliac crest is a frequent problem which appears to be associated with pin placement without fluoroscopic control, and iliac wing displacement from injury.

Pin penetration of the hip joint results from half-pins placed in the supra-acetabular region. A pin that inadvertently enters the hip joint that is recognized and removed at the time of the initial surgery is usually not a problem. However, a pin that is left in the hip joint can lead to septic arthritis secondary to bacterial seeding from pin tract infection.

Skeletal deformity after anterior external fixation of the pelvis has been documented. Dickson and Matta described an external fixator deformity with flexed and internally rotated hemipelvis [63]. Most patients also had an increase in posterior cephalad translation or posterior diastasis with placement of an anterior external fixator.

Re-displacement or continued displacement of pelvic injuries after pelvic external fixation is a common complication with a higher incidence of inability to maintain reduction reported in obese patients [64]. Loss of reduction should lead to the suspicion of a missed unstable injury at the time of initial evaluation, especially if the pin-bone interface is stable. Entrapment of the anterior bladder wall between the pubic rami following pelvic external fixation has been reported [65, 66]. A similar complication without a fistula was also described by Cass et al. [67]. Bladder entrapment from retrovesical pelvic hematoma occurred following closed reduction and external fixation of an open book pelvic fractures with pubic symphysis diastasis [68]. Due to the possibility of increased incidence of bladder involvement after closed reduction of symphysis disruptions, follow-up CT is recommended [68]. Small bowel obstruction, with a loop of herniated small bowel in the sacral fracture fragments, was reported as a complication from an external fixator used for a pelvic fracture [69]. It is sensible to place a Foley catheter prior to performing pelvic external fixation.

6.10 Aftercare

The care of damage control patients in the ICU has been encouraging with the advances in re-warming, reversal of coagulopathy, and determination of end points of prolonged resuscitation. Patients may be transferred from the bed to a chair the day following external fixation, provided their general condition allows mobilization. Follow-up radiographs at 2-week intervals are taken before the frame is removed.

Routine pin tract care is initiated the day after surgery with removal of the gauze packing around the skin-pin junction. The skin-pin junction is cleaned with half-strength hydrogen peroxide on a sterile applicator. Then, one or two drops of a benzalkonium chloride antiseptic solution are applied to each pin. The patient and family are taught how to clean each pin site daily (see Chap. 11). Oral antibiotics are routinely prescribed as a prophylactic measure to decrease the incidence of pin tract infection once the patient is off parental antibiotics [60]. Cephalosporins are used in subtherapeutic doses, which can be increased to higher doses if an active infection is detected or believed to be impending. Fluoroquinolones are the second line of antibiotic therapy [60]. Checketts et al. reported a classification system for pin tract infections and provided a suggested treatment in a stepwise fashion [70, 71]. Any major infection around a pin or loosening of a pin necessitates pin removal. The nuts of the fixator are monitored for loosening. Patients are discharged home when their condition is stable and they have the ability to manage the external frame.

The fixator is usually removed in the outpatient clinic using an ethylene hydrochloride topical cryorefrigerant spray for local anesthesia. The half-pins are removed, pin tracts cleaned and irrigated with Betadine solution, and a dry sterile dressing applied. Immersion in water (swimming or bathing) is not allowed until the half-pin site has sealed off.

6.11 Conclusion

External fixation has an important role in the resuscitation of hemodynamically unstable patients with unstable pelvic fractures. Additional open anterior approaches or percutaneous placement of iliosacral lag screws can be performed quickly and routinely after a patient is hemodynamically stable in the early treatment phase [72]. In the future, pelvic external fixation will be used less frequently for long durations, and more routinely as a temporary reduction device and bridge to staged open reduction of symphyseal disruptions based on biomechanical markers [73], percutaneous fixation of pelvic fractures, and percutaneous fixation of acetabular fractures. There will doubtless be material improvement both in the design and composition of the frames and the pins.

References

1. Van Vugt AB, Van Kampen A, Van Vugt AB, Van Kampen A. An unstable pelvic ring. J Bone Joint Surg Br. 2006;88-B(4):427–33.
2. Mears DC. Clinical techniques in the pelvis. In: Mears DC, editor. External skeletal fixation. Baltimore: Williams and Wilkins; 1983. p. 342.
3. Slatis P, Karaharju EO. External fixation of the pelvic girdle with a trapezoid compression frame. Injury. 1975;7(1):53–6.
4. Slatis P, Karaharju EO. External fixation of unstable pelvic fractures: experiences in 22 patients treated with a trapezoid compression frame. Clin Orthop Relat Res. 1980;151:73–80.
5. Giannoudis PV, Pape HC. Damage control orthopaedics in unstable pelvic ring injuries. Injury. 2004;5:671–7.
6. Ganz R, Krushell RJ, Jacob RP, et al. The antishock pelvic clamp. Clin Orthop Relat Res. 1991;267:71–8.
7. Heini PF, Witt J, Ganz R. The pelvic C-clamp for the emergency treatment of unstable pelvic ring injuries. A report on clinical experience of 30 cases. Injury. 1996;27 Suppl 1:S-A38–45.
8. Solomon LB, Pohl AP, Chehade MJ, et al. Surgical anatomy for pelvic external fixation. Clin Anat. 2008;21(7):674–82.
9. Vrahas MS, Wilson SC, Cummings PD, et al. Comparison of fixation methods for preventing pelvic ring expansion. Orthopedics. 1998;21(3):285–9.
10. Rommens M, Hessmann ML. External fixation for the injured pelvic ring. In: Tile M, editor. Fractures of the pelvis and acetabulum. 3rd ed. Philadelphia: Lippincott Williams & Wilkins; 2003.
11. Haidukewych GJ, Kumar S, Prpa P. Placement of half-pins for supra-acetabular external fixation: an anatomic study. Clin Orthop Relat Res. 2003;411:269–73.
12. Deridder VA, DeLange S, Popta JV. Anatomic variations of the lateral femoral cutaneous nerve and the consequence for surgery. J Orthop Trauma. 1999;13:207–11.
13. Hospodar PP, Ashman ES, Traub JA. Anatomic study of the lateral femoral cutaneous nerve with respect to the ilioinguinal surgical dissection. J Orthop Trauma. 1999;13:17–9.
14. Pohlemann T, Braune C, Gansslen A, et al. Pelvic emergency clamps: anatomic landmarks for a safe primary application. J Orthop Trauma. 2004;18(2):102–5.
15. Grimm MR, Vrahas MS, Thomas KA. Pressure-volume characteristics of the intact and disrupted pelvic peritoneum. J Trauma. 1998;44(3):454–9.
16. Bottlang M, Simpson T, Sigg J, et al. Noninvasive reduction of open-book pelvic fractures by circumferential compression. J Orthop Trauma. 2002;6(6):367–73.

17. Simonian PT, Routt Jr ML, Harrington RM, et al. Anterior versus posterior provisional fixation in the unstable pelvis. A biomechanical comparison. Clin Orthop Relat Res. 1995;310:245–51.
18. Gardner MJ, Kendoff D, Ostermeier S, et al. Sacroiliac joint compression using an anterior pelvic compressor: a mechanical study in synthetic bone. J Orthop Trauma. 2007;21(7):435–41.
19. Ponson KJ, van Dijke GA Hoek, Joosse P, et al. Improvement of external fixator performance in type C pelvic ring injuries by plating of the pubic symphysis: an experimental study on 12 external fixators. J Trauma. 2002;53(5):907–12; discussion 912–3.
20. Archdeacon MT, Arebi S, Le TT, et al. Orthogonal pin construct versus parallel uniplanar pin constructs for pelvic external fixation: a biomechanical assessment of stiffness and strength. J Orthop Trauma. 2009;23(2):100–5.
21. Garcia JM, Doblare M, Serai B, Serai F, Palanca D, Gracia L. Three-dimensional finite element analysis of several internal and external pelvic fixations. J Biomech Eng. 2000;122(5):516–22.
22. Rieger H, Brug E. Fractures of the pelvis in children. Clin Orthop Relat Res. 1997;336:226–39.
23. Noordeen MHH, Taylor BA, Briggs TWR, et al. Pin placement in pelvic external fixation. Injury. 1993;24:581–4.
24. Bone L. Emergency treatment of the injured patient. In: Browner B, Jupiter J, Levine A, Trafton P, editors. Skeletal trauma. Philadelphia: Saunders; 1992.
25. Huittinen V. Lumbosacral nerve injury in fracture of the pelvis. Acta Chir Scand. 1972; 429(Suppl):3–43.
26. Cook RE, Keating JF, Gillespie I. The role of angiography in the management of hemorrhage from major fractures of the pelvis. J Bone Joint Surg. 2002;84(2):178–82.
27. Tscherne H, Pohlemann T, Gansslen A, et al. Crush injuries of the pelvis. Eur J Surg. 2000;166(4):276–82.
28. Pohlemann T, Paul C, Gansslen A, et al. Die traumatische hemipelvectomie. Erfahrungen aus 11 Fallen. Unfallchirurg. 1996;99:304–12.
29. Bellabarba C, Ricci WM, Bolhofner BR. Distraction external fixation in lateral compression pelvic fractures. J Orthop Trauma. 2000;14(7):475–82.
30. Bellabarba C, Ricci WM, Bolhofner BR. Distraction external fixation in lateral compression pelvic fractures. J Orthop Trauma. 2006;20(1 Suppl):S7–14.
31. Kellam JF. The role of external fixation in pelvic disruptions. Clin Orthop Relat Res. 1989;241:66–82.
32. Pennig D, Gladbach B, Majchrowski W. Disruption of the pelvic ring during spontaneous child birth. J Bone Joint Surg Br. 1997;79(3):438–40.
33. Hoshino Y, Doita ML, Yoshikawa M, et al. Unstable pelvic insufficiency fracture in a patient with rheumatoid arthritis. Rheumatol Int. 2004;24(1):46–9.
34. Matta JM, Yerasimides JG. Table-skeletal fixation as an adjunct to pelvic ring reduction. J Orthop Trauma. 2007;21(9):647–56.
35. Burgess AR, Eastridge BJ, Young JWR, et al. Pelvic ring disruptions: effective classification system and treatment protocols. J Trauma. 1990;3Q:848–56.
36. Dalai SA, Burgess AR, Siegel JH, et al. Pelvic fracture in multiple trauma: classification by mechanism is key to pattern of organ injury, resuscitative requirements and outcome. J Trauma. 1989;29:981–1002.
37. Young JWR, Burgess AR, Brumback RJ, et al. Pelvic fractures: value of plain radiography in early assessment and management. Radiology. 1986;160:445–51.
38. Tile M. Pelvic ring fractures: should they be fixed? J Bone Joint Surg Br. 1988;70(B):1–12.
39. Duxbury MS, Rossiter ND, Lambert AW. Cable ties for pelvic stabilization. Ann R Coll Surg Engl. 2003;85:130.
40. Simpson T, Krieg J, Heuer F, et al. Stabilization of pelvic ring disruptions with a circumferential sheet. J Trauma. 2002;52(1):158–61.
41. Vermeulen B, Peter R, Hoffmeyer P, et al. Prehospital stabilization of pelvic dislocations: a new strap belt to provide temporary hemodynamic stabilization. Swiss Surg. 1999;5:43–6.
42. Schutz M, Stockle U, Hoffmann R, et al. Clinical experience with two types of pelvic C-clamps for unstable pelvic ring injuries. Injury. 1996;27 Suppl 1:SA46–50.

43. Buckle R, Browner B, Morande M. Emergency reduction for pelvic ring disruptions and control of associated hemorrhage using the pelvic stabilizer. Tech Orthop. 1995;9:258–66.
44. Reynolds JH, Attum B, Acland RD, et al. Anterior versus posterior pin placement of pelvic C-clamp in relationship to anatomical structures: a cadaver study. Injury. 2008;39(8):865–8.
45. Archdeacon MT, Hiratzka MS. The trochanteric c-clamp for provisional pelvic stability. J Orthop Trauma. 2006;20(1):47–51.
46. Holt GE, Mencio GA. Pelvic C-clamp in a pediatric patient. J Orthop Trauma. 2003;17(7):525–7.
47. Pohlemann T, Gansslen A, Bosch U, et al. The technique of packing for control of hemorrhage in complex pelvic fractures. Tech Orthop. 1994;9:267–70.
48. Yang A, Lannacone WM. External fixation for pelvic ring disruptions. Orthop Clin N Am. 1997;28(3):331–44.
49. Zinghi GF et al. Fractures of the pelvis and acetabulum. Stuttgard: Georg Thieme Verlag; 2004. p. 69–70.
50. Kim WT, Hearn TC, Saleem O, et al. Effect of pin location on stability of pelvic external fixation. Clin Orthop Relat Res. 1999;61:237–44.
51. Gardner MJ, Nork SE. Stabilization of unstable pelvic fractures with supraacetabular compression external fixation. J Orthop Trauma. 2007;21(4):269–73.
52. Solomon LB, Pohl AP, Sukthankar A, et al. The subcristal pelvic external fixator: technique, results, and rationale. J Orthop Trauma. 2009;23(5):365–9.
53. Ponsen KJ, Joosse P, Van Dijke GA, et al. External fixation of the pelvic ring: an experimental study on the role of pin diameter, pin position, and parasymphyseal fixator pins. Acta Orthop. 2007;78(5):648–53.
54. Lefaivre KA, Starr AJ, Barker BP, et al. Early experience with reduction of displaced disruption of the pelvic ring using a pelvic reduction frame. J Bone Joint Surg Br. 2009;91(9):1201–7.
55. Mason WT, Khan SN, James CL, et al. Complications of temporary and definitive external fixation of pelvic ring injuries. Injury. 2005;36(5):599–604.
56. Stewart MC, Little RE, Highland TR. Osteomyelitis of the ilium secondary to external pelvic fixation. J Trauma. 1986;26(3):284–6.
57. Hoffmann PR. Du danger des fixators externes et des moyens de le pallier. Acta Chir Belg. 1957;6:585–602.
58. Mahan J, Seligson D, Henry SL, et al. Factors in pin tract infections. Orthopedics. 1991;14:305–8.
59. Paley D. Problems, obstacles, and complications of limb lengthening by the Ilizarov technique. Clin Orthop Relat Res. 1990;250:81–104.
60. Parameswaran AD, Roberts CS, Seligson D, et al. Pin tract infection with contemporary external fixation: how much of a problem? J Orthop Trauma. 2003;17(7):503–7.
61. Magyar G, Toksvig-Larsen S, Moroni A. Hydroxyapatite coating of threaded pins enhances fixation. [Clinical Trial. Journal Article. Randomized Controlled Trial]. J Bone Joint Surg Br. 1997;79(3):487–9.
62. Moroni A, Aspenberg P, Toksvig-Larsen S, et al. Enhanced fixation with hydroxyapatite coated pins. [Clinical Trial. Journal Article. Randomized Controlled Trial]. Clin Orthop Relat Res. 1998;346:171–7.
63. Dickson KF, Matta JM. Skeletal deformity after anterior external fixation of the pelvis. J Orthop Trauma. 2009;23(5):327–32.
64. Hupel TM, McKee MD, Waddell JP, et al. Primary external fixation of rotationally unstable pelvic fractures in obese patients. J Trauma. 1998;45(1):11–5.
65. Bartlett CS, Ali A, Helfet DL. Bladder incarceration in a traumatic symphysis pubis diastasis treated with external fixation: a case report and review of the literature. J Orthop Trauma. 1998;12(1):64–7.
66. Chitale SV, Almeida A, Hadfield JIH. Urological complication of pelvic fracture treated by an external fixator. Br J Urol. 1997;80(4):681–2.
67. Cass AS, Behrens F, Comfort T, et al. Bladder problems in pelvic injuries treated with external fixator and direct urethral drainage. J Trauma. 1983;23(1):50–3.
68. Geracci JJ, Morey AF. Bladder entrapment after external fixation of traumatic pubic diastases: importance of follow-up computed tomography in establishing prompt diagnosis. Mil Med. 2000;65(6):492–3.

69. Tillman RM, Kenny NW. Small bowel obstruction as a complication of the use of an external fixator in a pelvic fracture. Injury. 1991;22(1):71–2.
70. Checketts RG, MacEachern AG, Otterburn M. Pin tract infection and the principles of pin site care. In: De Bastiani G, Apley AG, Goldberg A, editors. Orthofix external fixation in trauma and orthopaedics. London: Springer; 2000. p. 97–100.
71. Checketts RG, Otterbum M, MacEachem AG. Pin tract infection: definition, incidence and prevention. Int J Orthop Trauma. 1993;3:16–9.
72. Cole JD, Blum DA, Ansel LJ. Outcome after fixation of unstable posterior pelvic ring injuries. Clin Orthop Relat Res. 1996;329:160–79.
73. Pape HC, van Griensven M, Rice J, et al. Major secondary surgery in blunt trauma patients and peri-operative cytokine liberation: determination of the clinical relevance of biochemical markers. J Trauma. 2001;50(6):989–1000.

Chapter 7
External Fixation About the Wrist and the Forearm

Cyril Mauffrey, David Seligson, and Jonathan Yerasimides

7.1 Introduction

Fractures of the forearm and wrist are usually treated with direct osteosynthesis – plates, pins, and screws. These fractures and dislocation are important but unimportant. They do not cause loss of life. Patients with major, life-threatening injuries need life-saving treatments first and intricate limb repair later. The damage control strategy facilitates staged repair. A complex trans-scaphoid perilunate fracture dislocation with a dorsal marginal fracture of the distal radius is not well repaired while the patient's life is at risk from a high-grade bleeding liver laceration. Even in straightforward injures, like both bone forearm fractures it is a useful option to stage repair with external fixation for "traveling traction" followed by planning internal fixation when the forearm bones are at length and the swelling has subsided.

Delay is an opportunity. It is an opportunity for planning thoughtful review of the x-rays. It is an opportunity for additional studies like CT scans with 3D reconstruction. It is an opportunity to get exactly the right equipment that allows the case to be done beautifully. It is an opportunity to work with the family to get meaningful consent and to answer their questions about the injury, recovery, and late consequences.

In the forearm and wrist, strong ligaments connect skeletal elements. With traction in the direction of the mechanical axis of the limb, these ligaments can reduce or partially reduce displaced skeletal elements. The principle of aligning bone with axial traction is called "ligamentotaxis." No amount of traction, however, will restore displaced articular fragments, for example, which are driven into the shaft of a bone. Success in reduction depends on location, type of injury, and to a great extent on the force transmitted to the ligament and bone at the time of injury. With high-grade musculoskeletal injury, ligaments are torn from bone, the instability is greater, and the restoration that can be achieved by straightening the limb and applying external

C. Mauffrey (✉) • D. Seligson • J. Yerasimides
Department of Orthopaedics, University Hospital Louisville, Louisville, KY, USA
e-mail: cmauffrey@yahoo.com

D. Seligson et al. (eds.), *External Fixation in Orthopedic Traumatology*,
DOI 10.1007/978-1-4471-2197-8_7,

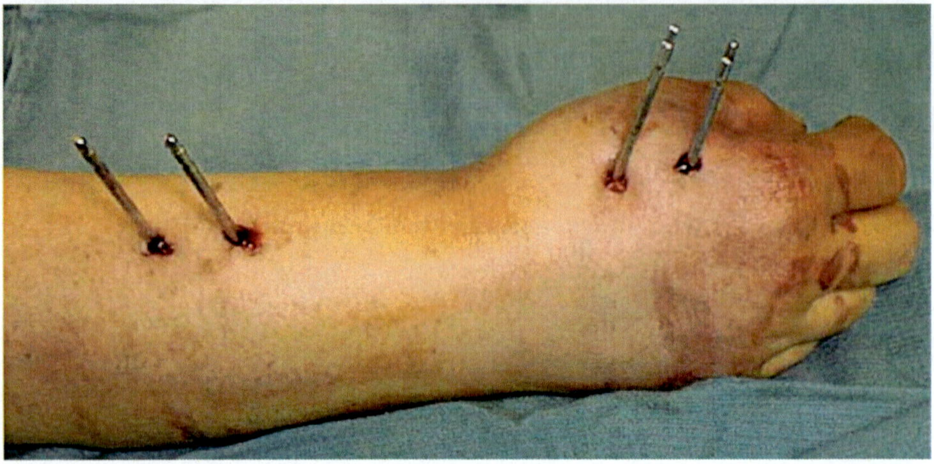

Fig. 7.1 Clinical photograph of a wrist with insertion of half-pins in the radial shaft and in the second metacarpal shaft

fixation is less predictable. Once external fixation is installed, reduction can often be improved with pressure around the displaced bone to attempt to restore its position. The initial closed reduction and external fixation facilitates later definitive surgery.

7.2 Basic Montage

External fixation about the wrist has two basic patterns – Hoffmann's Osteotaxis and the Mayo Clinic frame. The key principle is that the fixation should be balanced [1]. Equal holding power proximal and distal to the wrist joint reduces pin loosening [2]. The radius and ulna should not be linked by the frame. Connecting them together will result in pin loosening, or wire breakage from rotational forces [3].

7.2.1 The Osteotaxis Frame

The Osteotaxis frame has a pin group in the radius proximal to the fracture site connected to a pin group in the index metacarpal (Figs. 7.1 and 7.2) [4]. The pins are oriented midway between the lateral and the anteroposterior plane. The half-pins are 3 mm. Larger half-pins can fracture the index metacarpal. The easiest way to increase mechanical stability is to increase the diameter of the connecting rod [5]. Thus, a fixator with a stout connector like the monotube (Fig. 7.3) is more stable than one with a small 5 mm connecting bar [6]. Another strategy to increase the stability of the frame would be to place a second bar in a different plane. For example, the distal pin in the radius can be connected to the proximal pin in the metacarpal with a bar which will be perpendicular to the pin connecting the pin groups.

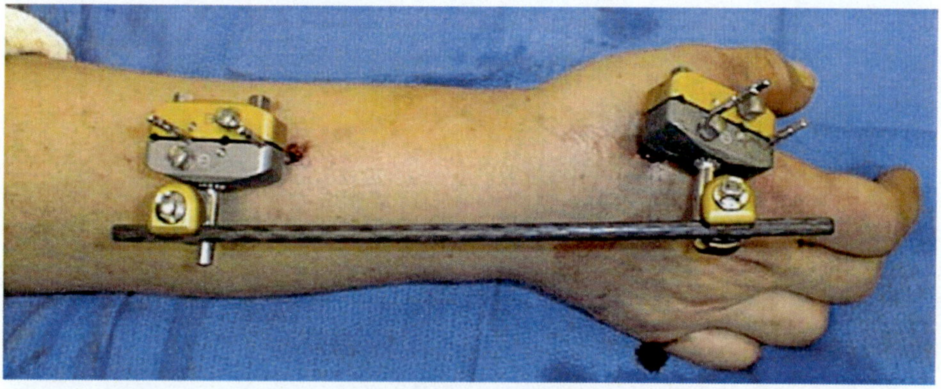

Fig. 7.2 Uniaxial external fixator bridging the wrist using the principle of ligamentotaxis for fracture reduction

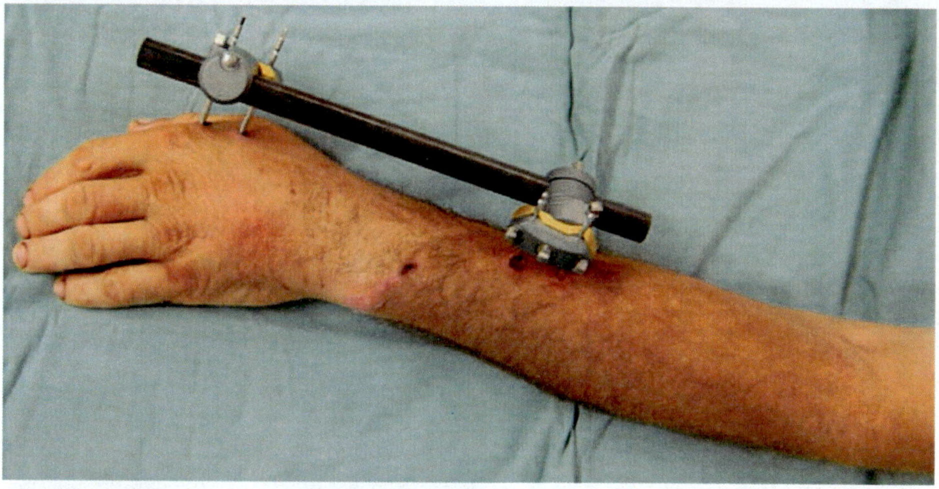

Fig. 7.3 Clinical photograph centered on a left forearm showing a monotube wrist-bridging external fixator

7.2.2 The Mayo Clinic Frame

The Mayo Clinic frame (Fig. 7.4) links the forearm to the hand with three pins in the radius and two in the hand. The distal pins are placed at the base of the index and ring finger metacarpals. Two pins are placed in a line in the radial side at the radius and the third between these two on the ulnar side of the radius [7]. The pins are connected using single pin-to-bar clamps to make a box on the dorsum of the hand. Use this frame when the patient is smaller or when there is marked instability at the wrist, since the orientation of the carpus to the distal radius can be adjusted better with pins radial and ulnar. The frame also avoids the pin in the narrow shaft of the index metacarpal which can be problematic if the bone is small.

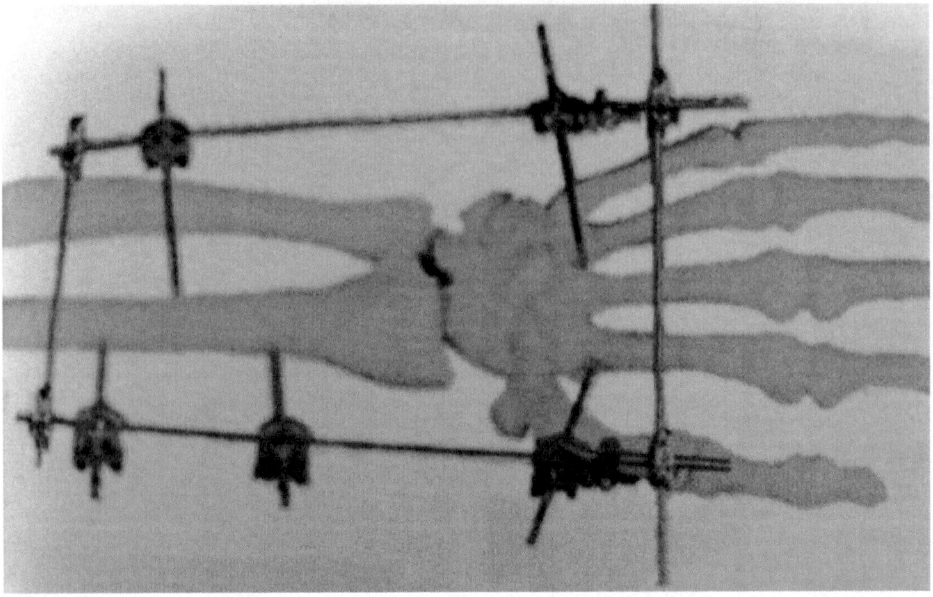

Fig. 7.4 Mayo Clinic frame for a distal radius fracture

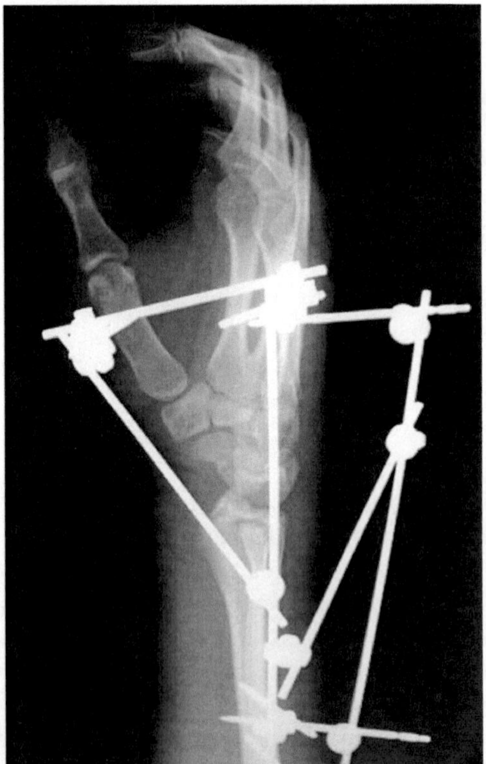

Fig. 7.5 Lateral radiograph showing an external fixator using a combination of the Strasbourg and the Mayo frame for a distal radius and a scaphoid fracture

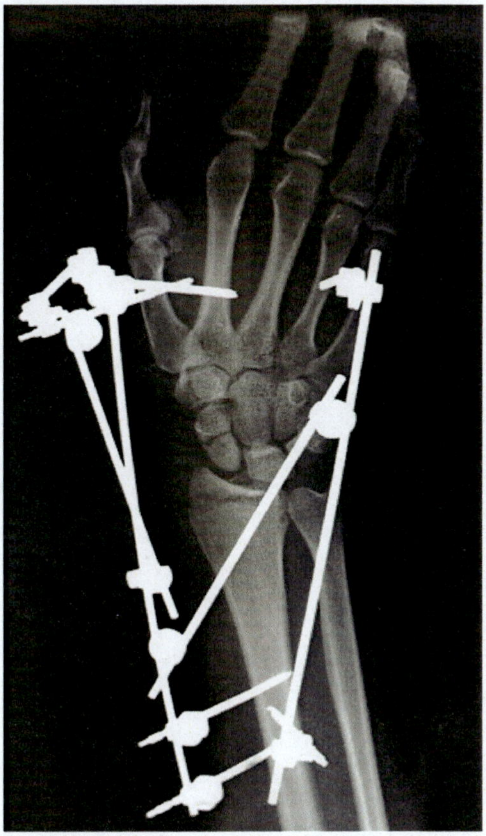

Fig. 7.6 AP radiograph centered on a wrist showing a scaphoid waist and a distal radius fracture stabilized using an external fixator in a Strasbourg/Mayo frame configuration

7.2.3 The Strasbourg Frame

The Strasbourg frame (Figs. 7.5 and 7.6) is an extension of the Mayo Clinic basic box frame to the thumb metacarpal. An additional 3 mm half-pin is placed in the proximal thumb metacarpal and a bar connects this pin to the radial bar of the Mayo Clinic frame. A second bar locks the position of the thumb in abduction and antepulsion [8]. The Strasbourg frame can be used to treat fractures of the scaphoid and injuries of the thenar eminence. It maintains the web space of the thumb.

Half-pins placed in fracture fragments are known as intrafocal pins. One strategy is to connect a pin group in the radius to a pin group in the distal radius. The fragments have to be large enough for fixation to be practical. Alternatively, a spanning frame is installed and supplemental half-pins attached to the connecting pods. A pin could be used to improve the alignment. In weeks prior to removal of a spanning frame, getting the pins out improves hand function and reduces the risk of infection [9].

In a Cochrane review published in 2008 [10], Handoll et al. reviewed all level I evidence for the management of distal radius fractures using different configurations of external fixators. Nine small trials involving 510 adults with unstable distal radius fractures were grouped into five comparisons. Two trials comparing a bridging

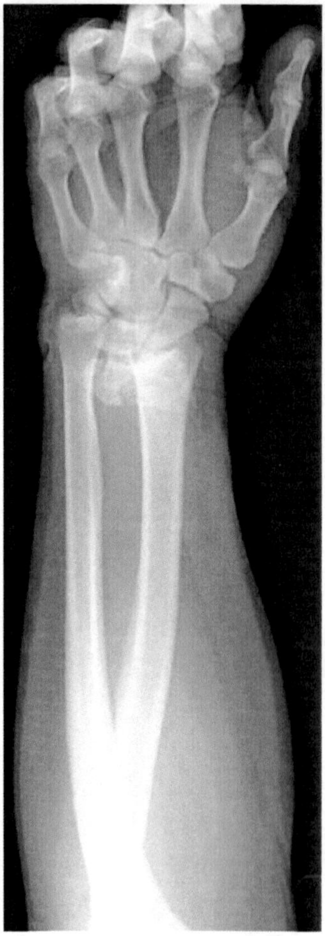

Fig. 7.7 Intra-articular distal radius fracture on AP wrist radiograph

external fixator versus pins and plaster external fixation found no significant differences in function or deformity. One trial found tendencies for more serious complications but less subsequent discomfort and deformity in the fixator group. Three trials compared non-bridging versus bridging fixation. Of the two trials testing uniplanar non-bridging fixation, one found no significant differences in functional or clinical outcomes; the other found non-bridging fixation significantly improved grip strength, wrist flexion, and anatomical outcome. The third trial found no significant findings in favor of multi-planar non-bridging fixation of complex intra-articular fractures. One trial using a bridging external fixator found that deploying an extra external fixator pin to fix the "floating" distal fragment gave superior functional and anatomical results. One trial found no evidence of differences in clinical outcomes for hydroxyapatite-coated pins compared with standard uncoated pins. Two trials compared dynamic versus static external fixation. One trial found no significant effects from early dynamism of an external fixator. The conclusion of the study was that the evidence toward one type of construct versus another was inconclusive for distal radius fractures managed with external fixation.

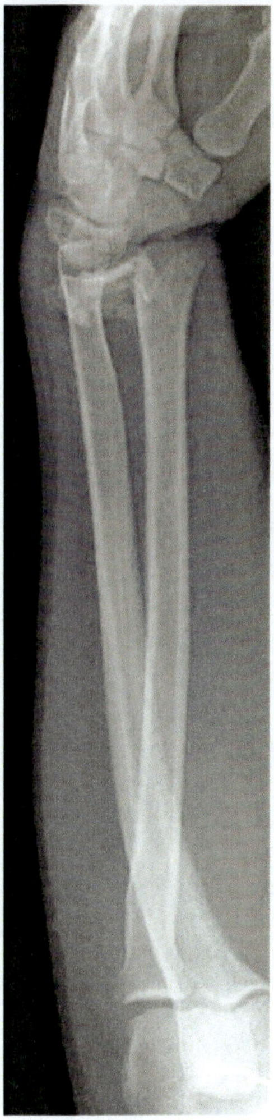

Fig. 7.8 Lateral radiograph of an intra-articular distal radius fracture

7.3 Case Studies

7.3.1 Case 1

A 50-year-old salesman was involved in a motor vehicle accident sustaining an anteroposterior compression pelvic injury, stable hemodynamically, associated with a 100% displaced extra-articular distal radius fracture with intact neurovascular status (Figs. 7.7 and 7.8). He was taken to the operating room on the same day for application of pelvic external fixator and a wrist bridging external fixator with half-pins in the radius shaft and distal pins in the shaft of the second metacarpal using the ligamentotaxis as a reduction means (Fig. 7.9).

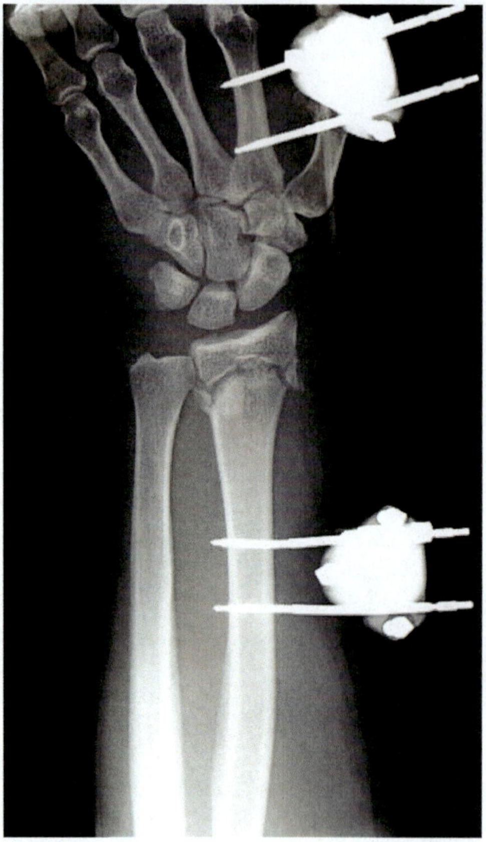

Fig. 7.9 AP radiograph following reduction of the distal radius and application of wrist-bridging external fixator

7.3.2 Case 2

A 54-year-old female teacher fell from a 12-ft-high ladder sustaining a right scapula blade fracture, and a right open distal intra-articular distal radius fracture extending to the DRUJ (Fig. 7.10). The neurovascular status of the right upper extremity was intact and the skin wound was 2 cm. Her treatment was staged with the first step involving debridement, lavage, closure of the wound over antibiotic beads, and application of a wrist-bridging external fixator (Figs. 7.11 and 7.12). This construct was left for 1 week until the swelling subsided. The definitive treatment consisted in open reduction and internal fixation of the fracture with removal of the antibiotic bead chain.

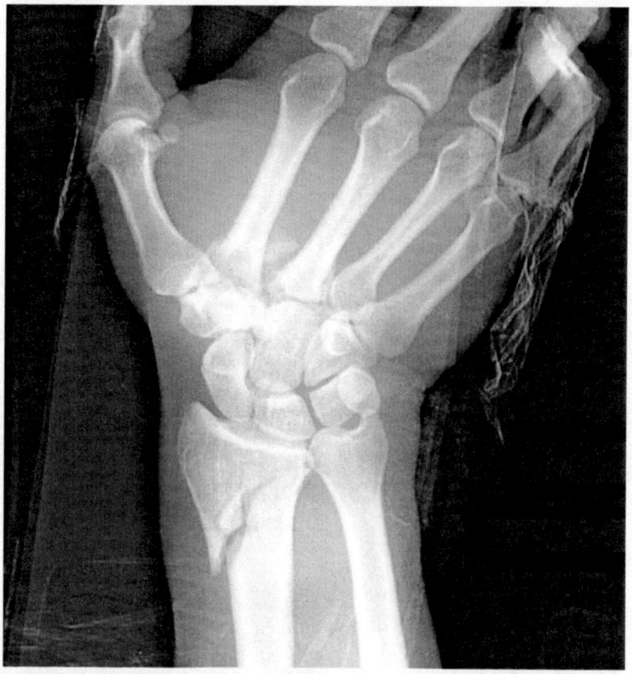

Fig. 7.10 AP radiograph of a distal radius fracture extending into the distal radioulnar joint

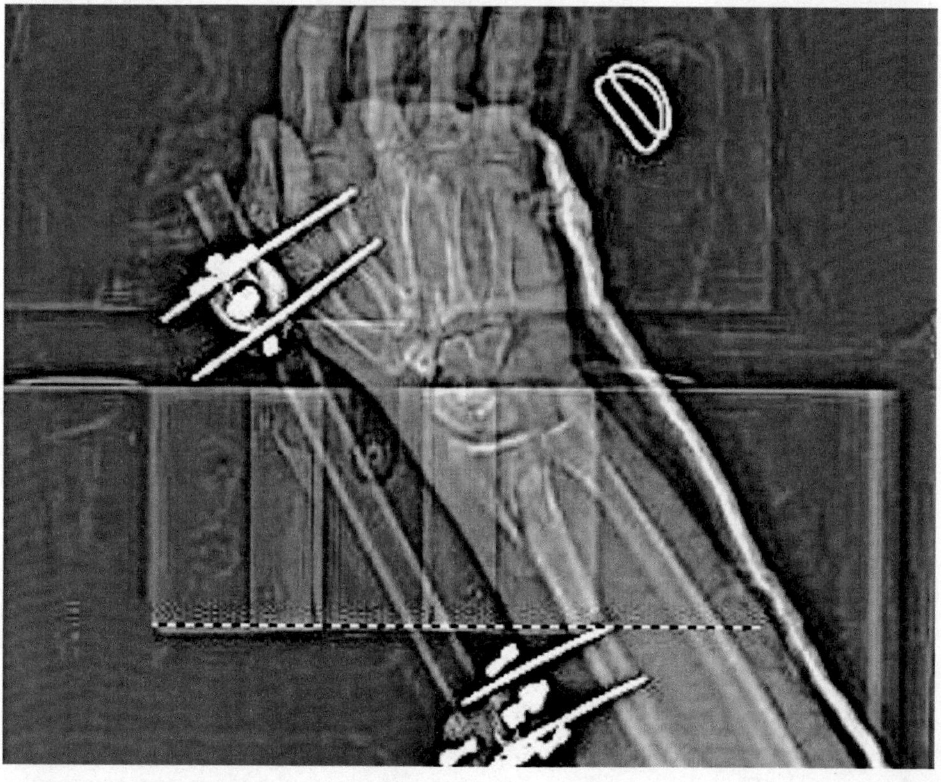

Fig. 7.11 AP radiograph of a distal radius fracture with extension into the DRUJ following reduction and fixation with a bridging monotubular external fixator

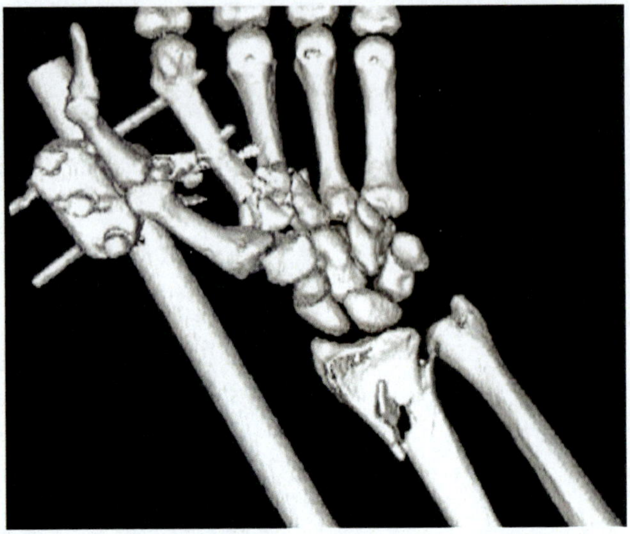

Fig. 7.12 3D CT reconstruction views of a distal radius with extension into the DRUJ. Closed reduction and temporary fixation using a monotubular external fixator

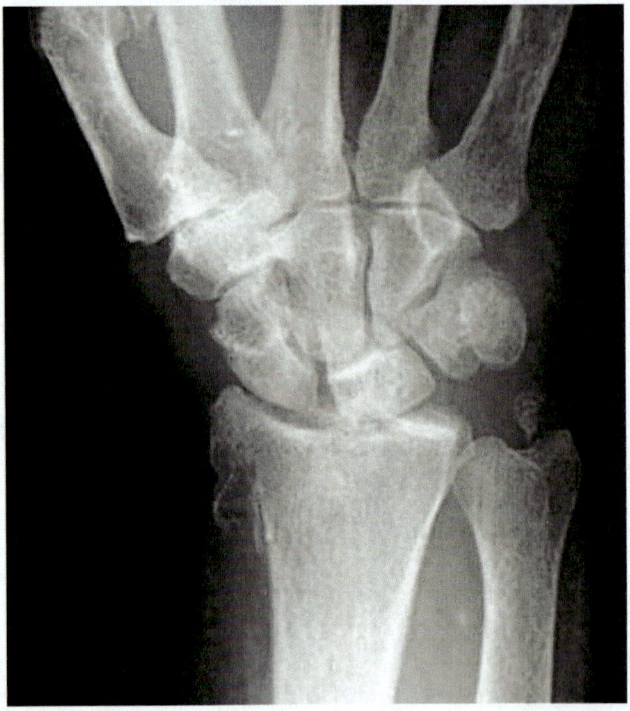

Fig. 7.13 AP radiograph of an intra-articular distal radius fracture associated with an ulnar styloid fracture

7.3.3 Case 3

A 72-year-old retired lady was involved in a motor vehicle accident sustaining head injuries requiring intubation, a femoral neck fracture, and an intra-articular distal radius fracture (Figs. 7.13 and 7.14). The neurovascular status of her upper extremity

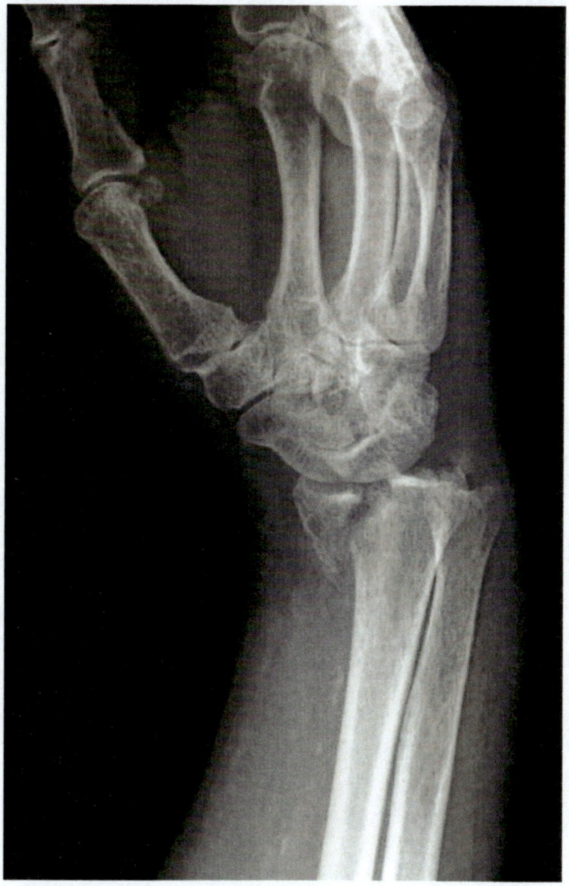

Fig. 7.14 Lateral radiograph of a displaced intra-articular distal radius fracture. Also noted is an oblique fracture of the proximal phalanx of the thumb

was intact and the skin was not breached. We elected to treat her wrist injury with a bridging external fixator supplemented by Kirshner wires (Fig. 7.15). We also noted a fracture of the proximal phalanx of the homolateral thumb treated at the same time with Kirshner wire. The frame and wires were left on for 5 weeks and the patient encouraged to mobilize at this stage.

7.4 Conclusion

Upper extremity injuries are important and potentially disabling. Today their care is increasingly specialized. With the exception of neurovascularly compromised limbs, hasty treatment has the potential for less than the best result. The particular problems of the case may not be entirely evaluated. The equipment may not be available. The surgeon may be tired. The patient and family may not be adequately prepared. Damage control strategies use external fixation to *bridge* the interval between the injury and the definitive treatment. Splinting is also a damage control technique.

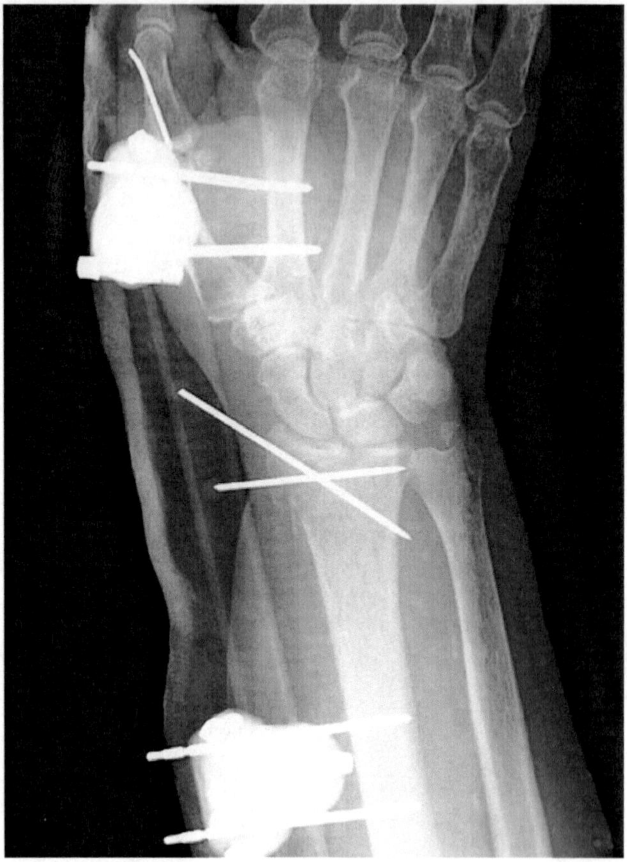

Fig. 7.15 AP radiograph centered on a wrist showing the reduction of the distal radius fracture and combined fixation using a monotubular bridging external fixator with two Kirshner wires

However, a splint does not provide traction and a splint does not give access to the limb for evaluation of the neurovascular status and for soft tissue care.

There are many montages for the arm and hand. Decide first if one wants to span either the elbow or the wrist. Intrafocal (non-spanning) frames are best for diaphyseal fractures; spanning frames work well for fractures near the elbow or wrist joint. With half-pin (Osteotaxis) frames, try not to connect the radius and ulna. The torque between the bones is so great that either the pin or the bone can fracture. On the other side, fine wire circular frames can be used from proximal ulna to distal radius to make a traction frame for the forearm. Wrist-spanning frames are particularly versatile since they can be extended to the thumbs and fingers for complex hand injuries.

The postoperative program for patients in upper limb external fixators is crucial. Awake patients should be trained to use their hands. Unconscious patients need passive mobilization to avoid contractures. Negative attitudes about external fixation such as the physical therapist telling the patient that they "cannot do anything until the frame is off" are not helpful. Patients with arm and hand fractures need to reintegrate their limbs into useful daily function. Frames that are sufficiently stable for functional use are therefore essential. Extra connecting bars can be added for stability and taken off temporarily for wound care. With a good postoperative program, the limb works well, grasp is restored, wounds heal, and swelling subsides. Then, osteosynthesis in a controlled, planned fashion can be performed expertly and beautifully.

References

1. Dodds SD, Cornelissen S, Jossan S, Wolfe SW. A biomechanical comparison of fragment-specific fixation and augmented external fixation for intra-articular distal radius fractures. J Hand Surg. 2002;27A(6):953–64.
2. Pope MH, Byrt W, Andrews G, Seligson D. Effect of cortical area on the holding power of Hoffman minipins. Tech Orthop. 1986;1(2):22–6.
3. Chang D, Kummer FJ, Egol K, Tejwani N, Wolinsky P, Koval KJ. Biomechanical comparison of five external wrist fixators. Bull Hosp Joint Dis. 2002–2003;61(1–2):40–4.
4. Schuind F, Donkerwolcke M, Burny F. External fixation of wrist fractures. Orthopedics. 1984;7:841–4.
5. McQueen MM, Hajducka C, Court-Brown CM. Redisplaced unstable fractures of the distal radius: a prospective randomized comparison of four methods of treatment. J Bone Joint Surg. 1996;78(3):404–9.
6. Sommerkamp TG, Seeman M, Silliman J, Jones A, Patterson S, Walker J, et al. Dynamic external fixation of unstable fractures of the distal part of the radius. A prospective, randomized comparison with static external fixation. J Bone Joint Surg. 1994;76(8):1149–61.
7. Frykman GK, Peckham RH, Willard K, Saha S. External fixators for treatment of unstable wrist fractures. Hand Clin. 1993;9(4):555–65.
8. Herrera M, Chapman CB, Roh M, Strauch RJ, Rosenwasser MP. Treatment of unstable distal radius fractures with cancellous allograft and external fixation. J Hand Surg. 1999;24(6):1269–78.
9. Wolfe SW, Austin G, Lorenze M, Swigart CR, Panjabi MM. A biomechanical comparison of different wrist external fixators with and without K-wire augmentation. J Hand Surg. 1999;24A(3):516–24.
10. Handoll HHG, Huntley JS, Madhok R. Different methods of external fixation for treating distal radial fractures in adults. Cochrane Database Syst Rev. 2008;23(1):CD006522.

Chapter 8
External Fixators in the Treatment of Tibial Plateau Fractures

V. Manakavala Perumal, Cyril Mauffrey, and Craig S. Roberts

8.1 Introduction

Despite advances in locked plating, internal fixation of high-energy tibial plateau fractures is associated with a high complication rate [1]. External fixation of tibial plateau fractures, used either temporarily or definitively, is a practical and powerful technique which can limit the risk of catastrophic complications (e.g., deep infection and osteomyelitis) associated with plating of tibial plateau fractures. This chapter will focus on indications, biomechanics, montages, techniques, and complications of temporary external fixators (knee joint spanning) and definitive external fixators (knee joint sparring) for tibial plateau fractures.

8.2 Indications

The general indication for external fixation of tibial plateau fractures is a complex, combined bony and soft tissue injury (e.g., severe open fracture) which makes open plating procedures unsafe because of an unacceptable risk of soft tissue complications and infection. Specific indications for external fixation for tibial plateau fractures are Schatzker type 5 and type 6 fractures, proximal tibial fractures with metaphyseal and subchondral comminution not amenable to routine plate and screw fixation, complex fracture patterns with soft tissue compromise (e.g., associated

V.M. Perumal (✉)
PWD Road, Chettikulam Junction, Nagercoil, 629002, Tamil Nadu, India

C. Mauffrey • C.S. Roberts
Department of Orthopaedics, University Hospital Louisville, Louisville, KY, USA
e-mail: cmauffrey@yahoo.com; craig.roberts@louisville.edu

D. Seligson et al. (eds.), *External Fixation in Orthopedic Traumatology*,
DOI 10.1007/978-1-4471-2197-8_8, © Springer-Verlag London Limited 2012

Table 8.1 Factors affecting stability of a fine wire frame

Wire diameter	Thicker wires increase stability (2 mm better than 1.5 mm)
Wire number	3 wires minimum in proximal segment
Wire crossing angle	Increase wire crossing angle (minimum 60°)
Wires tension	Increase wire tension (optimum of 140 kg)
Olive wires	Olive wires tensioned on both the ends and placement of the olive on the side of bending
Number of rings proximal segment	A second ring can be added proximally

compartment syndrome), mangled limbs, open fractures with soft tissue loss, and fractures in multiply injured patients who require a damage-control approach [2].

8.3 Biomechanics

The design and construction of an external faxator provides the opportunity to modulate the stiffness of the external faxator and customize it to the individual injury pattern. When constructing an external faxator for definitive fixation, a general rule is that increasing frame stiffness is associated with increasing frame symmetry. The stiffness of the definitive external fixation construct, commonly hybrid or circular external faxator, is also a function of several variables: transfixation wire diameters, half-pin diameter, wire crossing angle, wire tension, placement of olive wire, number of rings, and frame symmetry. Each of these variables can be adjusted to increase or decrease stiffness and, therefore, increase or decrease the overall stability of the faxator construct (Table 8.1). In general, a minimum of three transfixation wires is required in the proximal tibia for a tibial plateau fracture. Ideally, transfixation wires will span both the sagittal and coronal planes. In additional to three transfixation wires, a half-pin inserted in the anterior-posterior direction in the proximal tibia neutralizes sagittal plane shear forces from knee flexion and extension.

An increase in the crossing angle of the tensioned wires in the proximal tibia from 30° to 90° increases axial, torsional, and bending stiffness by 75% [3]. Practically speaking, the largest angle that can be formed by crossing wires at the proximal tibia level without altering safe corridors is about 60°. The positioning of the wires with regard to each other is also important. The construct of two wires crossed one centimeter posterior to the center of the tibia, and the third wire placed in coronal plane one centimeter interiorly from the center of the tibia increases overall stiffness of the faxator, predominantly in the sagittal plane [4]. Olive wire tensioned on both the ends and placing the olives on the side of bending also significantly increase bending stiffness of the external faxator [4]. Pugh et al. [5] compared the biomechanical properties of these constructs and concluded that frames with two levels of fixation in the periarticular segment were stiffer than those with one periarticular level of faxator in the bending mode.

The biomechanics of traditional knee spanning frames with half-pins and bars is less critical because of its temporary nature. Half-pin diameter, number of half-pins, multiplanar half-pin insertion, bar height relative to the bone, and faxator span (working length) are variables which can be adjusted to increase or decrease frame stiffness.

8.4 Technique

There are two main types of external fixators which are applied in the treatment of tibial plateau fractures: knee joint spanning (temporary damage-control fixators) and knee joint sparring (hybrid fixators or all ring fixators). In a recent survey performed by the OTA [6], the trends of orthopedic traumatologists' management of tibial plateau fractures were gathered. Two hundred and fifty surgeons responded to the questionnaires (50% of OTA members). The total duration of external faxator application before definite treatment was 8–14 days in 72% of respondents, while restoration of leg length was to their eye the most important factor during the acute management of patients with a tibial plateau fracture. Two thirds of surgeons favored anterior pin placements both in the femur and tibia while 1/3 favored lateral pins in the femur and medial pins in the tibia. Forty percent of surgeons disagreed with the monolateral rail.

8.4.1 Knee Spanning Frames

Knee spanning frames are temporary external fixators with a goal of converting fractures of immobility into fractures of mobility [7]. The concept of staged treatment of these fractures with initial external fixators followed by a period of rest which allows the soft tissues to heal and swelling to abate is usually necessary prior to open reduction and internal fixation. These fixators are the cornerstone of the damage-control orthopedics approach to fractures.

The femoral half-pins are placed laterally or anterolaterally to minimize injury to the quadriceps mechanism (Fig. 8.1). The tibial pins are placed anteromedially [8].

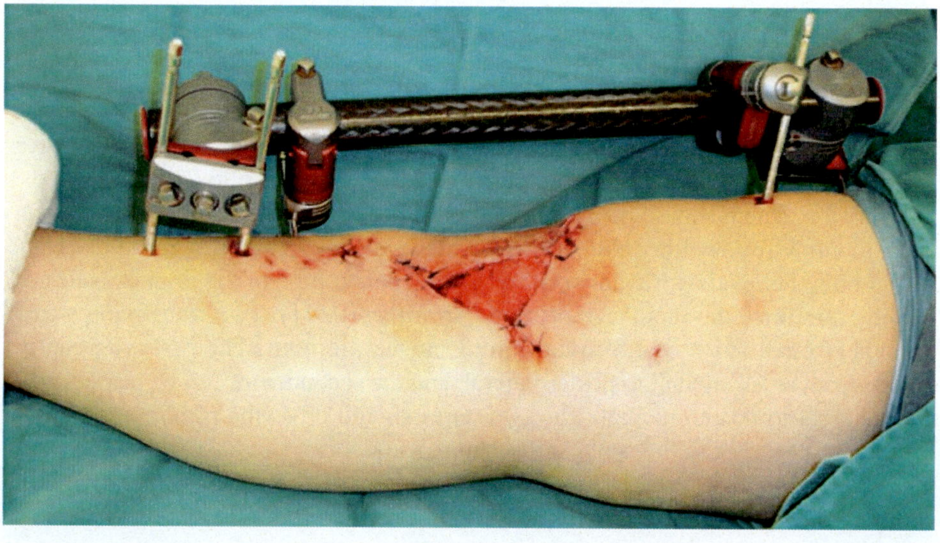

Fig. 8.1 Photograph of a temporary knee sparring faxator used for initial limb damage control for a complex tibial plateau fracture prior to anticipated staged locked plating in the next 2 weeks

Anglen and Aleto [9] inserted the femoral pins in the anterior direction. The placement of the pins in the femur and the tibia depends upon the fracture pattern; areas for future internal fixation should be spared. For spanning of tibial plateau fractures, the tibial pins should be placed in the distal tibia. The femoral pins should be placed in the supracondylar region or the distal third of the shaft. However, avoiding pin insertion into the zone of future internal fixation takes priority over the biomechanics of the faxator. The knee should be placed in slight flexion and gentle traction applied for realignment of the limb under fluoroscopic control. Excess traction should not be applied because increasing soft tissue tension may exacerbate soft tissue swelling and contribute to the development of increased compartment pressures. After faxator application, soft tissue swelling should be reassessed, compartment pressures measured as needed, and a thin cut CT of the tibial plateau obtained.

8.4.2 Knee Sparring Frames

Knee sparing frames do not span the knee joint and are fine-wire fixators (all ring or hybrid constructs), with the goal of using the faxator for definitive osteosynthesis. When it is unlikely that the soft tissue will present a favorable environment for plating procedures within 2–3 weeks, then definitive fixation with a fine wire frame should be considered. These fixators neutralize the metaphyseal component of the tibial plateau fracture and maintain the reduction of the articular surface. One advantage of these frames is that early knee motion can be initiated because the knee joint is not spanned. There are basically two types of configuration in this category: all ring construct or hybrid construct ring(s) proximally and pin clamp distally.

8.4.3 All Ring Constructs

This construct uses two ¾ rings for stabilizing the fracture (Fig. 8.2). First, the proximal ¾ ring is held over the proximal tibia such that the limb is in the center. The ring is placed with the open end positioned posteriorly to allow for unrestricted knee flexion. There should be a minimum of 3 finger breaths of space circumferentially to allow for swelling and soft tissue management. Wires should be placed at least 14 mm below the articular surface to avoid penetration of the joint capsule and thereby minimize the incidence of septic arthritis [10, 11]. Two transfixion wires, preferably olive wires of 1.5 to 2.0-mm diameter, are used. The first wire can be passed from anteromedial to posterolateral, and the second wire can be passed from anterolateral to posteromedial. The two wires should cross the proximal tibia one centimeter posterior to the center of the tibia, and a third wire, a smooth wire without an olive, should be placed in the coronal plane one centimeter anterior to the center of the tibia [4]. Three wires are a minimum, and four wires are preferable if

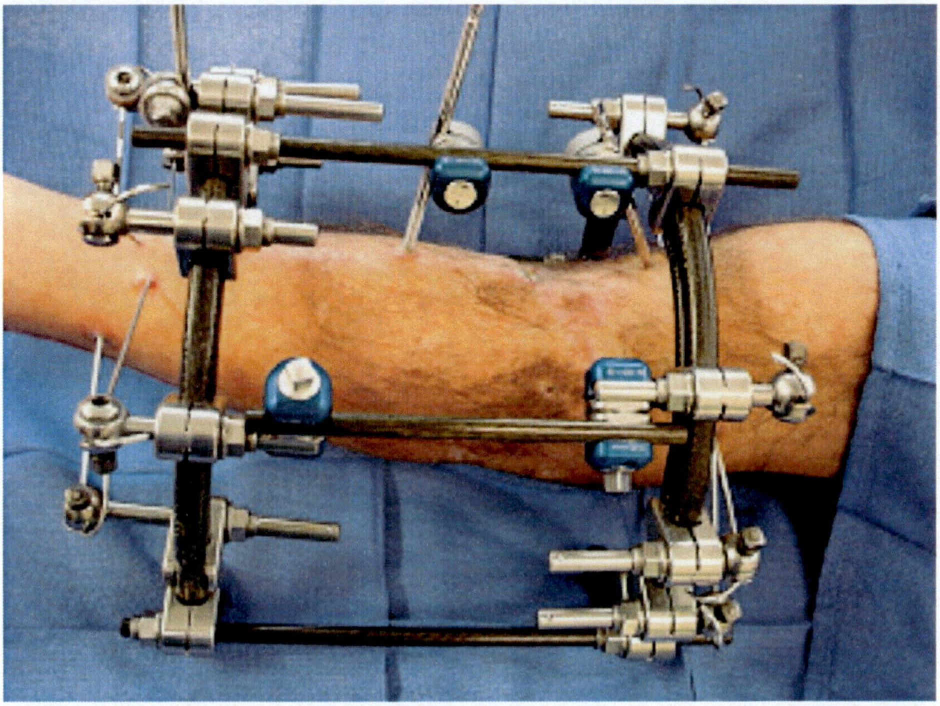

Fig. 8.2 Photograph of a two-ring fine-wire faxator for definitive fracture stabilization of a tibial plateau fracture with a complex soft tissue injury

space on the ring is available [12]. Distally, the rings are attached to the tibia with three wires or a combination of wire and half-pins. The girth of the distal tibia is smaller than the proximal tibia, so the distal ring size can be decreased accordingly to match the anatomy. One smooth wire is generally inserted first 90 degrees to the distal tibia and tensioned to the ring. This wire serves as a reference wire. Next, the alignment of the limb is reestablished, and the proximal and distal rings are attached with three bars. Additional wires are then placed in the distal ring followed by a half-pin 90 degrees to the smooth wire.

8.4.4 Hybrid Construct (Ring Bar Frames)

Hybrid external fixation, which we define as a combination of proximal periarticular ring(s) with tensioned fine wires connected by bars to half-pins distal to the fracture, has become increasingly popular for the fixation of fractures of the tibial plane.

The application of the proximal ring to the periarticular fracture is essentially the same as that of the all ring construct as discussed above. The distal component of the hybrid frame is different from the all ring frames. The distal pin cluster consists

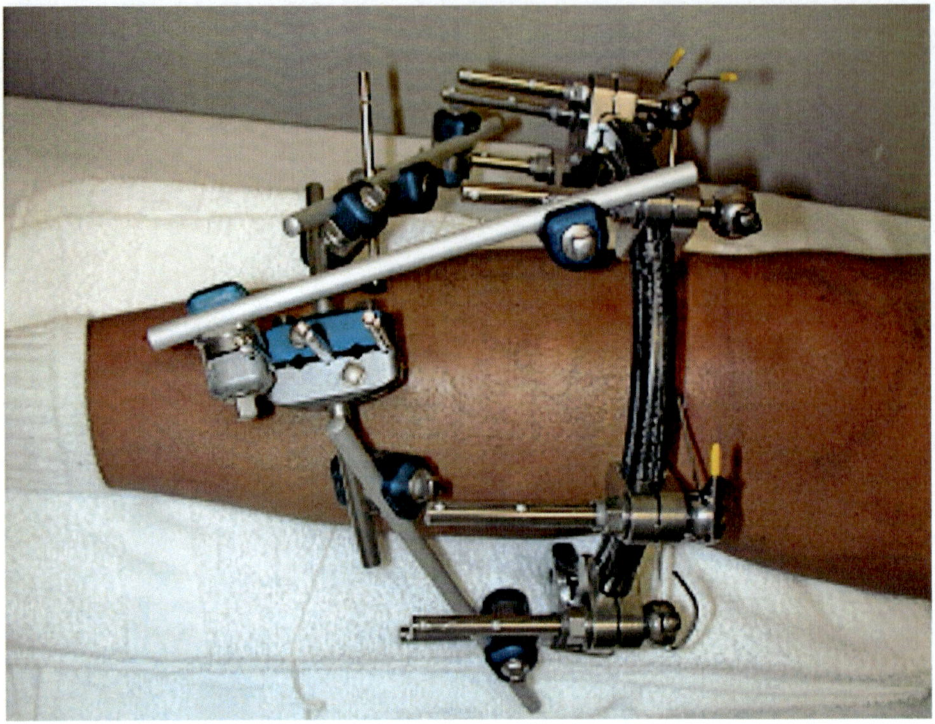

Fig. 8.3 Photograph of a hybrid faxator (ring-bar frame) for definitive fixation of a complex tibial plateau fracture

of a pin clamp with at least two five-millimeter half-pins (Fig. 8.3). A third half-pin in a different plane can also be added when necessary.

8.5 Postoperative Care

The postoperative course depends on the application of the external faxator for fracture management. If the frame is applied as a damage-control measure, the frame should be removed once the soft tissues are ready for open reduction and internal fixation. This waiting period is usually 1–2 weeks. If the frame is applied as definitive treatment protocol, the frame should be maintained until the fracture is united. Most patients who are in the frame are followed up every 2 weeks to monitor for pin tract infections. Patients are kept toe-touch weight-bearing for at least the first 6–8 weeks. Weight-bearing is then increased gradually with progression determined on a case-by-case basis for the rest of treatment. Patients are instructed on pin care and are kept on low-dose prophylactic oral antibiotics. Follow-up X-rays are taken once in 2 weeks to ascertain the fracture union. Stiffness of the fixators can sometimes be decreased gradually by removal of the medial and lateral struts from a V-shaped triple rod construct in order to improve load transfer to bone before the entire faxator is removed.

8.6 Complications

Complications of knee external fixators include pin tract infection, deep infection, malunion, non-union, knee sepsis, knee stiffness (adhesions), quadriceps weakness, and posttraumatic arthrosis.

Pin tract infection is the major complication of external fixation of fractures. The infection rate ranges from 0.5% to 30% [2, 13]. The incidence of infection depends upon the montage. The incidence of pin tract infection using ring fixators was 3.9% and with hybrid fixators, 20% [14]. Pin tract infection is defined as signs and symptoms of infection around pins or wires that require a change in antibiotic, pin removal, or surgical debridement. Although pin tract infection can be graded according to Checketts et al. [15], it is probably more practical to separate pin tract infection into superficial and deep. Superficial pin tract infections are treated with local pin care, antibiotics, and sometimes pin removal and curettage and debridement. Deep infections are treated with removal of the offending pin and sometimes even the entire faxator followed by aggressive debridement.

Deep infection, like chronic osteomyelitis after external fixation, has traditionally been reported to be about 4% [16]. However, chronic osteomyelitis after external fixation in our experience appears to be around 1%. Knee sepsis has been reported following placement of tensioned transfixing wires and half-pins near the knee [17]. Hutson et al. [11] reported an incidence of 2%. In the anterior plateau, a distance of 10–14 mm below the joint is considered safe [17]. In our experience, the capsule is usually disrupted in the presence of complex plateau fractures so that arbitrary distances from the joint line for insertion points for wires are probably a moot point. Nonetheless, it seems prudent to maximize distances from the joint line without compromising wire purchase in the proximal segment. The key is to recognize knee sepsis early and to treat it adequately with arthrotomy and intravenous antibiotics.

Fracture malunion is more common with external fixation in our experience (unpublished data) when we compared it to locked plating of Schatzker 5 and 6 tibial plateau fractures. However, this increased incidence may not be related to the fixation because formal open reduction was performed more commonly when plating than when using fine-wire fixation.

Loss of knee motion after tibial plateau fracture is common and results from extensor mechanism scarring, arthrofibrosis, and posttraumatic arthrosis. Extensor mechanism scarring is associated with prolonged across-the-knee fixation. Knee sparring fixators have lesser problems regaining a good range of motion. One study showed superior total arc of motion after treatment with an external faxator compared with open reduction and internal fixation [18]. The goal is 90° of knee flexion at 4 weeks after surgery. Patients with less than 90° of flexion at 4 weeks should have an accelerated rehabilitation program for range of motion. Quadriceps weakness is often associated with half-pin insertion through the quadriceps muscle and appears to be associated with subsequent muscle weakness and atrophy.

Honoken SE et al. [15] found the incidence of posttraumatic arthrosis after tibial plateau fracture was 44% at 7.6-yr follow-up. Numerous investigators have shown that articular incongruity and joint instability are the two main causes for posttraumatic arthrosis. Although anatomical reduction may have been achieved, significant joint arthrosis may result nonetheless as a result of the initial articular cartilage damage.

8.7 Discussion

External fixators have a definite role in treatment of tibial plateau fractures, especially Schatzker type 5 and type 6 fractures with soft tissue injury. Fixators can also be used as a temporary measure prior to staged open reduction and internal fixation. Alternatively, fine-wire fixation can be used as a definitive osteosynthesis when the combined soft tissue and bony injury make a plating procedure too risky. Locked plating is neither atraumatic, even with minimally invasive approaches, nor complication free. An infection rate of 22% with locked plating of proximal tibial fractures was recently reported [1].

The main advantages of using external fixation around the knee include the flexibility and increased options of treatment. Temporary spanning fixation allows the reestablishment of limb alignment, soft tissue healing, and optimization of soft tissue conditions for future staged locked plating. External fixators provide the opportunity and flexibility for the surgeon to modulate the biomechanical stiffness of the faxator to match the fracture while decreasing the likelihood of catastrophic complications such as deep sepsis and osteomyelitis.

When a definitive fine-wire faxator is selected, symmetrical frames with rings on both the sides of the fracture have the best biomechanical stability. Fine wires have a lower incidence of pin tract infection than half-pins. Variables that are under the surgeon's control include customizing the frame construct with regard to wire orientation, wire number, wire tension, and frame symmetry and adding a second ring (level of fixation). Temporary or definitive external fixation remains a powerful option for the treatment of tibial plateau fractures.

References

1. Phisitkul P, McKinley TO, Nepola JV, Marsh JL. Complications of locking plate fixation in complex proximal tibia injuries. J Orthop Trauma. 2007;21(2):83–91.
2. Mahan J, Seligson D, Henry SL, Hynes P, Dobbins J. Factors in pin tract infections. Orthopedics. 1991;14(3):305–8.
3. Roberts CS, Antoci V, Antoci Jr V, Voor MJ. The effect of transfixion wire crossing angle on the stiffness of fine wire external fixation: a biomechanical study. Injury. 2005;36(9):1107–12.
4. Antoci V, Raney EM, Antoci Jr V, Voor MJ, Roberts CS. Transfixion wire positioning within the bone: an option to control proximal tibia external fixation stiffness. J Pediatr Orthop. 2006;26(4):466–70.
5. Pugh KJ, Wolinsky PR, Dawson JM, Stahlman GC. The biomechanics of hybrid external fixation. J Orthop Trauma. 1999;13(1):20–6.

6. Cory Collinge MD, Jason Kennedy MD, Andrew Schmidt MD. Temporizing external fixation of the lower extremity: a survey of the orthopaedic trauma association membership. Orthopaedics. 2010;33(4):239.
7. Watson JR, Coufal C. Treatment of complex lateral plateau fractures usig Ilizarov techniques. Clin Orthop Rel Res. 1998;353:97–106.
8. Haidukewych GJ. Temporary external fixation for the management of complex intra- and periarticular fractures of the lower extremity. J Orthop Trauma. 2002;16(9):678–85.
9. Anglen JO, Aleto T. Temporary transarticular external fixation of the knee and ankle. J Orthop Trauma. 1998;12(6):431–4.
10. DeCoster TA, Crawford MK, Kraut MA. Safe extracapsular placement of proximal tibia transfixation pins. J Orthop Trauma. 1999;13(4):236–40.
11. Krupp RJ, Malkani AL, Roberts CS, Seligson D. Treatment of bicondylar tibia plateau fractures using locked plating versus external fixation. Orthopaedics. 2009;32(8):559.
12. Antoci V, Roberts CS, Antoci Jr V, Voor MJ. The effect of transfixion wire number and spacing between two levels of fixation on the stiffness of proximal tibial external fixation. J Orthop Trauma. 2005;19(3):180–6.
13. Hutson Jr JJ, Zych GA. Infections in periarticular fractures of the lower extremity treated with tensioned wire hybrid fixators. J Orthop Trauma. 1998;12(3):214–8.
14. Parameswaran AD, Roberts CS, Seligson D, Voor M. Pin tract infection with contemporary external fixation: how much of a problem? J Orthop Trauma. 2003;17(7):503–7.
15. Checketts RG, MacEachern AG, Otterburn M. Pin tract infection and the principles of pin site care. In: De Bastiani G, Apley AG, Goldberg A, editors. Orthofix external fixation in trauma and orthopaedics. London: Springer; 2000. p. 97–103.
16. Green SA, Ripley MJ. Chronic osteomyelitis in pin tracks. J Bone Joint Surg Am. 1984;66(7):1092–8.
17. Stevens MA, DeCoster TA, Barcia F, Sell JJ. Septic knee from Ilizarov transfixation tibial pin. Iowa Orthop J. 1995;15:217–20.
18. Canadian Orthopaedic Trauma Society. Open reduction and internal fixation compared with circular faxator application for bicondylar tibial plateau fractures. Results of a multicenter, prospective, randomized clinical trial. J Bone Joint Surg. 2006;88(12):2613–23.

Chapter 9
The Use of External Fixators in the Acute Management of Tibial Pilon Fractures

Cyril Mauffrey, David Seligson, and Jessica Heinsen

9.1 Background

A pilon fracture is a fracture into the articular surface of the distal tibia. The complexity of this injury and problem in its treatment are detailed in a fascinating monograph by the French radiologist Chaput. His name is memorialized in the eponym "Chaput's tubercle" for the important anterolateral corner of the distal tibia, which contains the origin of the anteroinferior tibiofibular ligament – the cinch for the tibiofibular syndesmosis [1]. Reassembly of the distal articular surface is detailed in Lambotte's books on fracture fixation [2]. It was, however, not until the Swiss Fracture group began their historic systematic approach to the operative treatment of fractures that the "pilon fracture" was categorized and regularly repaired surgically.

Pilon fractures come in three important varieties. There is the Pilon fracture due to rotational forces around the ankle that is a more severe type of ankle malleolar fracture [3]. These are the supination external rotation and pronation external rotation fractures with large articular fragments. Usually, the posterior malleolar piece is a substantial chunk of bone. More than a third of the articular surface is involved. These fractures were characterized by Lauge-Hansen and have been a normal and successful part of operative fracture care since their inception.

Lauge-Hansen recognized the injury to the ankle of axial loading with concomitant compression of the distal tibial metaphysis and added the type "pronation dorsiflexion" to his classification scheme for ankle injury. The importance of articular surface damage and compression was systemically explored by Ruedi and Allgower, who developed both a classification and a treatment program for the injury [4]. The teaching was to plate the fibula, restore the articular surface, graft the void left by compression, and plate the tibia to defend the axis of the tibia. Pilon fractures caused

C. Mauffrey (✉) • D. Seligson, • J. Heinsen
Department of Orthopaedics, University Hospital Louisville, Louisville, KY, USA
e-mail: cmauffrey@yahoo.com

D. Seligson et al. (eds.), *External Fixation in Orthopedic Traumatology*,
DOI 10.1007/978-1-4471-2197-8_9, © Springer-Verlag London Limited 2012

by low-energy axial loading in healthy individuals have good outcomes with this form of treatment. As North American orthopedists attempted to apply this program to high-speed injuries, the results were less successful. The dictum was to operate early because immediate motion of the ankle joint was considered important for a good result. With high-speed injuries, the results were not predictably good. The circulation to the soft tissues of the subcutaneous bones of the ankle joint is precarious. Tissue necrosis, infection, and osteonecrosis followed fracture treatment too often [5]. After all, the treatment for Pott's fractures in the nineteenth century was amputation, and they still shoot horses for acral fractures of the legs. To complete the picture, there is a variety of Pilon fracture that is an extension of a fracture of the distal tibial shaft into the ankle joint. These are often rotational injuries with and without disruption of the syndesmosis. The treatment of these "Spiral Extension" fractures can be nonoperative, particularly if the articular surface displacement is minimal. The spiral extension fracture is the third variety of pilon fracture.

Poor results in the operative treatment of pilon fractures led to the popularization of external fixation as an alternative treatment approach for this injury. Indeed, when the fracture is not too severe, an equally good outcome can be expected from either formal osteosynthesis with plates and screws, or external fixation, or external fixation combined with limited internal fixation. The real dilemma with the fixator is not so much of infection or skin necrosis, but recurrence of deformity and atrophy of bone, particularly if the fixator is left for an extended period [6]. The short-term use of external fixation decreases the incidence of immobilization osteoporosis and joint stiffness, but increases the likelihood of recurrent deformity. Therefore, neither immediate internal fixation nor cautious mobilization in a fixator provides predictable, good outcomes for this important injury to the ankle.

In this background, damage control techniques with immediate external fixation and delayed internal fixation appear to offer an excellent solution for the management of pilon fractures and seem to reduce the difficulties associated with their care, particularly when the injury occurs in a polytraumatized patient or is the result of high energy.

9.2 Initial Treatment: External Fixation

One can treat nearly every fracture of the distal tibial pilon, ankle, and/or hindfoot in a splint. However, there are important reasons not to do this. These reasons to not begin the care of a pilon fracture with splinting include:

1. The position in the splint may not be correct. Problems with splinting lead to deformities that are hard to overcome at the time of definitive surgery. Additional procedures such as an Achilles' tenotomy may be required.
2. Local complications caused by the fracture are hard to evaluate and manage in plaster. For example, a compartment syndrome may develop. It is hard to see developing fracture blisters. Skin necrosis may not be evident.
3. New complications can occur in casts. The worst of these may be pressure ulceration of the heel. A heel ulcer can cause greater morbidity than the fracture problem that is being treated.

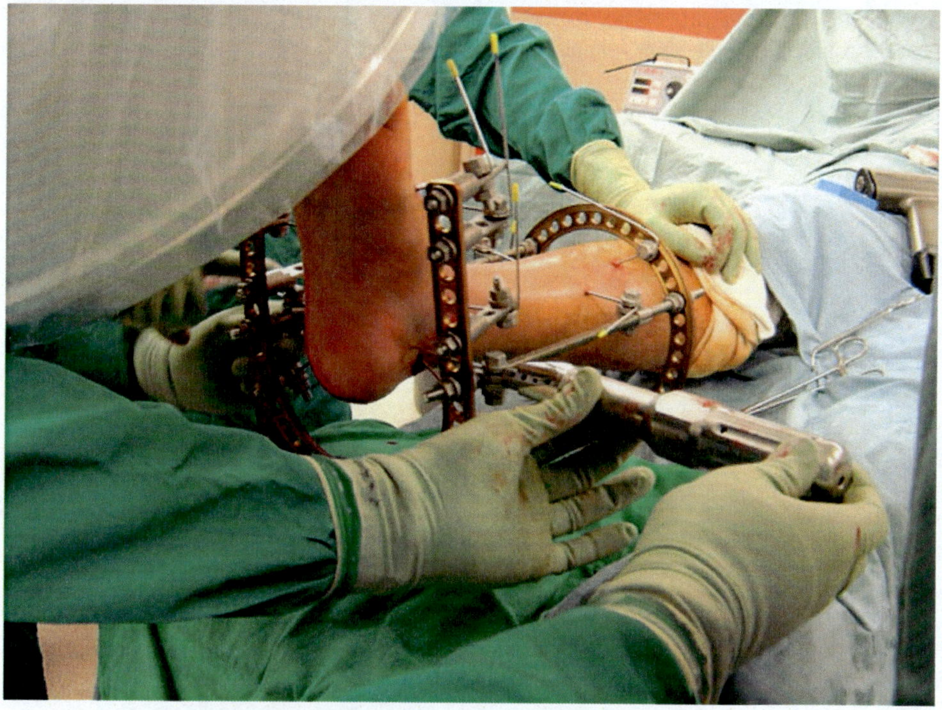

Fig. 9.1 Application of a fine wire frame to a closed high-energy pilon fracture

4. A plaster splint is a removable appliance. Anyone who so chooses can take it off. An unsplinted leg is a leg that needs to be resplinted. This can be not only hard to do but also inconvenient.
5. If the general condition of the patient is precarious, there may be considerable delay before an operative procedure is performed. The first chance may be the only chance for some days.
6. When the limb is placed in external fixation, the limb is placed in traction. This traction can lead to important information on subsequent X-ray and/or CT scan. This information helps in precision planning of definitive treatment for the fracture.

The frame types (montages) for treatment of a pilon fracture are intrafocal frames, half-pin frames, ring frames with either small wires or half-pins, and combinations of half-pin and ring frames. Choose a frame based on fracture type, soft tissue problems, and patient profile.

Use of an intrafocal frame is acceptable for a fracture of the distal tibial metaphysis, which does not have significant articular surface involvement. It can either be a large pin frame with a pin group in the tibia shaft connected to a pin group in the distal tibia just proximal to the ankle joint, or it can be a ring frame proximal and distal (Fig. 9.1). Sometimes, it is possible to use two opposing olive wires to maintain the articular surface congruence of a fracture which, though it enters the ankle joint, is not significantly displaced or can be reduced and held together by olive wires.

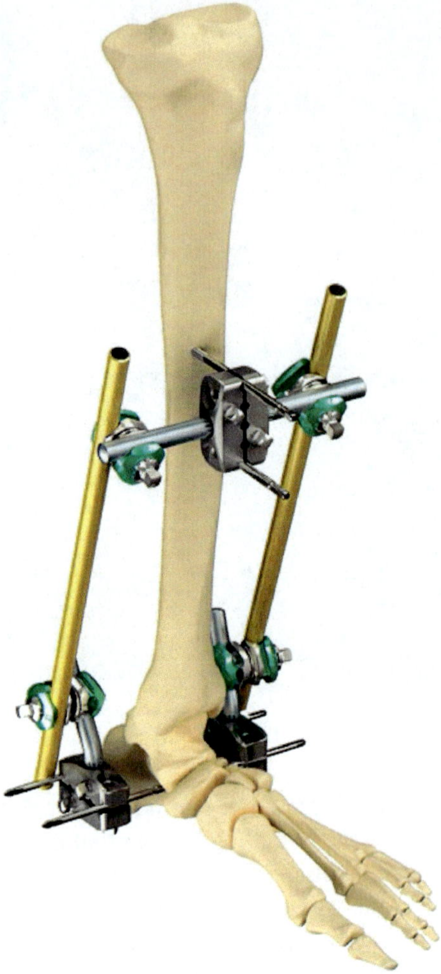

Fig. 9.2 External fixator Hoffmann type III spanning the ankle joint with half-pins in the tibia and the calcaneus

The simple large pin frame, based on a half-pin group in the tibia, connects to a pin(s) in the calcaneus. There are many variations of this simple frame (Fig. 9.2). Hoffmann used a pin group in the tibia connected to a pin group in the calcaneus. These pin groups were connected by a single connecting rod. The pin group and connection rod can either be medial or lateral. Alternatively, the tibia pin group is connected medially and laterally to a transfixion pin in the calcaneus. This triangular montage gives good control of varus and valgus position of the foot (Fig. 9.3). Addition of a pin in the forefoot or midfoot will control dorsiflexion and plantar flexion of the ankle in the simple frame (Figs. 9.4–9.6). The advantage of simple frames is that their construction can be varied to allow for soft tissue reconstructive procedures. The simple lateral frame gives good access to the medial side of the ankle and vice versa. The disadvantage of simple frames is that they do not suspend the heel and cannot protect against a pressure sore in the unconscious patient.

Ring frames are best for complex pilon fractures in severely injured patients. The footplate suspends the heel in the frame, which protects the heel from pressure

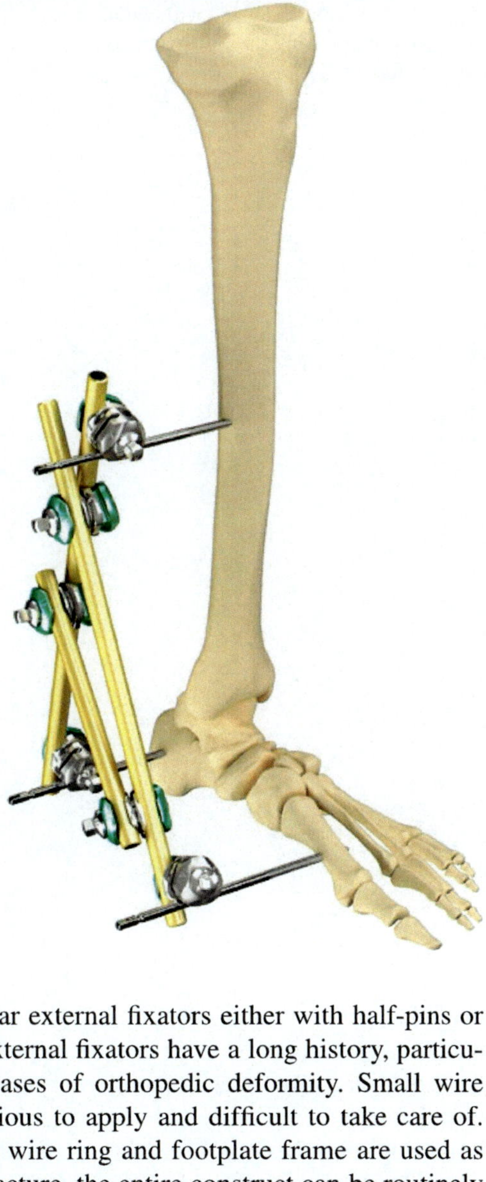

Fig. 9.3 Triangular montage using the Hoffmann III external fixator

sores. The surgeon can construct circular external fixators either with half-pins or with small wires. Small wire circular external fixators have a long history, particularly for complex reconstructions in cases of orthopedic deformity. Small wire frames have a reputation for being tedious to apply and difficult to take care of. Actually, when a straightforward small wire ring and footplate frame are used as damage control treatment for a pilon fracture, the entire construct can be routinely placed in less than an hour. To apply a damage control ring frame, it is useful to think of the frame placement in two phases.

9.2.1 Phase 1: Traction

Place one wire in the tibia perpendicular to the long axis of the bone. Tension the wire in a ring. The tibia should lie in the anterior one-third of the ring. Moderate tension (50Kgf) is enough (Fig. 9.7). The second wire is an olive wire passed through

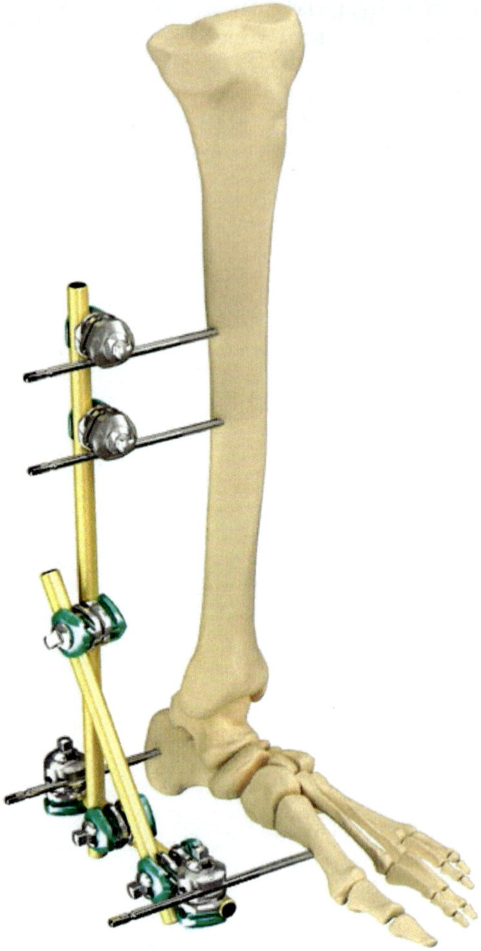

Fig. 9.4 Triangular montage with addition of a forefoot pin using the Hoffmann II external fixator

the calcaneus from anteromedial just posterior to the posterior tibial neurovascular bundle to posterolateral. This olive is tapped in place so it is on the medial cortex of the calcaneus. Then, fasten the olive to the footplate on the medial side. Now, the olive is lightly tensioned and fixed to the ring laterally. The next step is to line up the tibial ring with the footplate using connection bars. Now, place the foot in traction and tighten the connection bars (usually 3).

9.2.2 Phase 2: Frame Stabilization

In this phase, a second wire is added to the ring. This wire locks the ring so it cannot tip in the transverse plane. Placing the wire on drop posts so that it is not in the plane

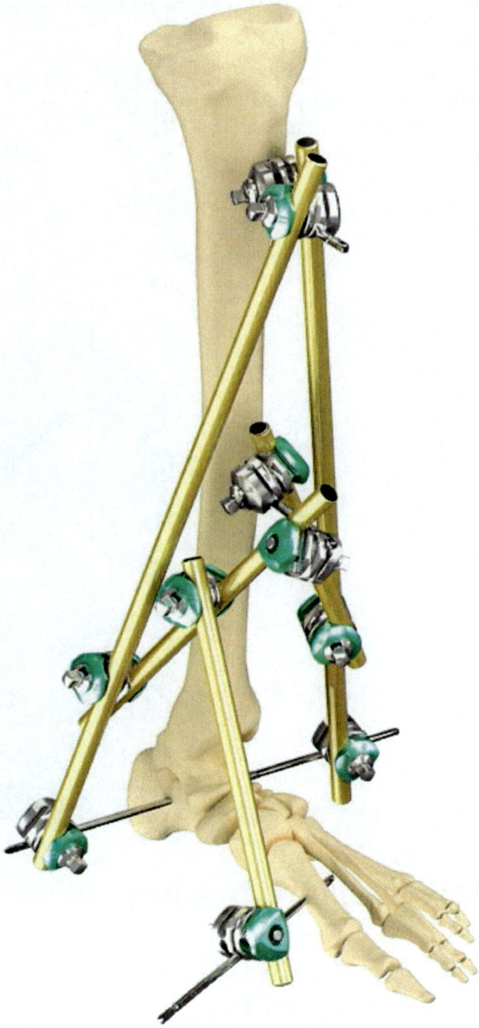

Fig. 9.5 Triangular montage for pilon fracture with frame mounted on both the medial and lateral side of the ankle using the Hoffmann III system

of the ring increases stability. Finally, crossing transverse wires are placed across the midfoot or forefoot and a second olive wire is driven from lateral to posteromedial across the calcaneus [7, 8]. This completes the simple 2-ring damage control frame.

Alternatively, a damage control frame utilizes half-pins instead of fine wires. Two half-pins hold the ring to the tibia and two pins stabilize the calcaneus. There are several options for holding the pins to the ring. Another possibility is a combination of pins and fine wires. In the calcaneus, drive the half-pins from medial and lateral angled toward the toes to suspend the heel and improve the anchorage.

Postoperatively, the patient needs a pin care program, additional X-rays or a CT scan, and local wound care. An antibiotic is given. If necessary, the patient gets thromboembolism prophylaxis.

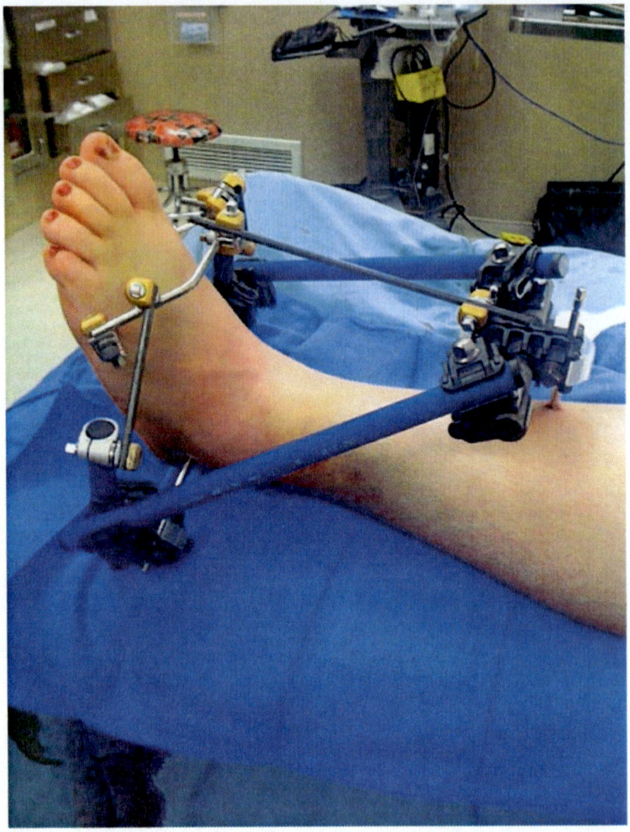

Fig. 9.6 External fixator (Hoffmann Express) for closed high-energy pilon fracture using half-pins in the tibia, calcaneus, first and fourth metatarsal

9.3 Definitive Treatment: Nails and Plates

External skeletal fixation is not a satisfactory method for the definitive treatment of pilon fractures. The frame must be non-weight-bearing. Pin breakage or pin bending is inevitable with fixation across the ankle. Perhaps this problem will be solved in the future; for the moment, it is not. Extended non-weight-bearing leads to osteopenia, stiff joints, and pain on walking; recovery is difficult. Shortening the time in the frame helps. However, the shorter the duration of external fixation, the more likely will be the recurrence of deformity.

Brief periods of skeletal fixation – a few weeks for example – do not cause significant morbidity. In the intermediate term, there is an annoying emergence of minor problems such as pin track drainage, pain, and loss of fixation. In the long-term, nearly all patients are dissatisfied with life in the external fixator.

The few weeks between the application of a damage control frame across the ankle and definite treatment are crucial. Care of the patient in the fixator is presented in Chap. 12. Meet with the patient between the application of the frame and definitive surgery. Assure that the condition of the pins and the skin of the foot are acceptable. Obtain further diagnostic studies to help with preoperative planning. Think over the alternatives and develop a step-by-step program for the procedure.

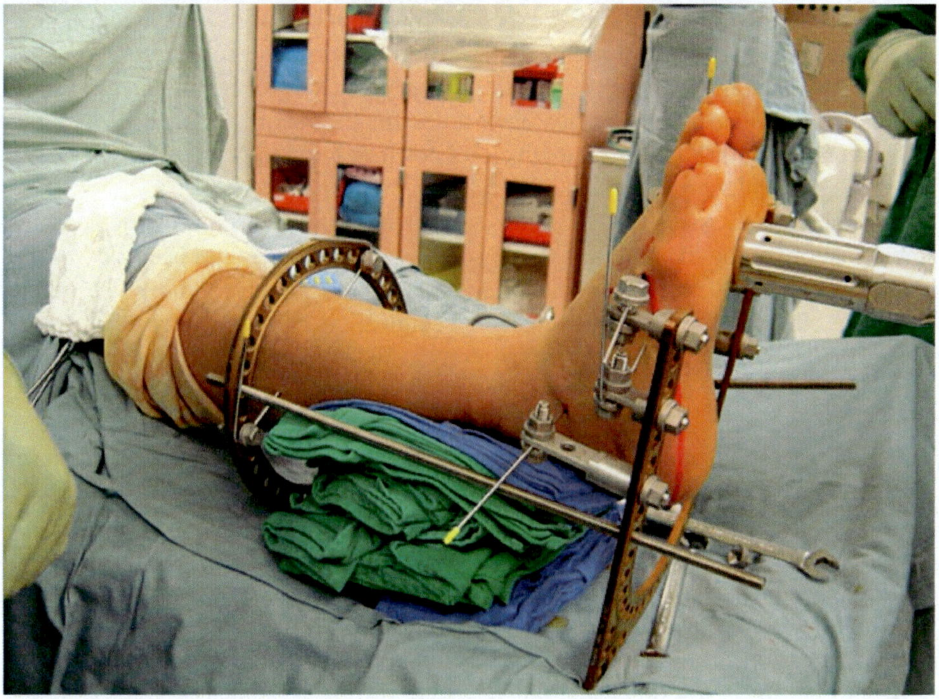

Fig. 9.7 Application of fine wire frame (LIMA frame)

Interlocking plating and tibial nailing are the two alternatives for definitive treatment of the pilon fracture after a damage control frame. Generally, frame removal and nailing or plating are done in a one-step procedure. It is usually not necessary to remove the frame and allow weeks to pass before the fracture is treated.

The plan for *plating* requires two important decisions. First, decide whether plate fixation of the fibula will assist the reduction; second, decide whether to use a medial or anterolateral plate. Modern locking plates have revolutionized the definitive treatment of tibial pilon fractures. With conventional plates, the axial length of the tibia is maintained with structural bone grafts. With locking plates, the need for bone grafts is less critical. The locking screws secure the osteosynthesis so that deformity is much less likely to recur. The transverse cuts of the CT scan or 3D CT reconstruction are useful in deciding where to place the implants. If the anteromedial border of the tibia is relatively intact, use the anterolateral plate. If the posterior wall of the tibia is intact with a good Volkmann's triangle, then the anterior plate works better. Reconstruct the articular surface with K-wires and then stabilize the tibia with an angle-stable locking plate. Finally, decide if syndesmosis screws should be placed to maintain the relationship between the fibula and tibia at the distal tibiofibular joint.

To conduct the procedure deliberately, prepare a drawing of the plan for the procedure. Not all of the details of the operation may work out, but the plan is useful in getting the fracture problem clearly in one's mind.

The operative procedure takes place under either regional or general anesthesia. The OR needs a good list of the equipment for the operation. Be certain that the surgical sets are complete and the power equipment works. Use a tourniquet. A bloodless field is helpful for an accurate articular surface reconstruction. Do the case under image intensification. The fluoroscopy helps to locate the plates exactly the first time. Most locking plates have holes for provisional K-wires. Place the plate, secure it with K-wires, and check its position with an X-ray. The lay of the plate in the lateral view is critical.

It is important to assess the syndesmosis. An intertibiofibular screw can add considerable stability to the fixation. It is usually necessary when there has been a complete rupture of the syndesmosis in the original injury. Generally, remove the screw 8–10 weeks later. This requires an additional surgical intervention. Unfortunately, the plastic, biodegradable screws that are currently available do not have enough strength to resist sheer forces and may break too soon. Another consideration is bone grafting to fill voids and assure fracture healing. The "gold standard" is autogenous cancellous bone for osteoinduction and corticocancellous autografts for structural support. Alternatives include a variety of synthetic and natural materials. These substances are not satisfactory for a variety of reasons. They lack compressive strength, do not reliably provoke fracture repair, are hard to handle, are costly, or simply do not have enough evidence to support the costs associated with their use. The morbidity of autogenous bone grafting has been overemphasized. Particularly, the proximal tibial metaphysis is a relatively easy place to get adequate bone graft with minimal morbidity [9, 10].

Tibial nailing is the other alternative strategy from a damage control external fixator to definitive osteosynthesis. A tibial nail should be considered when the articular surface is relatively intact and there is not significant compression in the pilon [11]. The fractures most amenable to external fixation are pilon fractures with large malleolar fragments and spiral extension fractures. Indeed, after two or three weeks of external fixation, there has been considerable healing in the distal tibia because of its good blood supply. The healing indicates that it is unlikely the fracture will displace with the introduction of a medullary nail. Additional screws placed through or around the nail can improve the fixation of the pilon. These screws are useful to either provide fixation for definite fracture fragments such as a fracture of the medial malleolus or give transmedullary support to guide the passage of the nail and maintain angular relationships of the short distal fragment. A nail usually provides enough stability that bone grafting is unnecessary. Retrograde tibial nailing from the calcaneus across the posterior subtalar joint and the ankle joint is usually a salvage strategy for failed osteosynthesis of the tibial pilon. The retrograde nail is also a useful strategy for high-risk patients where ankle joint and subtalar motion can be sacrificed for a reasonable functional result with low morbidity.

9.4 Recovery

After surgery, treat the patient in a posterior padded plaster splint with a heel cup. Close the wound with a few subcutaneous Vicryl sutures and simple sutures of 000 nylon. Dress questionable areas with an antibacterial gauze. The initial treatment is non-weight-bearing status for the patient. Change the dressings at 1 week. Skin sutures are removed 2–3 weeks postoperatively. Important priorities are to maintain the plantar grade position of the foot and have sufficient compression over the wound so that blood and serum do not collect under the edges of the incision and cause skin necrosis. Start ankle motion after the sutures are removed. For the first 6 months, the patient should be in a PTB brace. The brace cannot be fitted while the leg is still swollen because the brace will be too loose to protect the fixation during the first few critical weeks of weight-bearing. Off-the-shelf "walkers" – CAM or ROM – boots are not satisfactory because they do not control the position of the foot.

Application of a soft casting material with a reinforcing splint occurs once the wound is stable (soft cast – 3 M). This cast can be used for partial weight-bearing while the patient is waiting for a more permanent brace. The fixed ankle PTB brace with an extra-depth rocker-bottom shoe encourages weight-bearing and is more secure than a brace with a mobile ankle. The patient is encouraged to work on motion out of the brace and walk in the brace.

A syndesmosis screw placed in surgery limits weight-bearing until screw removal. A metal screw across the syndesmosis may or may not break. The broken screw in an accident case can become significant to the patient. These screws do not break with a few weeks of eggshell weight-bearing prior to their removal in day surgery. Therefore, the progression is from a plaster splint to soft cast. Sutures are usually removed by week 3. Next are brace fitting, eggshell weight-bearing, and finally, syndesmosis screw removal and full weight-bearing status in the PTB brace by 10–12 weeks. Follow the patient with X-rays at 2–3 week intervals. Since the healing of an acral fracture takes longer to observe with X-rays, take films to assure that the alignment of the talus in the mortise is correct and that the fixation devices are in the proper places. The X-rays are not taken to judge fracture healing. The X-rays are taken to judge position.

9.5 Conclusion

Pilon fractures are complicated injuries. Outcomes are the results not only of the care in treatment but also of the force delivered to the limb at the time of injury. Current technology does not take into consideration the health of cartilage cells in the ankle joint or the vitality of the subchondral plate. Collapse of the joint and arthrosis may be predestined.

There is some evidence that with very long-term follow-up (more than 5 or 10 years), results improve. It takes good judgment to determine which cases require additional procedures and when these procedures should be performed. What should the orthopedist do if a patient has pain, swelling, cannot walk, and may not be able to earn a living? The first option is always to improve footwear, try unloading the ankle, give anti-inflammatory medicines and elastic support, and then see if results do not improve. Secondary procedures include ankle fusion, tibiotalar arthrodesis, corrective osteotomy, or fusion of the syndesmosis.

Patients with complex regional pain syndromes (causalgias) are more manageable in a pain care setting. Most infections can be suppressed with oral antibiotic therapy, debridement, and intermittent or long-term use of antibiotic impregnated implants (PMMA bead chains). The treatment of recalcitrant infection is amputation.

Volgas [12] looked at the effect of a pilon fracture in a cohort of 22 patients. He assessed the patients' ability to cope in work and financially (in a US setting). All three white-collar workers returned to work at 1 year, but only 3 of 21 blue-collar workers did so. Five out of 8 college graduates returned to work compared with 2 of 14 nongraduates. Forty two percent of patients used social assistance and 37% had to sell possessions to meet financial obligations.

References

1. Chaput HV. Les fractures malléolaires du cou-de-pied et les accidents du travail. Paris, 1907.
2. Lambotte A. Chirurgie opératoire des fractures. Paris: Masson & Cie Éditeurs; 1913.
3. Muale G, Seligson D. Fractures through the distal weight-bearing surface of the tibia. Orthopedics. 1980;3:517–21.
4. Ruedi TP, Allgower M. Fractures of the lower end of the tibia into the ankle joint. Injury. 1969;1(2):92–9.
5. Smith W. Letters to the editor. Re: surgical options for the treatment of severe tibial pilon fractures: a story of three techniques. J Orthop Trauma. 2001;15(8):591.
6. Blauth M, Bastian L, Krettek C, Knop C, Evans S. Surgical options for the treatment of severe tibial pilon fractures: a study of three techniques. J Orthop Trauma. 2001;15(3):153–60.
7. Mauffrey C, Klutts P, Seligson D. Surgical techniques: how I do it? Mini open reduction and fixation of calcaneal fractures with fine wire circular frames. Eur J Orthop Surg Traumatol. 2010. doi:10.1007/s00590-010-0678-5.
8. Mauffrey C, Klutts P, Seligson D. The use of circular fine wire frames for the treatment of displaced intra-articular calcaneal fractures. J Orthop Traumatol. 2009;10(1):9–15.
9. Alt V, Nawab A, Seligson D. Bone grafting from the proximal tibia. J Trauma Injury Infect Crit Care. 1999;47(3):555–7.
10. Mauffrey CP, Seligson D, Krikler S. Surgical techniques: how I do it? Bone graft harvest from the proximal lateral tibia. Injury. 2010;41(2):242–4.
11. Newman SDS, Mauffrey CPC, Krikler S. Distal metadiaphyseal tibial fractures. Injury. 2010;41(7):693–702.
12. David Volgas J, DeVries G, Stannard JP. Short-term financial outcomes of pilon fractures. J Foot Ankle Surg. 2010;49(1):47–51.

Chapter 10
External Fixation of Long Bones

Dennis Beck and Charles Daniel Benson

10.1 Introduction

In polytrauma patients, the temporary stabilization of long bone fractures is critical to the effective sequencing of all of the patient's injuries. When faced with intrathoracic, abdominal, and other life-threatening pathology, temporarily controlling the movement of long bone fractures with external fixation facilitates the patient's mobility for other procedures, reduces blood loss, controls pain, and decreases the incidence of fat embolism syndrome. Moreover, temporary external fixation can be done quickly and by non-traumatologists at referring hospitals, thus enabling more-organized and efficient transfer in compliance with U.S. federal patient transfer regulations. Damage control treatment of femur fractures is not indicated for every patient with this injury. Pape et al. [1] have shown that subdivision of patients into injury severity groups and selective application of DCO vs. early fracture treatment can maximize the benefits outlined below.

10.2 Femur

Temporary external fixation of the femur reduces blood loss, reduces the incidence of fat embolism syndrome, controls pain, and enables more-efficient patient transfers and transport [2]. External fixation of the femur is almost never used as a final treatment option in adults, so time and expense can be reduced by employing simple techniques to stabilize this bone.

D. Beck (✉)
Orthopaedics Associates, Evansville, IN, USA
e-mail: indianatrauma@yahoo.com

C.D. Benson
Department of Orthopedic Surgery, Resident in Orthopedic Surgery,
University of Kansas Medical Center, 3901 Rainbow Boulevard, Kansas City, Kansas, USA
e-mail: cdanbenson@aol.com

D. Seligson et al. (eds.), *External Fixation in Orthopedic Traumatology*,
DOI 10.1007/978-1-4471-2197-8_10, © Springer-Verlag London Limited 2012

10.2.1 Bleeding

About 1–2 units of blood can be lost into the quadriceps and hamstring compartment with a simple midshaft femur fracture [3]. About 1 cm of increase in the radius of the compartment roughly equates to 1 unit of bleeding into the muscle. This blood loss occurs from not only the initial trauma, but also the soft tissue damage from the fractured femur ends tearing the compartment. Bleeding caused by femur fracture is accentuated by destruction of the high-pressure artery system of the thigh. By reducing fracture site motion and restoring adequate anatomical alignment, bleeding can be reduced, or even eliminated, and arterial tamponade created. In a recent retrospective review [4], two cohorts (462 patients with 481 femoral shafts) were identified to compare multiple-injured patients with femoral shaft fractures treated with early total care and damage control orthopedic surgery. Primary outcome measures included mortality, pulmonary complications (adult respiratory distress syndrome [ARDS] score), transfusion requirements, and multiple organ failure (MOF score). Operative time, estimated blood loss, intensive care unit length of stay (LOS), and hospital length of stay (LOS) were also compared. Fracture fixation method did not have an impact on the incidence of systemic complications, and DCO was noted to be a safer initial approach, significantly decreasing the initial operative exposure and blood loss.

10.2.2 Pain Control

There are no adequate noninvasive methods to control femur fragment motion during transportation of a patient. Currently, prehospital services use some version of a Thomas splint, Hare traction, or even manual traction during transport. The pain experienced by the conscious patient, or even the autonomic stimulus from fracture site motion in the severely injured patient, can aggravate the overall physiological response to the injury, thus making airway, breathing, and circulation more difficult to maintain. While nonoperating room application of external fixators for the femur is not advocated, a short, safe, minimally invasive operation to apply a simple frame can significantly reduce pain and facilitate patient management in the trauma victim.

10.2.3 Fat Embolism Syndrome

The fat embolism syndrome is accepted as a major contributing factor to patient morbidity and mortality after long bone fractures, especially in the femur [5]. The pathology arises from the release of a bolus of fatty bone marrow from the post-injury patent intramedullary canal into the general circulation. The fat tissue and marrow circulates into the right heart and impedes the proper oxygenation of venous blood in the lungs, thereby causing increased patient oxygen requirements, positive end expiratory pressure, and tidal volumes on the ventilator and making management more difficult.

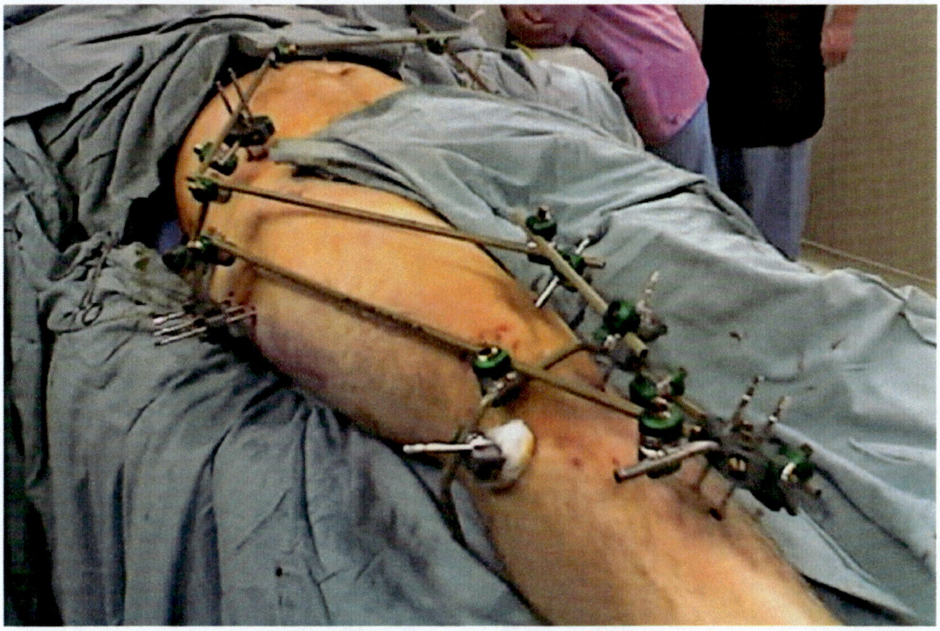

Fig. 10.1 A bridging external fixator for an open-book pelvic injury associated with ipsilateral femoral shaft and proximal tibia fractures

Wolinsky [6] visualized these fat globules on experimental dogs using transesophageal ultrasonography. Restoring adequate, not necessarily anatomic, alignment and reducing fracture site motion by fixing femur fracture fragments can reduce this unwelcome complication. Fat embolism syndrome causes increased length of stay in the intensive care unit, increased incidence of multisystem organ failure, and increased duration of mechanical ventilator dependence [7]. At our institution, arterial blood gases while breathing room air are routinely obtained before making any decision as to early fracture treatment (IM nailing) vs. DCO (external fixation). Patients with diminished pO_2 levels on room air after initial stabilization proceed into a DCO protocol, and temporizing external fixation is used until there is recovery from the initial hit phenomenon.

10.2.4 Femur Montages

External fixation of the femur should remain simple as with all effective orthopedic surgical techniques. Multiplanar fixation should be used employing the biomechanical knowledge basic for all orthopedic surgeons and referenced elsewhere in this text. At least two half-pins on either side of the fracture site are needed, with external fixation bars close to the skin (at least a fingerbreadth away) and pins close to and far from the fracture site (Fig. 10.1). Multiplanar fixation can be achieved by placing one pin out of the plane of the fixator on either side of the fracture site to significantly improve stability [8]. Pins in the femur should be placed strictly laterally in the proximal half of the bone; should a pin be required medially, place it as perpendicular to the floor as possible (Fig. 10.2). Additionally,

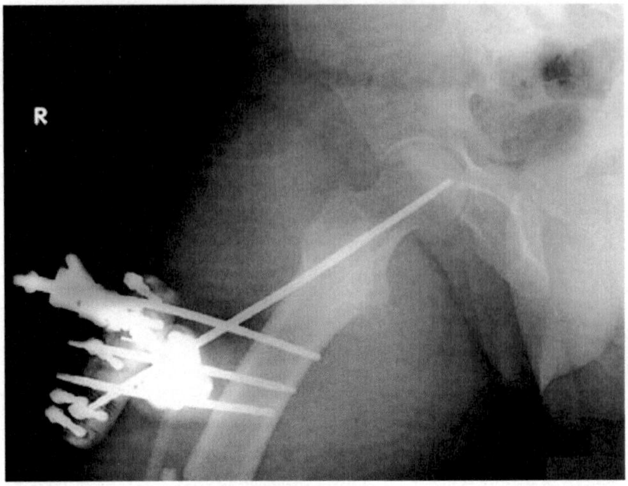

Fig. 10.2 External fixator for an open femoral shaft fracture using a half-pin in the femoral neck

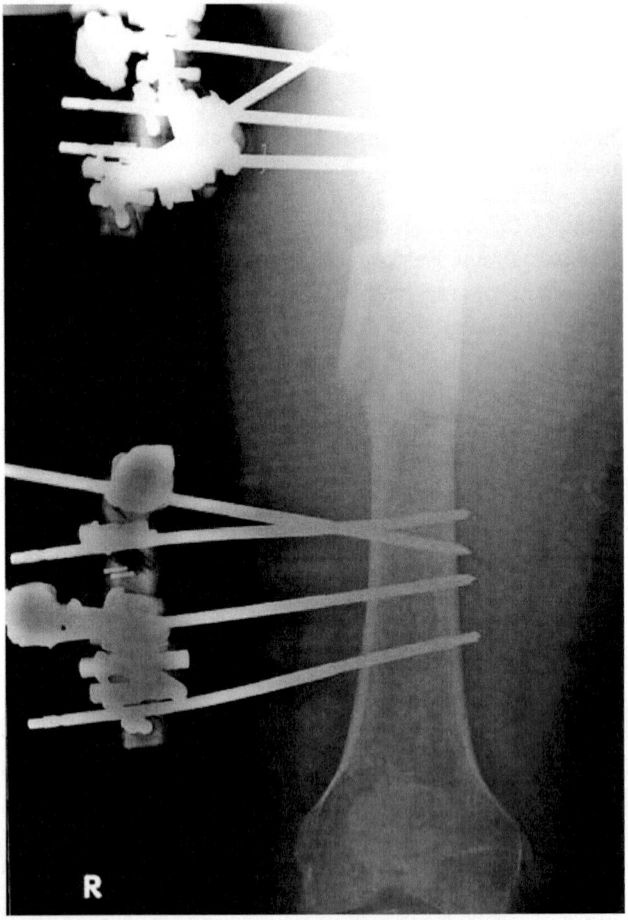

Fig. 10.3 External fixation for a femoral shaft fracture; note the pins pointing away from the fracture

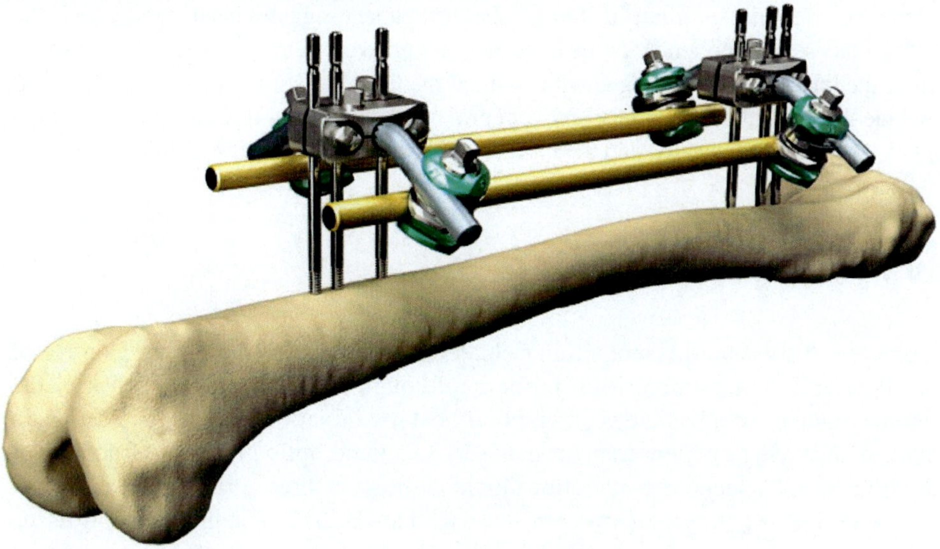

Fig. 10.4 Anterior frame for midshaft femoral fracture with pins placed in the anterior to posterior direction and 2 bars, one medial and one lateral using the Hoffmann III system

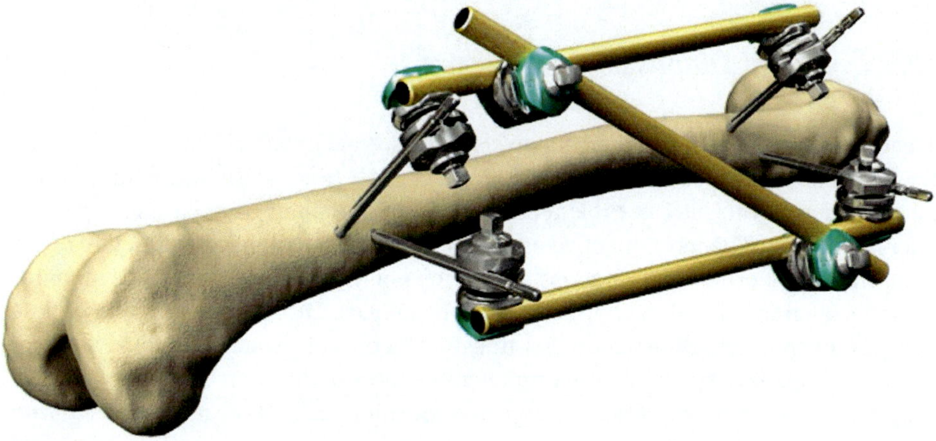

Fig. 10.5 Lateral femoral frame for a femoral midshaft fracture using the Hoffmann III system

after application of an external fixator to any part of the femur, the knee, if possible, should be manipulated to its full range of motion. This releases the fascial planes of the quadriceps, which probably reduces the incidence of post-injury arthrofibrosis of the knee. Proximal femur fractures can be fixed with at least two pins into the femoral neck, which are placed identically to screws for femoral neck fractures (Fig. 10.3). By using the femoral neck, with adequate image intensification, almost any level of diaphyseal fracture can be fixed externally. Midshaft fractures are fixed with simple lateral frames or anterior frames and pins placed in areas of intact bone (Figs. 10.3–10.5). Distal femur fractures should be fixed like midshaft fractures if the distal intact segment is large enough. If the distal intact segment is small, or the fracture is assumed or seen to be intra-articular to the knee, the knee should be bridged with external fixation. Structures at risk near the femur include the femoral nerve, artery and vein proximally, the distal branches of the femoral artery medially and distally, and the intra-articular section of the knee distally.

10.3 Tibia

Fractures of the tibia present similar challenges to those of the femur. Control of bleeding and the fat embolism syndrome (although not as significant a risk as the femur) remain two advantages of temporary external fixation of the tibia. Also, pain control and ease of patient transfer make DCO a good option for some fractures of the tibia. Some special considerations include the structures at risk (peroneal nerve and posterior neurovascular structures), as well as the lack of significant soft tissue covering the tibia most pronounced distally. For the purposes of this section, DCO tibia treatment will be divided into the diaphysis and both the distal and proximal metaphyses because of the specific issues involved in each.

10.3.1 Tibial Diaphysis

Treatment of fracture of the tibial diaphysis with external fixation is generally reserved for compound injuries, fractures with significant soft tissue destruction, or multiple injury patients who may not tolerate a formal tibial nailing or open reduction and internal fixation. The most effective use of DCO for the uncomplicated fracture of the tibial shaft is for orthopedic surgeons at outlying non-trauma centers who are unfamiliar or inexperienced with nailing or plating techniques. DCO techniques allow these surgeons to apply traveling traction for transfer to a referral center. Also, external fixation of the tibia is most widely used for open fractures of the tibia. Some authors have suggested that open tibia fractures (up to a Gustilo grade 3B) can be treated with appropriate irrigation and debridement, and initial intramedullary nailing or plating with no significantly increased risk [9]. There remains, however, a small subgroup of patients in whom initial external fixation of the tibial shaft should be used.

When fixing extra-articular fractures of the tibial shaft with half-pin, non-ring fixators, the same principles applied to the femur should be considered. The pins should be placed on the anteromedial face of the tibia when possible with special care taken to avoid penetration into the deep posterior compartment causing injury to neurovascular structures. At least two pins are necessary on either side of the fracture [10] (Figs. 10.6 and 10.7); if possible, a multiplanar fixator should be used [11]. Newer ring fixators can be used for damage control of the tibia. However, ring fixators may prove to be more complex and time-consuming for the limited indications we have outlined. If ring fixators are used, thin wires should be placed,

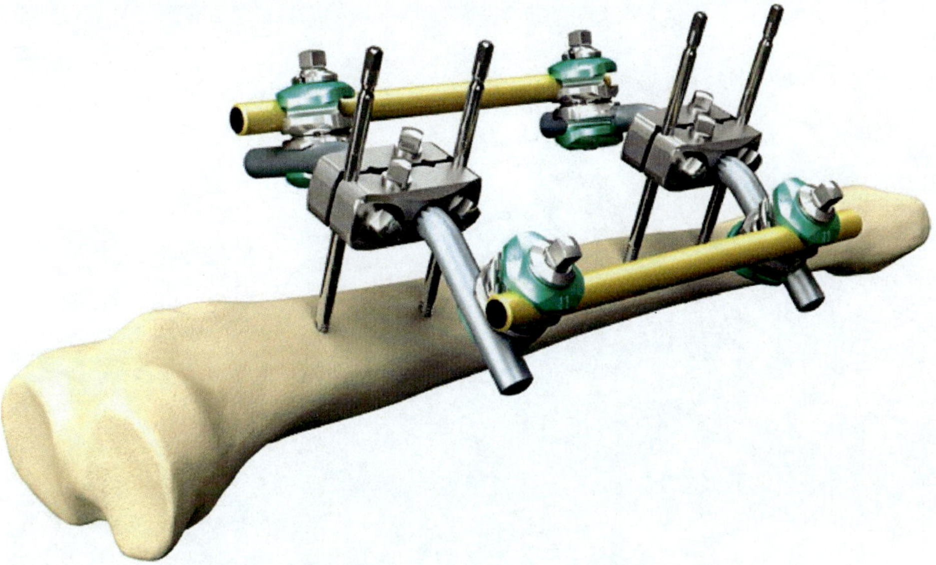

Fig. 10.6 Tibia shaft external fixator using a double-bar construct with the Hoffmann III external fixator

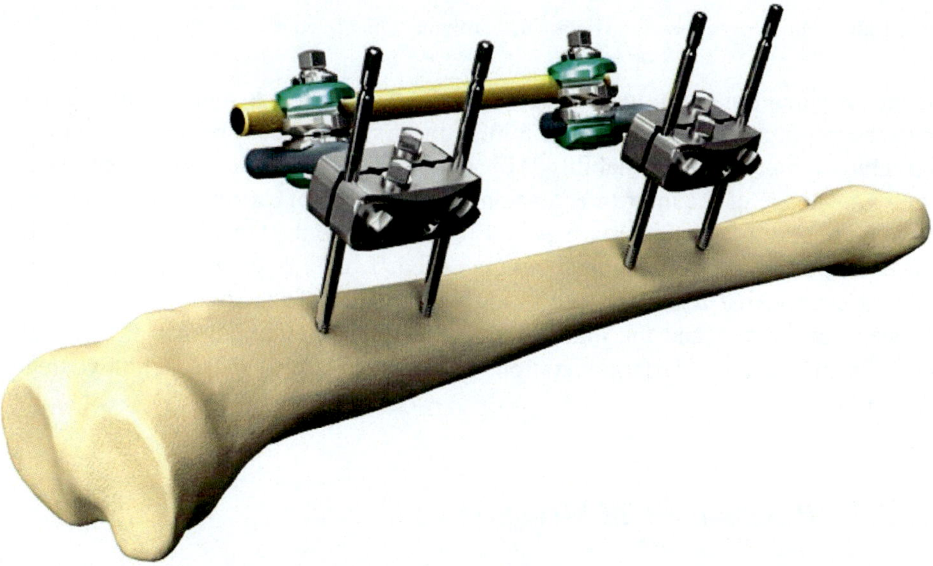

Fig. 10.7 Tibia shaft fixator using a single-bar construct with the Hoffmann III external fixator

generally mediolaterally, with a pin drilled into the tibia on the side of the structure at risk. A moist sponge can be used to control the thin wire as it penetrates the bone and to guide it in the direction necessary to intersect the ring on the contralateral side. The wires are placed with their mutual acute angle as close to 30° as possible.

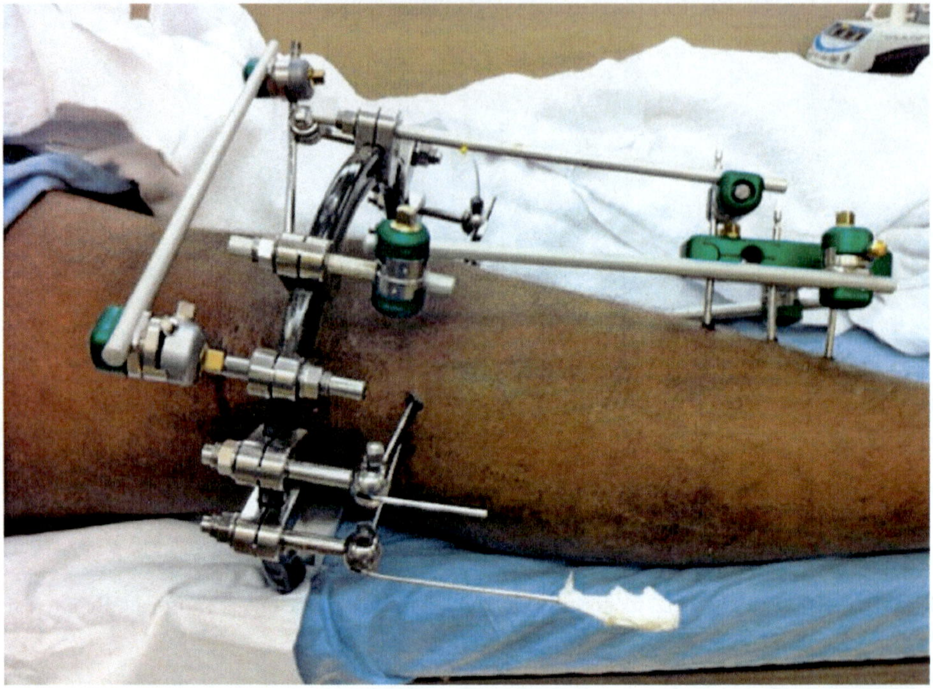

Fig. 10.8 Hybrid frame used for a right-sided proximal tibial fracture

In the proximal tibia, full rings should be avoided if possible to reduce impingement into the popliteal fossa of the knee joint. Ring fixators should be as symmetric as possible to improve frame stability [12] (Fig. 10.8). Ring fixators should be placed with knowledge of the inferior extension of the knee joint capsule. Bono et al. [13] have outlined this to be approximately 14 mm distal to the bony knee joint. Septic knee arthritis from ring fixation about the knee is from 4.2 [14] to 16.1 [9] percent. Others believe that if the fracture is intra-articular, there is already a connection between the fixator and the joint through the fracture site, and the joint capsule consideration is moot. External fixation of the tibia is rarely used as definitive treatment of the fracture.

10.3.2 Proximal Tibial Metaphysis

DCO of the proximal tibia metaphysis can either be a temporary technique or definitive treatment. For the purposes of this book, the indication will be DCO. Temporary external fixation of the proximal tibia almost always should be bridging fixation across the knee to control joint movement and fracture fragments. Bridging knee joint fixation also protects the neurovascular structures about the knee and allows for easier transport and intensive unit care (Fig. 10.9). With all fractures, the surgeon should have a high suspicion for compartment syndrome in fractures about the

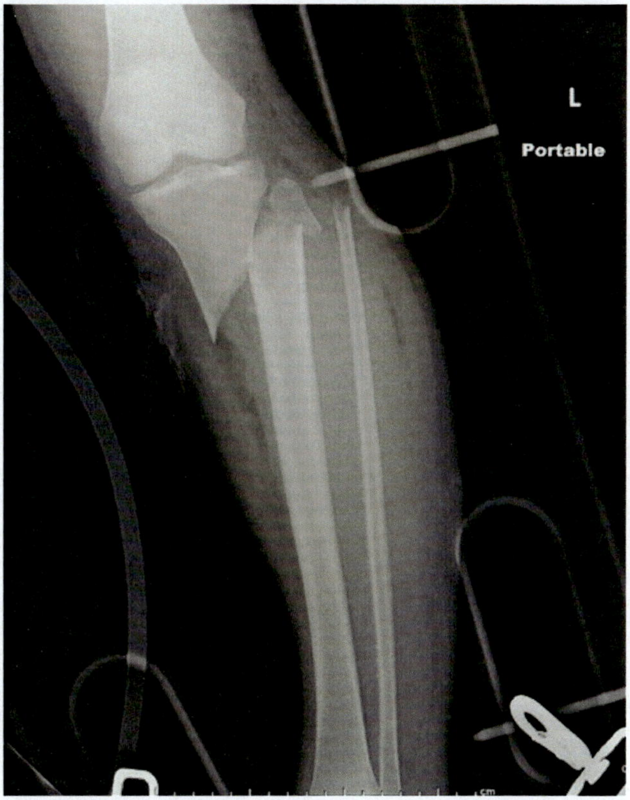

Fig. 10.9 Knee bridging external fixator using the Hoffmann III device

proximal tibia although the overall incidence is still debated with a reported range from 1.6% [15] to 11% [16]. For any question or even consideration of vascular injury, the authors recommend urgent angiography of the lower extremity to rule out occult injury (Figs. 10.10–10.12). In addition, angiography consideration for penetrating periarticular wounds of the tibia as well as distal femur is appropriate.

Bridging external fixation of the knee dates to Raoul Hoffmann in the 1940s and 1950s, and his original descriptions still provide the best techniques for this type of fixation, although the devices have improved. Pins in the tibia should be placed in the anteromedial face and in the femur, the lateral side. The most commonly encountered difficulty of bridging the knee is crossing the normal angle of the knee joint with proper pin placement. We recommend a sturdy joint in the fixator construct at the level of the knee joint to appropriately navigate this curve (Fig. 10.13). The external fixator bars and connecting clamps should never be less than one fingerbreadth from the skin at any point to allow for swelling and small changes of position. The knee should be fixed in a semi-flexed position (approximately 30°) and in the appropriate valgus position [10] with attention paid to reduction of the knee joint by fluoroscopic evaluation if the internal knee ligaments are also injured. Assumptions about timing of return to the operating room should never be made, and malreductions or subluxed joints should not be accepted if at all possible.

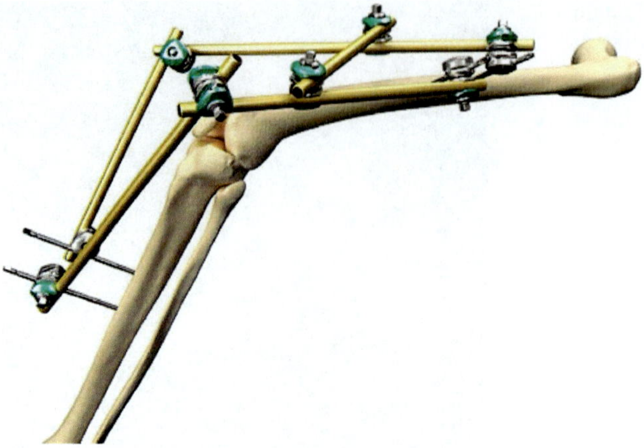

Fig. 10.10 Open left-sided metaphyseal proximal tibial fracture with significant displacement consistent with an angiography request

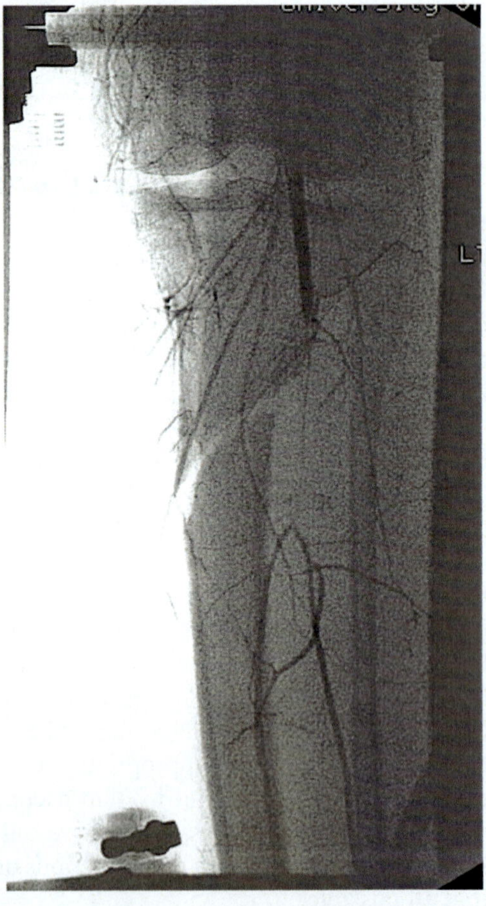

Fig. 10.11 Angiogram of left lower leg showing interruption of the flow through the posterior tibial artery at the level of the fracture

Fig. 10.12 3D reconstruction of the angiogram confirming interruption of blood flow through the posterior tibial artery

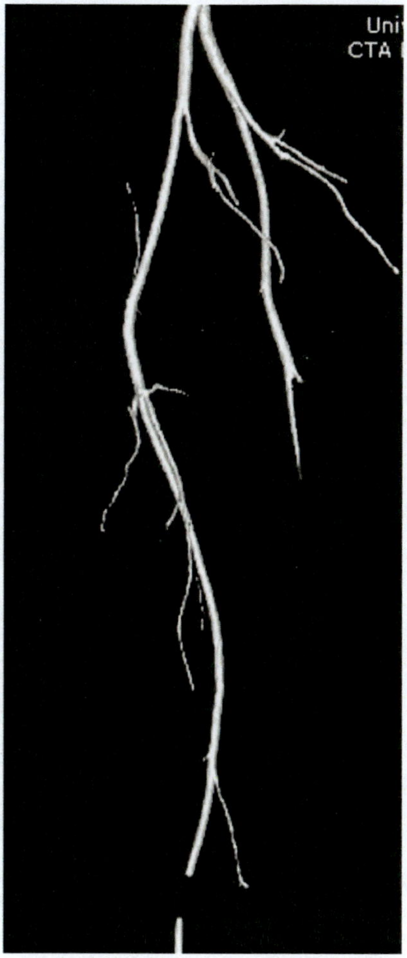

10.3.3 Distal Tibial Metaphysis

Definitive treatment of the distal tibial metaphysis with external fixation has been significantly supplanted recently by fixed or variable angle locked internal fixation and anatomic plating. Many authors [10] now agree that DCO should be used for a majority of distal tibial metaphyseal fractures for a limited time with some minimal internal fixation, staging the final treatment for a time when the soft tissue envelope permits locked anatomic plating. Restoration of the distal tibial articular surface for joint injuries and anatomic alignment for non-articular fractures remain paramount to successful patient outcomes. Complications of overly aggressive early fracture treatment include serious wound complications requiring free tissue transfers and sometimes amputations. Fractures occurring in the distal tibial metaphysis requiring DCO treatment prior to internal fixation or intramedullary nailing should be externally fixed across the ankle joint to include the foot. This will reduce ankle joint

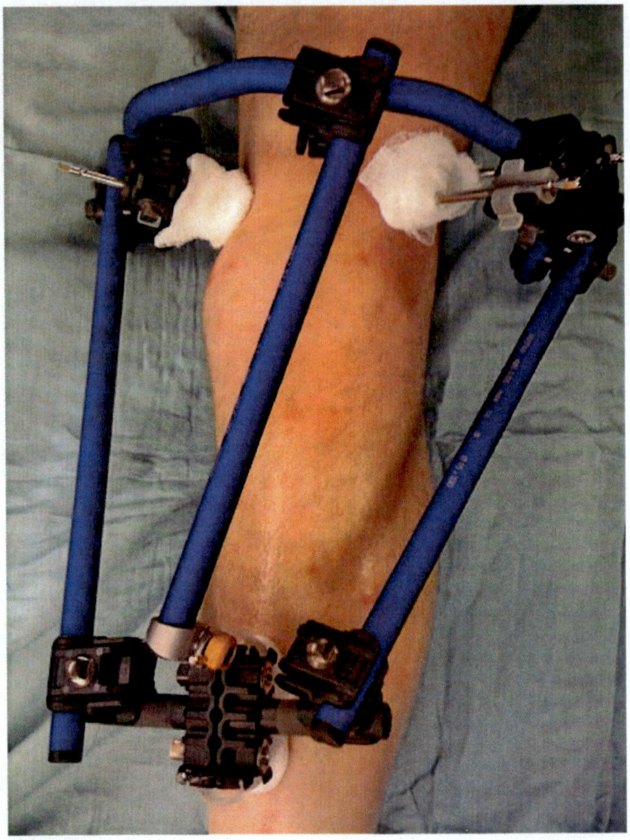

Fig. 10.13 Bridging external fixator across the knee joint for left proximal tibia fracture

micromotion, maintain alignment, and control any eventual tendency toward equinus deformity. Moreover, frame montages controlling the distal tibia that include the foot and ankle should provide elevation of the heel from the bed or resting surface to reduce the incidence of heel ulcers and control the midfoot position. A commonly missed problem with ankle and foot frames is maintaining toe position. We control this by placing small straps on each toe attached with elastic couplings to the frame to maintain neutral position and constant stretch on the toe flexors. Two commonly used frame montages in our institution are the ones shown on Figs. 10.14 and 10.15. These constructs can be used for any fracture within 10 cm of the tibial plafond as well as combined fractures of the tibia and talus or calcaneus. Pins should be placed in the anteromedial surface of the tibia distally (Fig. 10.9), and some combinations of two pins in the calcaneus and thin wires or half-pins in the first and fourth metatarsal or across the midfoot are effective in controlling midfoot motion and preventing equinus and toe flexion contracture. Effective initial DCO fixation of distal tibia fractures with supplemental limited internal fixation, proper staging of the final open reduction, and proper soft tissue maintenance can effectively improve and control the very complicated treatment of these potentially devastating injuries. For fractures that are proximal enough to enable pin placements in the distal tibial metaphysis, two

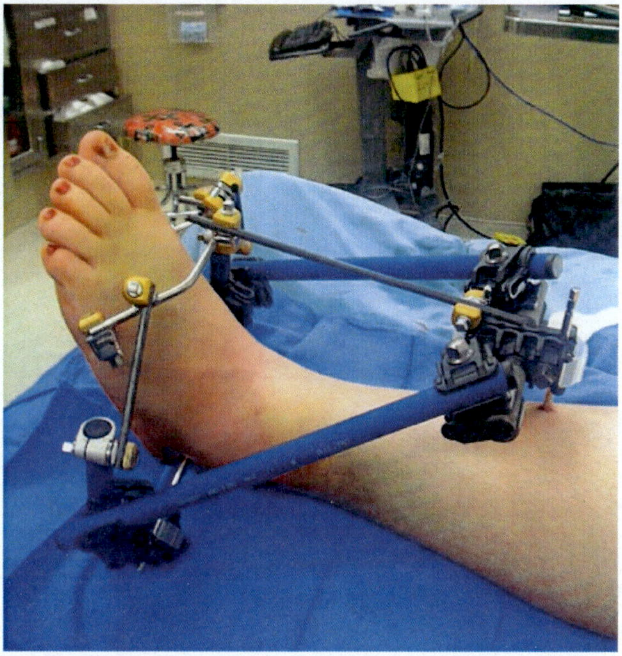

Fig. 10.14 Bridging external fixator across the ankle joint used for a left pilon fracture

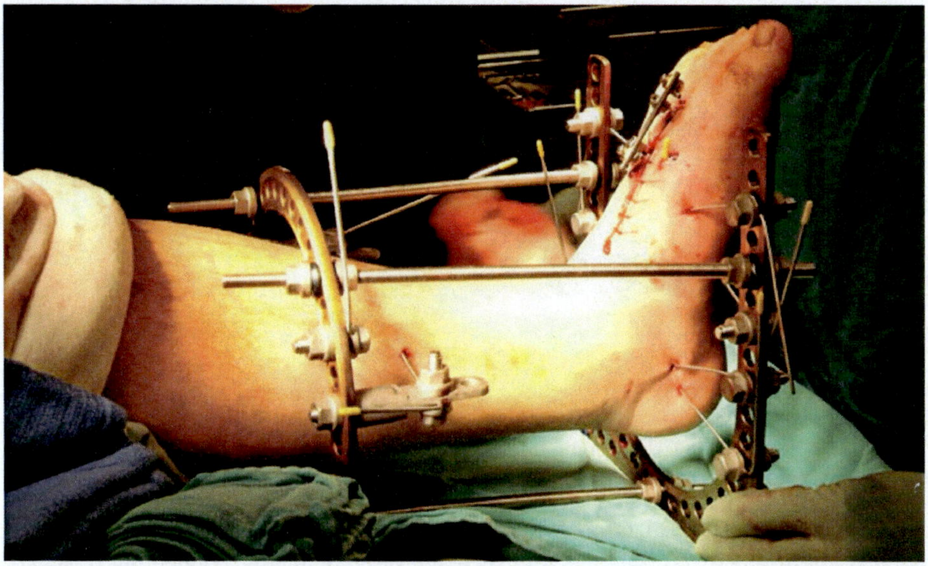

Fig. 10.15 LIMA frame (Lualdi Industria Meccanica Anduins) used to treat a pilon fracture with associated forefoot injuries

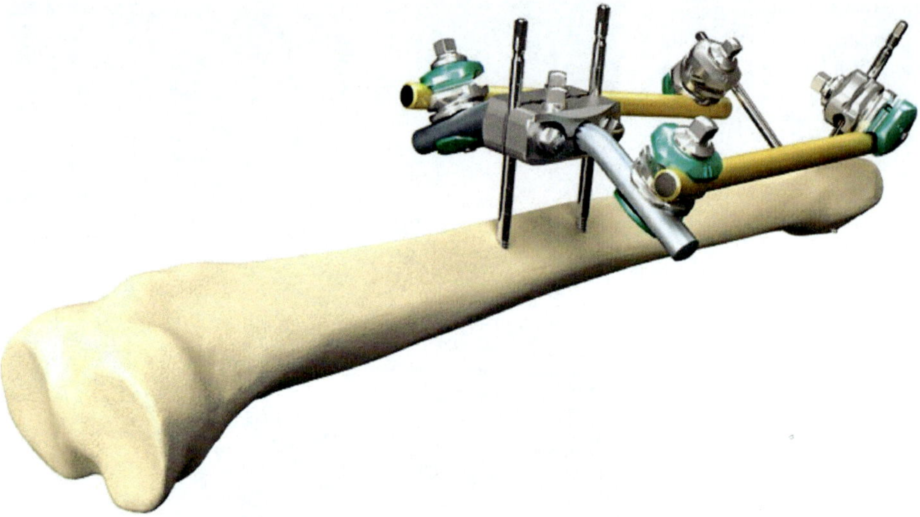

Fig. 10.16 Use of the Hoffmann III external fixator to create a circular frame with half-pins in the distal tibia metaphysis

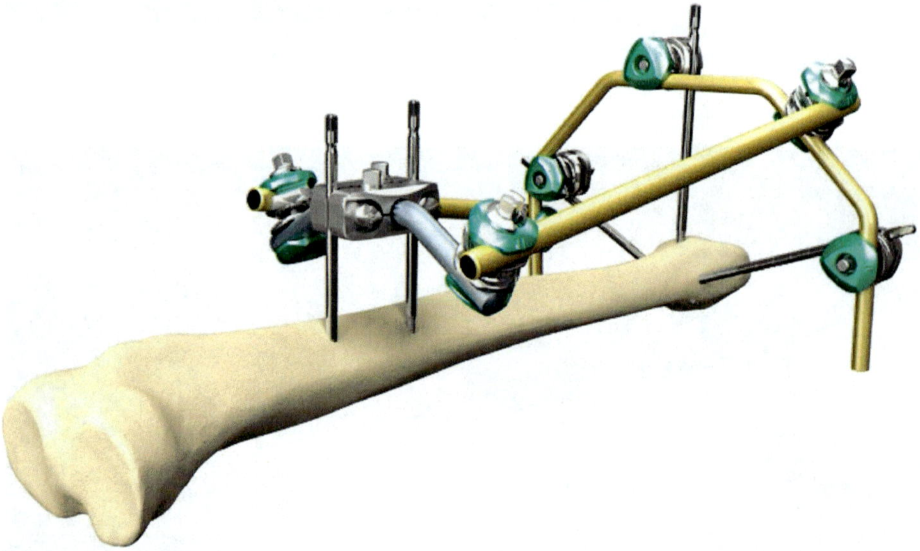

Fig. 10.17 Distal tibia independent pin frame for a distal tibia fracture proximal enough to avoid bridging the ankle

main types of constructs can be utilized. The first one involves the creation of a circular frame in the distal tibia metaphysis using three half-pins, connecting it to two proximal tibial half-pins (Fig. 10.16). The second technique involves the creation of two independent pin frames (Fig. 10.17).

10.4 Humerus and Forearm

The humerus and forearm are less commonly treated with initial DCO fixation. This is due to the generally forgiving nature of the soft tissue envelope and better rates of healing with early fracture treatment (internal fixation) [17]. However, there are indications for external fixation of either the humerus or forearm. These include irreparable soft tissue injury requiring delayed free tissue transfer, fractures involving vascular injury, fractures in patients so unstable their condition will not permit lengthy soft tissue or reconstructive procedures, and segmental fractures or blast injuries with large bony defects requiring multiple operations to reconstruct.

10.4.1 Humerus

The humerus can be externally fixed similarly to other long bones. Simple frames with at least two half-pins on either side of the fracture site(s) usually are adequate fixation for these injuries. Unfortunately, thin wire fixators in the humerus are less commonly used because of location relative to the chest and medial neurovascular structures. In the proximal humerus, half-pins should be placed laterally to avoid injury to the radial nerve. Distally, half-pins should be placed posteriorly up to about 10–15 cm proximal to the elbow joint to avoid injury to the radial nerve (Fig. 10.18). Any frame montage can be created around pin placement with modular fixators to allow access for soft tissue, vascular, or other reconstructive procedures to take place (Fig. 10.19).

The proximal humerus can be fixed with half-pins into the humeral head, much in the same way as the femur with adequate fluoroscopic guidance. Fractures of the proximal humerus not amenable to pin placement in that area can even be fixed with half-pins placed in the distal or midshaft clavicle for short-term control.

Fractures about the distal humerus usually require fixation across the elbow joint either with fixed or hinged devices to control elbow joint and distal humeral fracture site motion. Pin placement in the humerus should be posterior distally, and pin placement in the forearm is easily achieved in the relatively subcutaneous ulna shaft. Elbow position should first optimize fracture or elbow joint stability, and be placed in a slightly flexed position to maintain patient comfort and mobility. When using hinged fixators, the hinge may be initially locked at initial treatment with delayed gradual return of the elbow range of motion as the injury permits. The axial alignment of the elbow should maintain as close to anatomic valgus as possible.

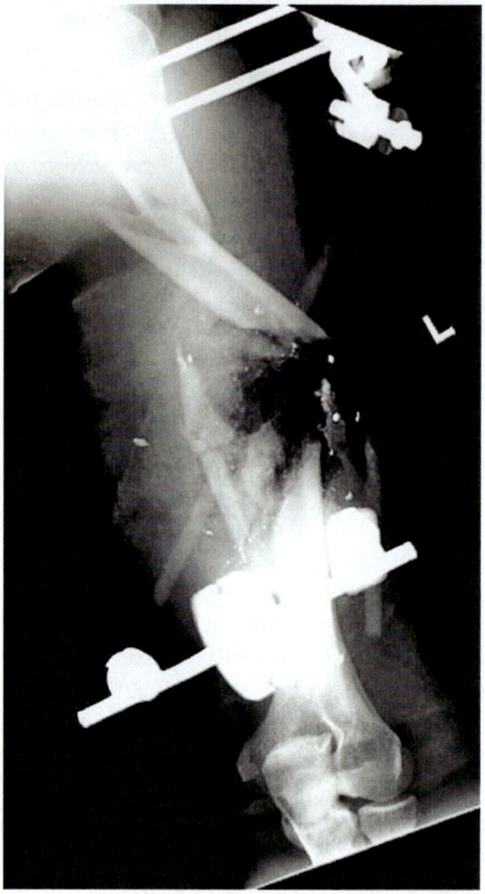

Fig. 10.18 Comminuted open segmental fracture of the humerus treated with external fixation using lateral proximal pins and posterior distal pins

10.4.2 Elbow and Forearm

DCO of the forearm is even less common than the humerus. Many [18] authors suggest acute internal fixation even in the presence of extensive soft tissue or neurovascular injuries. When necessary, forearm external fixation can and should be done with the intact ulnar segments due to its relative subcutaneous position and lack of structures at risk when placing half-pins (Fig. 10.20). The forearm can also be fixed temporarily with ring fixators applying the same principles to pin placement and ring placement outlined previously (Fig. 10.21). When the ulna is not accessible for half-pin placement, careful limited dissection of the radius should be done to avoid iatrogenic neurovascular damage. Forearm external fixation can restore length, maintain stability, and facilitate patient transfer very adequately for specific indications and should be used when necessary.

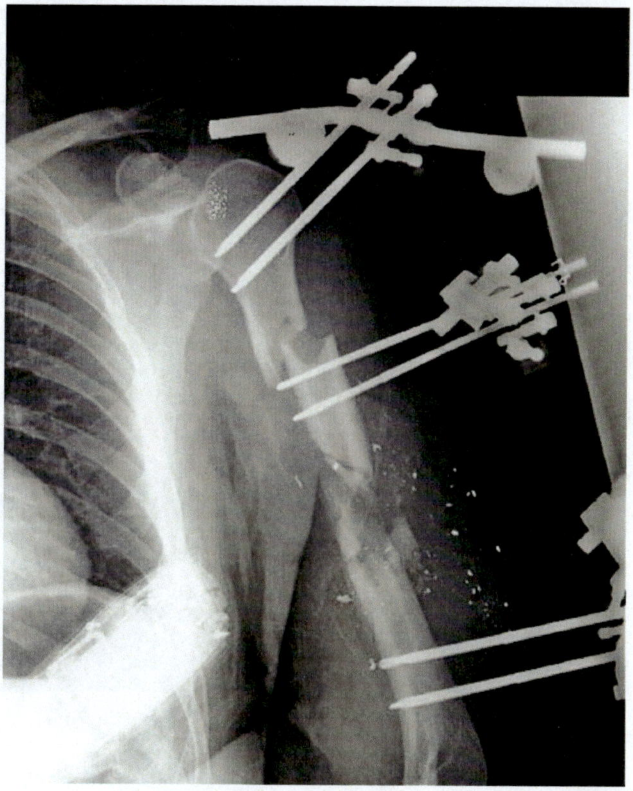

Fig. 10.19 Comminuted segmental open humerus fracture treated with external fixator using 2 pins to control the segmented fragment

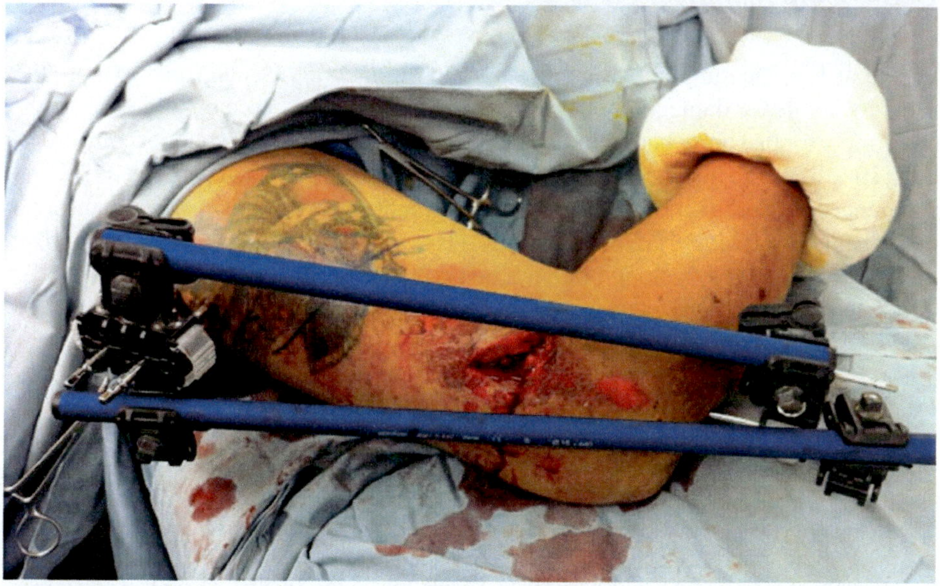

Fig. 10.20 Elbow frame used for an open distal humerus fracture. The distal pins are inserted in the intact ulna

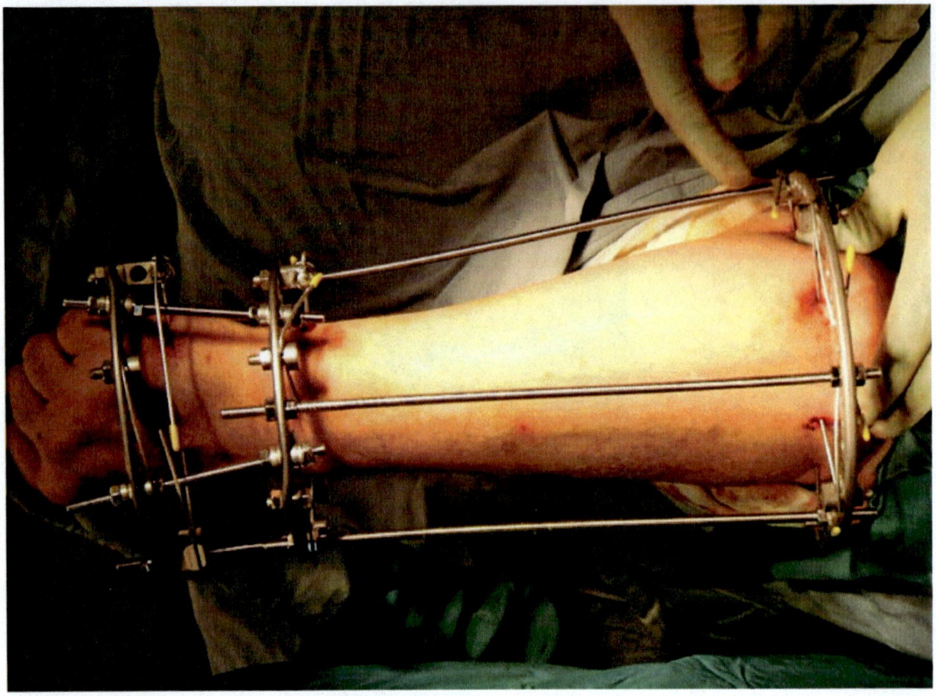

Fig. 10.21 Ilizarov frame for an open forearm fracture

10.5 Conclusion

In conclusion, the long tubular bones – femur, tibia, humerus, and forearm – are the usual locations for damage-control simple external frames based on large pins gathered into groups (bone handles) and connected with bars. This temporizing treatment simplifies the management of the multiply injured patient. There are important differences for the fixation of each limbs segment, but two pins proximal and two pins distal to a fracture are often enough. External fixation is an essential tool in modern fracture care for long bone fractures.

References

1. Pape HC, Hildebrand F, Pertschy S, Zelle B, Garapati R, Grimme K, et al. Changes in the management of femoral shaft fractures in polytrauma patients: from early total care to damage control orthopedic surgery. J Trauma Inj Infect Crit Care. 2002;53(3):452–61.
2. Bone LB, Johnson KD, Weigelt J, Scheinberg R. Early versus delayed stabilization of femoral fractures. A prospective randomized study. J Bone Joint Surg. 1989;71:336–40.
3. Lieurance R, Benjamin JB, Rappaport WD. Blood loss and transfusion in patients with isolated femur fractures. J Orthop Trauma. 1992;6(2):175–9.

4. Tuttle M, Smith W. Safety and efficacy of damage control external fixation versus early definitive stabilization for femoral shaft fractures in the multiple-injured patient. J Trauma. 2009;67:602–5. July 2003 – 17(6):415–20.
5. Tsai I-Tzun, Hsu C-J, Chen Y-H, Fong Yi-Chin, Hsu H-C, Tsai C-H. Fat embolism syndrome in long bone fracture – clinical experience in a tertiary referral center in Taiwan. J Chin Med Assoc. 2010;73(8):407–10.
6. Wolinsky P, Twjwani N, Richmond J, Koval K, Egol K, Stephen DJG. Controversies in intramedullary nailing of femoral shaft fractures. J Bone Joint Surg. 2001;83A:1404–15.
7. Nicholas B, Toth L, Van Wessem K, Evans J, Enninghorst N, Balogh ZJ. Borderline femur fracture patients: early total care or damage control orthopaedics? ANZ J Surg. 2010;81(3):148–53. doi:10.1111/j.1445-2197.2010.05582.
8. Schettler N, Ogden J, Seligson D. Temporary external fixation of femur fractures: new half frame applications with the "tower Pin" augmentation. Osteo Trauma Care. 2003;11(1):21–3.
9. Bhandari M, Guyatt G, Swiontkowski M, Schemitsch E. Treatment of open fractures of the shaft of the tibia. J Bone Joint Surg (Br). 2000;82B:62–8.
10. Schmidt A, Finkemeier C, Tornetta P. Treatment of closed tibial fractures. J Bone Joint Surg. 2003;85A:352–68.
11. Behrens F. A primer of fixator devices and configurations. Clin Orthop Relat Res. 1989;241:5–14.
12. Roberts CS, Dodds JC, Perry K, Beck D, Seligson D, Voor MJ. Hybrid external fixation of the proximal tibia: strategies to improve frame stability. J Orthop Trauma. 2003;17(6):415–20.
13. Bono C, Levine R, Rao J, Behrens F. Nonarticular proximal tibia fractures: treatment options and decision making. J Amer Acad Orthop Surg. 2001;9:176–86.
14. Rommens P, Gielen J, Broos P, Gruwez J. Intrinsic problems with the external fixation device of Hoffmann-Vidal-Adrey: a critical evaluation of 117 patients with complex tibial shaft fractures. J Trauma. 1989;29:630–8.
15. Park S, Ahn J, Gee AO, Kuntz AF, Esterhai JL. Compartment syndrome in tibial fractures. J Orthop Trauma. 2009;23(7):514–8.
16. Finkemeier CG, Schmidt AH, Kyle RF, Templeman DC, Varecka TF. A prospective, randomized study of intramedullary nails inserted with and without reaming for the treatment of open and closed fractures of the tibial shaft. J Orthop Trauma. 2000;14(3):187–93.
17. Schuind FA, Burny F, Chao EY. Biomechanical properties and design considerations in upper extremity external fixation. Hand Clin. 1993;9(4):543–53.
18. Putnam MD, Walsh TM. External fixation for open fractures of the upper extremity. Hand Clin. 1993;9(4):613–23.

Chapter 11
The Care and Management of Patients with External Fixators

David Seligson and Janet Macphaden

11.1 Introduction

Elective bone surgery requires consent: the surgeon is expected to explain the procedure preoperatively, and the patient signs a document stating that the proposed surgery has been explained, questions answered, and the patient agrees to the operation. In urgent trauma surgery, there may not be a fully documented consent. The patient with a skeletal injury treated in a damage control frame usually does not have information or experience with external fixators. Furthermore, fixators are generally considered to be awkward and inconvenient. Surgeons have limited experience and therefore adverse outcomes with external fixation. Close friends look with horror at the pins penetrating the skin. The case managers order wheelchairs, and physical therapists tell the patient that they will be able to begin treatment "once the frame is removed." Better appreciation for and better results with the use of fixators is a matter of education, experience, and marketing. The surgeon, therefore, must not only make the decision to use an external fixation system, get the equipment into the operating room, and install it reasonably, but must also attend to the details of postoperative care. The program includes explaining to the patient why the device was selected, how it functions, and how to take care of it. Typically, patients are fearful about frame removal [1, 2]. At follow-up examinations, they may hear the cries of preceding patients and become unreasonable about frame removal. The frightened patient will insist on being "put to sleep" in order to have the external fixator removed. When patients with fixators gather in the waiting room of the surgeon experienced in the use of external skeletal fixation, the device becomes normal for the management of accidents. The patients talk with each other,

---

D. Seligson (✉)
Department of Orthopaedics, University Hospital Louisville,
Louisville, KY, USA
e-mail: seligson@louisville.edu

J. Macphaden
Department of Orthopaedics, Nurse Practitioner, University Hospital Louisville,
Louisville, KY, USA

D. Seligson et al. (eds.), *External Fixation in Orthopedic Traumatology*,
DOI 10.1007/978-1-4471-2197-8_11, © Springer-Verlag London Limited 2012

compare appliances, and discuss their experiences. When the programs are consistent and the atmosphere is one of success, external fixation is an accepted and useful technique for fracture care and produces good outcomes [3, 4].

11.2 Elements of the External Fixator

The elements of an external fixation frame are (1) bone pins, (2) pin holders, and (3) connecting rods. This basic concept has been followed for more than a century.

The fixator pins are inserted through the skin and serve as the fixation points to bone. This anchorage to be is usually achieved by threading the pin into the bone. Other approaches are thin tensioned wires or pins placed at an angle and tensioned against each other. The pins are then held together outside the skin and soft tissue envelope using pin-holding clamps and connecting rods to form a self-contained traction/stabilization unit.

All external fixators are based on the same principle of connecting bones with rods. An external fixation frame has a number of advantages:

- Good access for wound care
- Early joint motion to prevent stiffness
- A low rate of infection in the fracture
- Easy removal of the fixator in clinic or day surgery
- Motion for uninjured muscles and neighboring joints

Each of the elements of the fixator has its own care requirements. The pin–skin and pin–bone junctions are the critical interfaces between the environment and the skeleton. For the patient with the fixator, pin care programs are directed at preventing loosening of the pin, preventing infection of skin and bone, and preventing pin breakage. Unfortunately, there is little critical research on what factors are actually effective. In one pin care program, all the secretions are removed, and the pin–skin junction is kept meticulously clean and dry. In another, the secretions are allowed to collect until they look like wax dripped from a candle. There is little information about which treatment regime produces the greatest protection from cellulitis at the pin–skin junction [5]. On the other hand, it is known that excessive use of hydrogen peroxide and saline can yield to colonization of the soft tissue surrounding the pin with *Serratia marscens*.

Most orthopedists believe that daily care of the fixator postoperatively is necessary to avoid complications. At first, hospital personnel take care of the fixator. As soon as the patient's health allows, if at all practical, the patient should learn how to care for the fixator.

Cleaning instructions for the patient:

- Wash hands and sanitize before starting.
- Clean the shaft of the pin where it enters the skin with cotton-tipped applicators moistened with saline/clean water.
- Clean the fixator (when wounds are sealed in 3–4 days) with a quick daily shower.
- Dry the pin site.
- Dry the frame.
- If there is drainage, dress the pins with gauze.

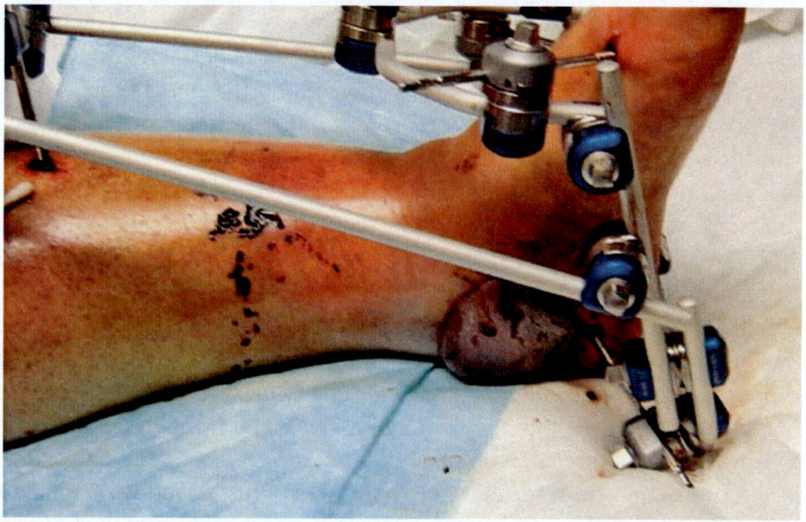

Fig. 11.1 External fixator for pilon fracture of the right ankle showing a fracture blister around the pin site with associated swelling and erythema

In the hospital, sterile cotton applicators and sterile dressings are used. When the patient goes home, clean applicators and dressings are sufficient. The rationale is that the hospital population of organisms is more invasive, and the risks of contamination from health care workers and other patients are greater than the flora that the patient will encounter at home.

11.3 Pin Site Drainage

The body drains around most external fixation pins. Drainage can be specific to the location of the fixation and the extent of injury, drainage can be related to patient variables such as skin colonization by invasive organisms, and drainage can be caused by technical variables which occur as the pins are installed by the surgeon (Fig. 11.1). Factors associated with increased drainage include the thickness of the soft tissue which the pin traverses, local skin hygiene, tenting of the skin over the pin, and pin loosening. Raoul Hoffmann's "three laws" of fixator care were skin preparation, skin incision, and skin relaxation – préparez la peau, ponctionnez la peau et relachez la peau! After the hospital, drainage from the pins is a major source of confusion and unhappiness. Concerned patients do not infrequently go to immediate care centers or emergency rooms where they are examined by doctors with little background in external skeletal fixation and even less common sense. The patient may be in a state of excitement from a diagnosis of a "staph" infection which it is alleged has the potential to complications. Hospitalization is insisted on. Bone scans are requested. Infectious disease is consulted. The postoperative care of the patient in the fixator requires patient and family education, patience, and even tolerance. The patient and family need a strategy for pin care. Some pin tract drainage is accepted. Patients often ask "is this normal." Best to say, there is nothing normal about pins screwed into bone through the skin. The question is does pin tract drainage happen, and is it a problem. In general, some tolerable mild weeping from pin tracts is usual. This drainage should not be confused with accelerating erythema, local warmth, and pain which are signs of the infrequent major pin tract infection [6]. Significant pin tract infection is usually controlled when the pin is removed. This is seldom an emergency. Osteomyelitis with chronic drainage caused by thermal necrosis of bone at the time of pin insertion can be difficult to manage. Common causes of this problem are placement of a pin only through cortex particularly in the tibia. Here the path the pin takes is through dense bone, and this generates heat which coagulates bone. The pin should pass from the cortex into the medullary cavity and through the cortex on the far side. A pin placed at too much of an angle from the perpendicular can cause bone necrosis and ring sequestrum for the same reason [7]. Pins placed with a hand brace are less likely to overheat than pins placed with a power drill. Pins with sharp drilling tips are better than dull ones [8].

Oral antibiotics have an empiric role in the care of the patient in an external fixator. One motto is "pins in the body, pills in the mouth." The choice of antibiotic is usually simple – trimethoprim sulfa, a tetracycline, or a quinolone.

In the clinic, increasing problem with pins is often associated with failure to continue oral antibiotics. A good evidence-based study is not available, so this use of antibiotics is empiric.

11.4 Approach to Patients Before and After Application of External Fixator

In the nineteenth century, surgical texts had tables about the healing time of fractures. In our more complex world, skeletal injures that would have been fatal in the past are survived, treated, and led for the most part to good outcomes. Patients have little information about their injury and often ask relatives and friends about what will be the course of their recovery. The fracture surgeon therefore has an educational function. The patient should understand that the healing of a particular fracture is different for each patient. This is part of the art of fracture treatment and depends on, among other factors, the extent of damage to the tissue surrounding the bone, the general condition of the patient, and the method of treatment. The doctor should in so far as possible keep the patient informed about the progress of the fracture healing or at least share uncertainty about the likely progress of the injury.

Following placement of an external fixator, follow-up x-rays are usually taken. These x-rays are generally performed every 2–3 weeks after fixator placement. The study of these x-rays allows the orthopedist to check the fracture site to be sure that the pins in the fracture site are in the correct position and not loose. The films also show whether or not the position of the fracture in the frame is being maintained.

Later, the x-ray gives information about fracture healing and helps determine the time to remove the fixator. It happens from time to time that the x-rays show unexpected findings – the fracture is not reduced, the pins are not in bone, or worse the pins are broken. As a matter of course, x-rays should be looked at with the patient, the findings should immediately be disclosed, and a plan to correct problems that would adversely affect outcome formulated. Defensiveness, concealment, and patronizing are not infrequently in the background of the legal difficulties that can arise in fracture care. On the other hand, x-rays taken in surgery do not always disclose complications that are found on the postoperative films either because the projections are not the same or because operative fluoroscopy is a real-time activity, and it is not uncommon to fail to see everything as clearly as it can be seen in a quiet office setting with plain films. It is also worth bearing in mind that our patients do not always do as they are told. It could be they were somewhere where they should not have been, doing something they should not have been doing (part of the reason they were injured in the first place), and indeed, they are fearful that there has been an adverse event and will be relieved that the surgeon has a solution.

11.5 Weight-Bearing Status and Physical Therapy

Physical therapy is essential for the recovery of the patient in an external fixator and for definitive healing of the fracture. The best story to keep in mind is the example of Raoul Hoffmann who fractured his own tibia, had his assistant install a tibial frame, and then bicycled to work until the fracture healed. Key points of this story are (1) the frame was stable enough for functional activity, (2) the fracture was a closed fracture, and (3) the patient was mobile in the frame.

Clearly, the surgeon is responsible for constructing frames that facilitate rehabilitation – "friendly frames." When patients come to clinic with frames that are poorly conceived and poorly constructed, the patients are confined to wheelchairs and apprehensive about moving around. The limb may be covered with a blanket or preciously perched on a pillow. Clearly, these "unfriendly frames" were the product of other doctors in clinics elsewhere.

Today, the surgeon and patient face dissociation between surgeon and therapist. Mandated by law in our state is the concept that the therapist is to "evaluate and treat." In some European countries, postoperative care is relegated to a generalist. It is indispensible to assess the stability of the fracture and the fixation at the end of surgery in order to intelligently prescribe the therapy. For example, a pelvic external fixator for a lateral compression injury with an intact symphysis pubis and no vertical instability can be full weight-bearing while patient in the identical fixation but with vertical instability can be only eggshell weight-bearing until posterior stability is restored. The surgeon works with the therapist to increase activity and the activity and function of the patient. Patients who appear in the office saying that the therapist has told them "nothing more can be done until the frame is removed" need someplace else to go for rehabilitation.

The fixation pins which go through the skin are a significant feature of the external fixator. These pins can hinder the patient's use of the injured limb. At the conclusion of the placement of the external fixator, the surgeon should move the limb to be sure that the soft tissue slides easily around the external fixation pin. Where the skin is tight, the skin needs to be released to facilitate motion of the extremity. Since motion and muscle strength are essential for fracture healing, exercises are important during recovery.

Through physical therapy, the range of motion of joints can be restored and muscle strength rebuilt. This will hasten tissue and bone healing. In order to get the patient back to a normal life, it is important that the injured limb be moved in a controlled fashion as soon as possible. Rehabilitation must be performed within the material constraints of the external fixation device. For example, with fine wire fixation around the foot and ankle, normal weight-bearing will break the pins in several weeks. It is possible, however, to take advantage of the concept of minimal effective strain. Thus, if the patient is instructed to full weight-bearing 6–10 times twice daily and the rest of the time to be on eggshell weight-bearing (40–60 pounds), the strain on the fracture will be sufficient to optimize fracture healing but not enough to break the construct.

Important aspects of the return to function are the control of pain and the control of swelling. Gentle but limited range of motion protects against joint stiffness. This motion with the assistance of a reassuring therapist will help to restore muscle function and reduce pain. Massage, gentle stretching, and sometimes transcutaneous nerve stimulation (TENS) can be of terrific assistance in restoring the use of an injured limb in an external fixator.

11.6 Postoperative Care of the Frame and Pins

Following discharge from the hospital, the patient will be responsible for the daily care of his/her external fixator. If necessary, advise the patient to have a friend or family member help. He/she will need the following for daily care:

- Clean 4×4 gauze pads or a clean cloth
- Plain soap and clean water
- Clean towels
- Shower or hand sprayer

Cleaning instructions for patient:

1. Go to the bathroom where one can use the shower, a faucet sprayer, or a spray bottle.
2. Lay out all necessary materials on a clean towel.
3. Either sit on a stool in the shower, or use the spray faucet, or spray bottle in the sink.
4. Wash hands with soap and water and/or sanitize before beginning.
5. Wet down the fixator pins and skin with clean, lukewarm water.

6. Clean the pin sites with soap and water using a 4×4 gauze pad or one part of the cloth for each pin. Gently push skin away from the pin as it is cleaned.
7. Remove any crusts around the pins using the gauze pads or cloth – the skin around the pins should be mobile.
8. Wash everything again.
9. Dry the pin sites with the gauze pads or a hair dryer. Use the cool or warm, not hot settings.
10. Dry the fixator with a clean towel or hair dryer.
11. Let any remaining secretions dry.
12. If there is drainage, wrap 4×4 gauze pads around the pin entrance sites.

Depending on the type of injury, try to do as many normal activities as possible. Keep certain precautions in mind: The bone is not fully healed; therefore, the patient has to avoid falling. Remind him/her to be particularly careful about steps, rugs, and loose shoelaces.

- Avoid contact with animals.
- Avoid contact with dust and dirt.
- Avoid unnecessary handling of the fixator.

If the physician gives permission, the patient can go swimming with the fixator. Instruct the patient not to change the components or the arrangement of the fixator. Remember to follow the instructions of the orthopedic team with regard to:

- Mobilization
- Weight bearing
- Physical therapy

The doctor will give specific orders to the physical therapist regarding the patient's particular treatment. Orders are best changed in the office when the clinical situation can be reviewed with the patient and x-rays available and a record written as to what has been decided.

11.7 Pin Tract Infection

Pin tract infections are probably more related to performance variables at the time the pins are placed than to the program of postoperative care, so that even if the patient follows all the precautions, it is still possible to have a pin tract infection. The patient may know that an infection is developing by the following signs:

- Local reddening of the skin
- Pain
- Swelling of the skin
- Unpleasant sensations from the pin entry sites
- Fever
- Loosening

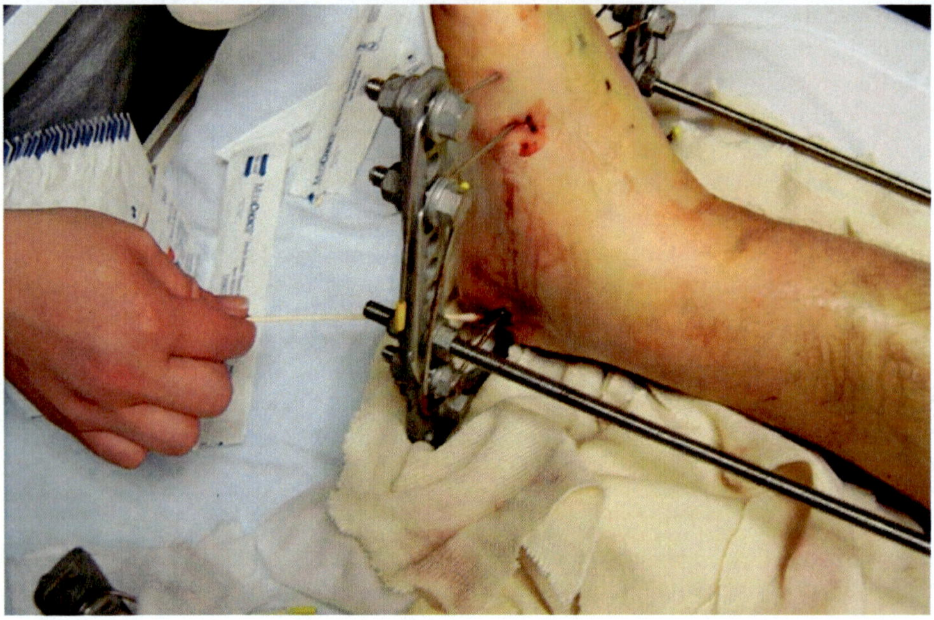

Fig. 11.2 Microbiological swabbing of a suspicious pin site

If the patient begins to get progressive symptoms, he/she should be instructed to contact the attending doctor or a member of the doctor's team. Sometimes, oral antibiotics are helpful in infection control. However, once a pin has lost anchorage in bone, it cannot become stable again (Fig. 11.2). It is also possible to change pins and put them in different locations. Statistics show that changing pins is only necessary in about 2% of all patients. If the x-rays show that there is a ring of dead bone surrounding where the pin was placed – ring sequestrum – drainage may persist until this dead bone is removed surgically. In the Checketts-Otterburns classification of pin track infections, grade six is for a major infection after fixator removal – really a post pin tract infection [9, 10]. The concept usefully identifies that it is the injury to bone and not the pin that is responsible for the continued clinical problem. Indeed, curettage of a persistent draining bone sinus can lead to quite a large hole in bone which may cause mechanical problems such as fracture through the defect. Considerable skill is required successfully to treat a late major pin tract infection.

11.8 Removal of the External Fixator: Where and When?

When to take the frame off and where? That is the question. The two major variables are the fracture and the soft tissue. Side plots include how the patient has adapted to external fixation and how the folks involved in patient care are managing the concept. When a frame is used for damage control of a significant skeletal fracture, the external fixator will be exchanged for definitive fixation – usually a nail or a plate from a few days to a few weeks after the injury. In practice, the frame can be removed and definitive fixation performed in one operative sitting. Indeed, removing the frame and delaying before performing osteosynthesis results in motion at the fracture site with inflammation and deterioration of the soft tissue condition which had been improved by the control of fracture site motion with the external frame.

In the situations where half-frame fixation is used for definitive fracture care, for example, treatment of a hand fracture with a mini-frame, treatment of a distal radius fracture with a wrist spanning frame, treatment of a pelvic fracture with an anterior half-pin frame, the fixator can be removed as an office procedure if the patient will accept the idea [11]. It is useless to struggle against negative attitudes which feed patient fear of frame removal. The hospital outpatient charges and waste of professional time are exorbitant. Nonetheless, it is better to take off the frame under anesthesia than to have a patient incident (vomiting, screaming, fainting, chest pain) in the office. A half-inch external frame can be removed without anesthesia. However, nitrous oxide administered by nasal mask is a possible method for dealing with patient apprehension at the time of external fixator removal. To sort out which patients can have office removal of a frame and which would benefit from an operative procedure, evaluation of x-rays for pin tract problems is helpful. In particular, pin tracts can be curetted in the operating room. This gentle curettage and irrigation will reduce the incidence of late pin tract problems. Small wire ring frames are more difficult to remove since the pins can seize in bone, so ring frames with thin transfixing wires are usually removed under a general or regional anesthetic. It may be better not to cut the wires but simply to wipe them off with alcohol and pull them through the bone. Cutting the wire makes an end which is flat and sharp which will damage the tissue around the tract as the pin is pulled out.

Following removal of the fixator, the pin tracts will have dressings for a few days. Usually, there is some drainage, but this rapidly subsides. After the dressing is taken off, the patient can shower and clean the skin. The pin tracts rapidly become sealed.

11.9 Conclusion

External fixation is a valuable tool for the care of skeletal trauma. It has significant advantages and serious drawbacks. As the technique became accepted in the latter part of the twentieth century, there was a hope that external fixation would be a definitive treatment for broken bones. Real doctors, it was opined, could carry fractures to union using just an external frame. Various sophisticated devices that promoted increased cyclic loading of fracture sites were proposed and tried clinically. In practice, the prudent traumatologist recognizes that splints, braces, crutches, bandages, and progressive physical therapy routines are rational adjuncts to improving outcomes with fixators and avoiding the disappointment and discouragement associated with refracture.

References

1. Rowe S. A review of the literature on the nursing care of skeletal pins in the paediatric and adolescent setting. J Orthop Nurs. 1997;1:26–9.
2. Santy J. Nursing the patient with an external fixator. Nurs Stand. 2000;14:47–52.
3. Coombs R, Green S, Sarmiento A. External fixation and functional bracing. London: Orthotext; 1989.
4. Jauernig P. Organizing and implementing an Ilizarov program. Orthop Nurs. 1990;9:47–55.
5. Davies R, Holt N, Nayagam S. The care of pin sites with external fixation. JBJSB. 2005; 87:16–9.
6. Carlino H. The child with an Ilizarov external fixator. Pediatr Nurs. 1991;17(4):355–8.
7. Hedin H, Larsson S. Technique and considerations when using external fixation as a standard treatment of femoral fractures in children. Injury Int J Care Injured. 2004;35:1255–63.
8. Alcivar E. A new method of external fixation for proximal fractures of the femur. Injury Int J Care Injured. 2001;32(4):SD107–14, 354.
9. W-Dahl A, Toksvig-Larsen S. Pin site care in external fixation sodium chloride or chlorhexidine solution as a cleansing agent. Arch Orthop Trauma Surg. 2004;124:555–8.
10. Green S. Patient management during limb lengthening. Instructional Course Lectures. AAOS. 1997;46:547–54.
11. Egol KA, Paksima N, Puopolo S, Klugman J, Hiebert R, Koval KJ. Treatment of external fixation pins about the wrist: a prospective, randomized trial. JBJSA. 2006;88:349.

Chapter 12
Complications of External Fixation

G. Zych

12.1 Introduction

External fixation has assumed an important role in damage control orthopedics. Common indications include open fractures, bridging juxta-articular fractures or dislocations, and pelvic external fixation. Complications may ensue from external fixation as with other surgical treatment. It is important for the surgeon to be aware of these potential complications and to manage them appropriately to achieve a successful outcome.

12.2 Pin Track Problems

External fixation systems function by external anchorage to the bone via various types of pins. The pins are connected to an external frame through various couplings. All of these systems are visible as frameworks surrounding the extremities or pelvis.

It has been shown that the most important determinant of frame stiffness, and therefore the ability to resist elastic deformation of the bone, is the fixation of the pin to bone [1, 2]. Mechanical loosening or infection can affect the integrity of the pin–bone interface. Either of these factors may produce loss of frame stability. There is controversy whether loosening occurs first and then infection, or vice versa. Pins that must pass through a large thickness of soft tissue, as would be found in the thigh and pelvis, tend to have a higher prevalence of infection. Some patients will

G. Zych
Department of Orthopaedic Trauma, University of Miami Leonard M Miller School of Medicine, Miami, FL, USA
e-mail: gzych@med.miami.edu

D. Seligson et al. (eds.), *External Fixation in Orthopedic Traumatology*,
DOI 10.1007/978-1-4471-2197-8_12, © Springer-Verlag London Limited 2012

develop a condition termed "pan-pin cellulitis" in which all fixation pins become simultaneously infected without antecedent loosening. The etiology of this is unknown but can be treated with several days of intravenous antibiotics.

12.2.1 Pin Drainage

Any metallic pin that traverses soft tissue before entering a bone has the potential to have wound drainage. This potential is increased in body regions that have more soft tissue thickness, such as the thigh and pelvis. Pins inserted into a subcutaneous surface, such as the anteromedial tibia, will rarely drain unless infected. Pins that are adjacent to joints will develop drainage with joint motion due to the soft tissue movement. Some drainage is to be expected from almost any fixation pin, but when the amount increases progressively, this is a good indication that there is either loosening or infection.

Many methods of pin–skin interface care have been recommended, and all have been reported to have good results [3–8]. Various cleansing agents, such as dilute hydrogen peroxide, normal saline, povidone, and soap, have been suggested. What seems to be important is to avoid the buildup of a crust (composed of desiccated tissue fluids) around the pin–skin interface. The goal should be to maintain the same degree of cleanliness of the skin as any other body region.

12.2.2 Pin Infection

The prevalence of external fixation pin infection varies from 2% to 83% [9–16]. Factors implicated to be associated with infection are improper pin insertion technique, poor maintenance of the pin–skin interface, mechanical loosening, and compromised host. Prevention of infection is key and can be subdivided into preoperative, intraoperative, and postoperative interventions [17]. These interventions can include preference of fine wire pins over half pins in patients with higher risk of infection (obese, immunocompromised, diabetics), insertion of pins in areas well covered by soft tissue, cooling of pins during insertion, avoiding tension on the skin around pin sites, and having a good interface between pins and bone, among other well-described prevention measures. The postoperative care of pin sites will be reviewed in Chap. 12.

The spectrum of pin infection ranges from mild superficial to deep with osteomyelitis [3].

Early pin infection usually presents with subjective complaints of increasing pain and pin drainage. Physical examination demonstrates pin-track drainage with local signs of inflammation: erythema, tenderness, and, possibly, induration (Fig. 12.1). Focal radiographs of the pin site should be done but usually have negative findings. Treatment should consist of culture of the pin track if the drainage is copious and administration of antibiotics. *Staphylococcus aureus* is the most common cause of pin infection and, therefore, empirical therapy should begin with an antibiotic effective against this organism and be adjusted if necessary, according to

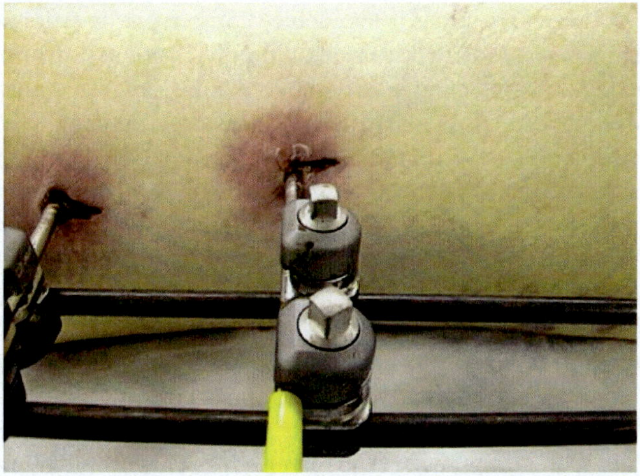

Fig. 12.1 Pin-track drainage with local signs of inflammation: erythema, tenderness, and, possibly, induration

the sensitivity. If an outpatient, many surgeons will prescribe an antibiotic to take as soon as the first signs of infection appear. The duration of antibiotic is at least several days and dependent on the clinical response.

Patients that have more advanced pin infection present with gross purulent drainage and signs of a typical local abscess. This degree of infection will only respond to aggressive treatment consisting of pin removal and local debridement of the soft tissue and bone with relocation of the pin, if needed. Focal osteomyelitis is present, and bone debridement is crucial to eradicate the infection. At this stage, it is not uncommon to see loosening of the pin–bone interface, which will be visualized radiographically as lysis around the pin (Figure of pin loosening and advanced pin infection). In a recent randomized control trial [18], 120 wrists managed with the placement of an external fixation device for a displaced, unstable, distal radial fracture were randomized into weekly dry dressing changes without pin-site care; daily pin-site care with a solution of one-half normal saline solution and one-half hydrogen peroxide; and treatment with the placement of chlorhexidine-impregnated discs (Biopatch) around the pins, with weekly changes of the discs by the treating surgeon. Twenty-three patients (19%) had a complication related to the pin track, with twelve of these patients requiring oral antibiotics for the treatment of a pin-track infection. There were no significant differences among the three groups with regard to the prevalence of pin-site complications. The age of the patient was found to be significantly associated with an increased risk of postoperative pin-track complications ($p=0.04$).

12.2.3 Pin Loosening

Stability of external fixation frames is dependent on the purchase of the fixation pins in the bone. Mechanical loosening of a pin will compromise this stability. The most frequent reason for pin loosening is pin-track infection, which has already been addressed in a previous section. Other causes are osteopenia, thermal necrosis of the bone during pin insertion, and inadvertent direct force applied to the pin.

Thermal necrosis is avoidable if proper pin insertion technique is used. The bone should be predrilled if the fixation pin is not self-drilling, or if the bone density is exceptional, manual insertion of the pin is suggested unless the specific pin has been designed to allow insertion with power equipment. The pin should be held steady during bone insertion to prevent expansion of the pin track from wobbling. Soft tissue protection with drill guides and cannulas is preferable.

Osteopenic bone presents challenges to maintenance of pin–bone integrity. Transfixation pins, those that pass through both sides of the bone and extremity, are more suitable for low-density bone. Pins should be inserted in the best available bone, which is usually found in the diaphysis or shaft. Hydroxyapatite-coated pins have been shown to have superior pullout strength in metaphyseal locations and represent an alternative for compromised bone [19–22]. Fixation pins that are located in the feet and hands are particularly vulnerable to being struck unintentionally with normal use of the extremities. This problem may be partially prevented by cutting these pins as short as possible, in the given bone, to resist these bending forces.

Regardless of the cause, pins that become loose do not contribute to frame stability and will often become infected. Loose pins should be removed as soon as recognized and new ones inserted, if clinically indicated.

12.3 Loss of Fracture or Joint Position

Generally in damage control orthopedics (DCO), external fixation is utilized for fracture or joint immobilization [24]. The injured tissues are stabilized from without and can undergo resuscitation prior to secondary surgical repair or are treated definitively with the external fixation frame. At anytime during this course, the initial fracture reduction or joint position can be lost. Minor degrees of loss may be tolerated and be dependent on the clinical situation. More significant degrees of change may be unacceptable and demand repeat surgical intervention.

The most common reason for the loss of reduction is inadequate frame stability caused by poor external fixator construction with too few fixation pins or stabilizing connecting rods. Generally, a minimum of two pins in each bone segment is needed in the diaphysis and at least one (preferably two) in most metaphyseal segments. The type of pin clamps used determines the distance between the pins. Multiple pin clamps are somewhat limited in the placement of pins far apart, and independent pin clamps are more able to spread the pins apart in the bone. Stable fixation blocks, consisting of two pins attached to a connecting rod, are then linked to each other via additional connecting rods, creating the external fixator. The concept is applicable regardless of the anatomic location of the external frame. When the injury site is close to the adjacent joint, it is better to extend the frame across the joint for improved stability.

Some pin clamp connections will become loose within the first 48 h after initial application due to mechanical creep. All clamps should be checked for tightness in the early postapplication period.

Typically, the most stable position for a fracture or joint is the normal anatomic position. The surgeon should strive to obtain an anatomic reduction since in many patients, another operative procedure to correct loss of reduction may be delayed due to the trauma patients' worsening medical condition. Femoral and tibial fractures that will have definitive secondary intramedullary nailing need slight distraction for maintenance of length and ease of reduction. Joint dislocations that have been bridged with an external frame and are still unstable will benefit from the passage of a transarticular smooth Steinmann pin. Either fluoroscopic or plain radiographs of the injury site reduction and all pin insertions are mandatory before leaving the operating room in all cases. Once the frame has been applied, it is imperative to test the stability by manually stressing the frame. Any excess motion of the segments needs to be addressed by additional pins or connecting rods. Frame stability and fracture reduction will never be better than at the conclusion of the initial application. All fixation frames should be checked for clamp tightness within 48 h of application.

Patients that are voluntarily or involuntarily noncompliant pose special challenges. Thrashing of the externally fixed extremities about the hospital bed can produce mechanical loosening of the pins or clamps or even plastic deformation of the pin (bending). Aside from physical restraints, the only other strategy is to "overbuild" the frame to counteract the unusual forces from this activity. These types of patients should have weekly radiographs to check the reduction.

12.4 Joint Contractures

Joint contractures of the externally fixed extremities arise from two scenarios. One, the joint was immobilized in an undesirable position, and two, an adjacent joint was not immobilized with the frame.

In most cases, joints should be immobilized in the resting neutral position, with the knee at 0° of extension and the ankle at 0° of flexion (Fig. 12.2). In some extraordinary situations, the joint may be positioned in some amount of flexion to maintain the reduction. Extremes of flexion should be avoided.

Equinus deformity, fixed plantar flexion, of the ankle is exceedingly common with any type of lower extremity trauma. Patients with neurological deficits, traumatic brain injury, and pain are especially susceptible to this complication. It is, for the most part, completely avoidable by extension of the external fixation frame to bridge across the ankle. This may be accomplished by a single half pin inserted into the first metatarsal base or combined with either a half or transfixation pin inserted

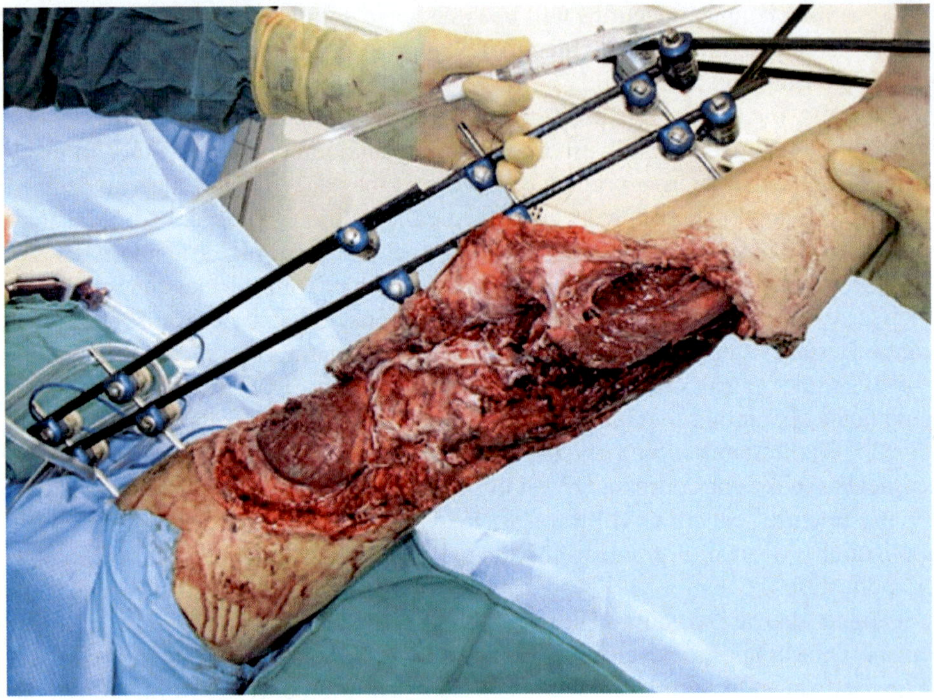

Fig. 12.2 A typical bridge or "spanning" external fixator for a open knee fracture dislocation

into the calcaneus. The bridging part of the frame can be used temporarily until the patient is able to actively move the ankle. Some patients will benefit from toe loops, which prevent the toes from developing flexion contractures.

12.5 Neurological and Vascular Injuries

Neurological and vascular structures are at risk for injury from improper fixation pin placement [23]. There are numerous articles and textbooks that define and illustrate the "safe" pathways for pin placement, and these should be reviewed prior to application of an external fixation system.

Care should be taken during pin insertion to avoid wrapping soft tissue around drills or pins through the use of appropriate soft tissue protectors. Drill or pin depth should be controlled to prevent excessive penetration into an extremity compartment. Peripheral pulses should be checked after fixator application.

Signs of vascular injury after pin insertion may be excessive bleeding from the pin site or expanding hematoma within the involved compartment. If either of these is present, then a CT angiogram or formal arteriogram is indicated.

If a neurological deficit is detected after fixator application, suspicion should be raised that a fixation pin may have injured a nerve. The suspected pin should be removed immediately, and consideration be given to nerve exploration, the importance of which will be directly proportional to the function of the compromised nerve. The area of the proximal fibula below the knee is especially prone to nerve injury due to the location of the peroneal nerve. Special care is needed with insertion of transfixation wires, which traverse the entire extremity width.

12.6 Delayed Union and Nonunion

External fixation may be chosen to be the definitive management for periarticular fractures and some diaphyseal fractures. As such, the external fixator will serve as the primary stabilization for the fracture until complete bone healing. Premature removal of the external fixator is one of the most common causes for delayed and nonunion of the fracture. The fixation must be maintained until there is radiographic evidence of bridging callus across three of the four cortices in the diaphysis and obliteration of the fracture lines in the metaphysis. In lower extremity fractures, the external frame can be partially loosened and the patient permitted full weight bearing for several days. Absence of pain with weight bearing usually is indicative of clinical fracture union. In cases where plain radiographs are not diagnostic, focal CT scans of the fracture are excellent for visualization of fracture healing.

It is difficult to state exact time to union but most fractures have an average healing time, with outliers in both directions. Progressive fracture healing should be seen in serial radiographs along with symptomatic improvement. Gradual loss of reduction can indicate a delayed union. Most extra-articular lower extremity fractures will derive benefit from early weight bearing to maintain bone density and stimulate fracture healing. External fracture stimulation with either ultrasound or electromagnetism could be a useful adjunct in delayed fracture healing.

Patients that have intact soft tissues or those that have had successful soft tissue coverage are potential candidates for early aggressive surgery in the form of an autogenous bone graft. External fixation could be converted to intramedullary nailing in suitable fractures.

Delayed union or nonunion – these are some of the factors that are thought to be associated with a delay of fracture healing:

- Subclinical infection
- Fracture distraction
- Fracture characteristics
- Lack of weight bearing
- Excess frame rigidity or instability

12.6.1 Subclinical Infection

Patients that have had open fractures are at risk for a low-grade occult infection at the fracture site. Clinical symptoms or signs may be absent. White blood cells, sedimentation rate, or C-reactive protein may be elevated. The diagnosis may only be confirmed by deep bone or soft tissue culture. If cultures are positive, then appropriate antibiotics are indicated. Fracture site debridement is rarely needed.

12.6.2 Fracture Distraction

Ligamentotaxis or distraction has been an effective method of obtaining fracture reductions by traction of intact soft tissues. Excessive distraction, however, can lead to delay of fracture healing, especially in the diaphysis. If this is recognized, then compressing the fracture surfaces in those fractures that are amenable to axial compression should eliminate the distraction. Compression enhances stability and perhaps contributes to bone healing. Fractures with comminution or those with less than 50% cortical contact should be maintained at anatomic length or even a few millimeters of shortening to avoid distraction.

12.6.3 Fracture Characteristics

Open fractures and those caused by high-energy mechanisms are prone to develop delayed union and nonunion. Bone loss and interference with the osseous blood supply are thought to be the reasons for this problem. Prompt soft tissue coverage of open wounds will prevent bone necrosis and provide the optimal milieu for fracture healing. Bone grafting must be considered early in the treatment of these problematic fractures, especially those with bone loss.

12.6.4 Patient Characteristics

Those with nutritional deficits, those who are smokers, and those that are immunocompromised will have a greater prevalence of dysfunction with fracture healing. Many trauma patients are catabolic for prolonged periods and are protein deficient. Cigarette smoking has been recognized as a significant factor in delay of fracture healing, and patients should be counseled to stop this injurious habit.

12.6.5 Lack of Weight Bearing

The beneficial effects of weight bearing on fracture healing have been documented in several studies. As Wolff's law states, bone responds to stress, and the accompanying strain produced by the application of stress contributes to fracture healing. All patients in lower extremity external fixators should be permitted at least toe touch weight bearing gait. In stable fractures, patients are encouraged to weight bear as tolerated.

12.6.6 *Excess Frame Rigidity or Instability*

It is not exactly known which type of stress is favorable for fracture healing. Some studies have suggested that shearing forces are detrimental and this has been observed clinically. Too much rigidity, on the other hand, deprives the bone of stress, and minimal, if any, callus forms. Some flexibility in the fixator is thought to be the best compromise. The overall goal is to maintain the fracture reduction and still transfer sufficient stress to the bone to achieve fracture healing.

The weakest point, for stiffness, in an external fixator is the pin–bone interface. The external frame or superstructure is considered to be secondary in importance. Therefore, additional fixation pins and then construction of additional planes of fixation are the best strategies to obtain increased frame stability. This applies mainly to external fixators that utilize straight connecting bars, as opposed to the circular frames.

12.7 Deep Infection at the Fracture Site

Fracture site deep infection occurs through two mechanisms: original contamination in open fractures or, rarely, secondarily from an infected pin track. Prevention of this complication is most important. Open fractures require thorough debridement, and the more severe the open fracture type, the greater the necessity for serial debridement and subsequent soft tissue coverage. Despite this regimen, deep infection has a definite prevalence in open fractures.

Infection from an infected pin track is, for the most part, avoidable. Fixation pins must not be in close proximity to a fracture or violate a joint capsule. Care must be exercised, especially with a bridging knee fixator in which violation of the suprapatellar knee pouch is a real possibility. This occurs most often with half pin fixation that is oriented in the sagittal plane (anterior to posterior) and too distal in the femur. A pin inserted in the lateral to medial direction is much less likely to enter the knee capsule.

A deep fracture infection is a surgical problem with almost no role for medical treatment alone. There is much to lose if this infection is treated expectantly. Any suspicion of infection requires aggressive treatment with surgical debridement and culture-specific antibiotics. Local pharmacotherapy via antibiotic-impregnated cement beads should be employed whenever feasible.

12.8 DCO Complications from the Literature

There are relatively few studies that have addressed the complications encountered in the utilization of DCO.

Nowotarski et al. [11] did a retrospective review of fifty-nine femoral shaft fractures that were treated initially with external fixation followed by conversion to an intramedullary nail. Four fractures developed pin drainage and required fixator removal, skeletal traction for a mean of 10 days, then intramedullary nailing. The rate of deep infection was 1.7%.

Another retrospective review from the same institution compared 284 patients treated with primary intramedullary nailing versus 43 with primary external fixation of femoral shaft fractures [24]. Two complications were stated: one patient with bleeding from an external fixation pin site and another with deep infection after conversion to an intramedullary nail.

Mason et al. reported 100 patients with pelvic ring injuries that were treated with both temporary and definitive external fixation [15]. The overall complication rate for temporary fixators was 21%, with 13% pin-track problems, which "rarely led to more serious complications." More recently, 195 periarticular complex fractures were treated with temporary bridging external fixators. The total rate of complication was 11%. Problems related to the achievement of length were observed in 5% of cases. Half pin–related infection was observed in 4%. Neurovascular injury (medial calcaneal nerve injury in a distal tibia fracture) was observed in 2% of cases [25].

In 2005, Lerner et al. published their series of 198 fractures treated with definitive external fixation [14]. 135 fractures were noted to be from high energy, and 39 patients were considered to be multiply injured. The complications were superficial pin-track infections, 165 (83%); soft tissue infections requiring systemic antibiotics, 12 (6%); and pin breakage, 5 (2.5%). This series does not strictly relate to short-term usage of external fixation but does illustrate that pin problems are the predominant complication.

12.9 Conclusion

DCO has been established as a guiding principle in the management of the multiply injured patient. However, the ultimate and definitive fracture treatment should be considered prior to application of the type of DCO initially selected. The surgeon should have the long-range plan in mind (the big picture) and perhaps not jeopardize subsequent management or produce a worse outcome due to poor selection of the initial treatment. For example, placement of multiple external fixation half pins in a very short metaphyseal fracture segment may compromise definitive internal fixation. Bridging the short metaphyseal segment and the adjacent joint would permit fracture stabilization and not invade the limited bone stock [26].

Another example is a femoral shaft fracture treated initially with external fixation. If the surgeon is reasonably certain that more than 2 weeks will elapse before the patient could undergo intramedullary nailing, external fixation may become definitive treatment. The most appropriate frame configuration would be to insert the external fixation pins in a lateral to medial direction, in the coronal plane, to minimize mechanical binding of the quadriceps mechanism. This frame is ideally suited for definitive treatment of the femoral shaft fracture [27].

In general, shortening of any fracture is undesirable at the time of initial external frame application, especially in diaphyseal and juxta-articular fractures. Later attempts at restoration of anatomic length are often rather difficult.

Elaborate frame configurations are to be avoided as state-of-the-art external fixation systems are designed to provide sufficient stability with a minimal number of components. The surgeon needs to understand the distinction between DCO frames and the more complex frames that are often utilized in trauma reconstruction.

The surgeon should remember that DCO with external fixation could be the first phase in treatment followed by other types of fixation or be continued as definitive management.

References

1. Chao EY, Kasman RA, An KN. Rigidity and stress analyses of external fracture fixation devices – a theoretical approach. J Biomech. 1982;15(12):971–83.
2. Pettine KA, Chao EY, Kelly PJ. Analysis of the external fixator pin-bone interface. Clin Orthop Relat Res. 1993;Aug;(293):18–27. J Trauma. 2001(Jun);50(6):1008–14.
3. Checketts RG, MacEachern AG, Otterburn M. Pin track infection and the principles of pin site care. In: De Bastiani A, Graham Apley A, Goldberg A, editors. Orthofix external fixation in trauma and orthopaedics. Berlin/Heidelberg/New York: Springer; 2000. p. 97–103.
4. Gordon JE, Kelly-Hahn J, Carpenter CJ, Schoenecker PL. Pin site care during external fixation in children: results of a nihilistic approach. J Pediatr Orthop. 2000;20(2):163–5.
5. W-Dahl A, Toksvig-Larsen S, Lindstrand A. No difference between daily and weekly pin site care: a randomized study of 50 patients with external fixation. Acta Orthop Scand. 2003;74(6):704–8.
6. Temple J, Santy J. Pin site care for preventing infections associated with external bone fixators and pins. Cochrane Database Syst Rev. 2004;(1):CD004551.
7. Camilo AM, Bongiovanni JC. Evaluation of effectiveness of 10% polyvinylpyrrolidone-iodine solution against infections in wire and pin holes for Ilizarov external fixators. Sao Paulo Med J. 2005;123(2):58–61. Epub 2005 Jun 8.
8. Davies R, Holt N, Nayagam S, Temple J, Santy JJ. The care of pin sites with external fixation. J Bone Joint Surg Br. 2005;87(5):716–9.
9. Van den Bossche MR, Broos PL, Rommens PM. Open fractures of the femoral shaft, treated with osteosynthesis or temporary external fixation. Injury. 1995;26(5):323–5.
10. Hutson Jr JJ, Zych GA. Infections in periarticular fractures of the lower extremity treated with tensioned wire hybrid fixators. J Orthop Trauma. 1998;12(3):214–8.
11. Nowotarski PJ, Turen CH, Brumback RJ, Scarboro JM. Conversion of external fixation to intramedullary nailing for fractures of the shaft of the femur in multiply injured patients. J Bone Joint Surg Am. 2000;82(6):781–8.
12. Parameswaran AD, Roberts CS, Seligson D, Voor M. Pin tract infection with contemporary external fixation: how much of a problem? J Orthop Trauma. 2003;17(7):503–7.
13. Stavlas P, Polyzois D. Septic arthritis of the major joints of the lower limb after periarticular external fixation application: are conventional safe corridors enough to prevent it? Injury. 2005;36(2):239–47.
14. Lerner A, Chezar A, Haddad M, Kaufman H, Rozen N, Stein H. Complications encountered while using thin-wire-hybrid-external fixation modular frames for fracture fixation. A retrospective clinical analysis and possible support for "Damage Control Orthopaedic Surgery". Injury. 2005;36(5):590–8. Epub 2005 Jan 21.
15. Mason WT, Khan SN, James CL, Chesser TJ, Ward AJ. Complications of temporary and definitive external fixation of pelvic ring injuries. Injury. 2005;36(5):599–604.
16. Egol KA, Tejwani NC, Capla EL, Wolinsky PL, Koval KJ. Staged management of high-energy proximal tibia fractures (OTA types 41): the results of a prospective, standardized protocol. J Orthop Trauma. 2005;19(7):448–55, discussion 456.
17. Bibbo C, Brueggeman J. Prevention and management of complications arising from external fixation pin sites. J Foot Ankle Surg. 2010;49:87–92.

18. Egol K, Paksima N, Puopolo S, Klugmam J. Treatment of external fixation pins about the wrist: a prospective, randomized trial. J Bone Joint Surg (Am). 2006;88:349–54.
19. Moroni A, Orienti L, Stea S, Visentin M. Improvement of the bone-pin interface with hydroxyapatite coating: an in vivo long-term experimental study. J Orthop Trauma. 1996;10(4):236–42.
20. DeJong ES, DeBerardino TM, Brooks DE, Nelson BJ, Campbell AA, Bottoni CR, et al. Antimicrobial efficacy of external fixator pins coated with a lipid stabilized hydroxyapatite/chlorhexidine complex to prevent pin tract infection in a goat model. J Trauma. 2001;50(6):1008–14.
21. Pommer A, Muhr G, David A. Hydroxyapatite-coated Schanz pins in external fixators used for distraction osteogenesis: a randomized, controlled trial. J Bone Joint Surg Am. 2002;84-A(7):1162–6.
22. Cimerman M, Cor A, Ceh M, Kristan A, Pizem J, Tonin M. Microstructural analysis of implant-bone interface of hydroxyapatite-coated and uncoated Schanz screws. J Mater Sci Mater Med. 2005;16(7):627–34.
23. Green SA. Complications of external skeletal fixation. Springfield: Charles C. Thomas; 1981. p. 12–42.
24. Scalea TM, Boswell SA, Scott JD, Mitchell KA, Kramer ME. External fixation as a bridge to intramedullary nailing for patients with multiple injuries and with femur fractures: damage control orthopedics. AN J Trauma. 2000;48(4):613–21, discussion 621–3.
25. Oh JK, Hwang JH, Sahu D, Jun SH. Complication rate and pitfalls of temporary bridging external fixator in periarticular comminuted fractures. Clin Orthop Surg. 2011;3:62–8.
26. Dickson KF, Montgomery S, Field J. High energy plafond fractures treated by a spanning external fixator initially and followed by a second stage open reduction internal fixation of the articular surface – preliminary report. Injury. 2001;32 Suppl 4:SD92–8.
27. Sabharwal S, Kishan S, Behrens F. Principles of external fixation of the femur. Am J Orthop. 2005;34(5):218–23.

Chapter 13
Timing and Strategies for Definitive Fixation After a Damage Control Frame

Thomas De Coster

13.1 Introduction

Damage control orthopedics is a technique to maximize patient survival in the short term. The techniques associated with damage control typically are not the most effective for producing good long-term outcomes. Effective damage control (DC) requires techniques that are effective in the short term and the long term. The treatment pattern typically requires conversion of the initial external fixation frame to some other form of definitive fixation. This chapter describes timing and strategies for that conversion.

13.2 General Principles

External fixation can typically be applied rapidly to a wide variety of skeletal injuries with minimal soft tissue injury, minimal blood loss, and minimal systemic consequence to the cardiovascular, CNS, and pulmonary systems. Avoidance of these problems is particularly important in the immediate post-injury period. Although definitive treatment with external fixation may be possible, it is typically associated with a wide variety of long-term problems. These problems include pin track infections, delayed and nonunions, late angulation and loss of reduction, impaired mobility, and psychiatric problems. The stability of the fixation is typically insufficient to allow full weight bearing. Even when external fixation is applied thoughtfully, the frame stability as well as tethering of the muscular envelope may preclude full active range of motion.

Definitive fixation options include conversion to an intramedullary nail, plating, or conversion to a more complex external fixator frame. Problems with this conversion include infection risk, difficulty obtaining reduction, and delayed fracture healing.

T. De Coster
Division of Trauma, Department of Orthopaedics, University of New Mexico, Albuquerque, NM, USA
e-mail: tadabq@aol.com

D. Seligson et al. (eds.), *External Fixation in Orthopedic Traumatology*,
DOI 10.1007/978-1-4471-2197-8_13, © Springer-Verlag London Limited 2012

One of the biggest concerns with conversion from external to internal fixation is the potential for infection. The pin tracks of external fixation are a pathway for osteomyelitis. All external fixation pins are at least contaminated. Established pin track infections are a more severe problem and are associated with a greater risk of infection of secondary internal fixation. Fortunately, the early incidence of pin track infections is low and conversion to internal fixation within 2–4 weeks has been associated with a low incidence of infection.

With delayed internal fixation, reduction of the fracture may be impaired by the early formation of callus. Impacted fragments may be very difficult to reduce. Shortening of major fracture sites is particularly difficult to overcome. For articular fractures, a CT scan in the frames helps define the major fragments. Then a strategy can be developed for the stepwise reduction and accurate fixation of the fracture. Although exact fracture reduction is difficult with external fixation, length is relatively easy to obtain and maintain in the DC frame. Distraction is typically applied. Although distraction may impair fracture healing and joint function in the long run, it is typically quite helpful in the short term. It helps to restore normal soft tissue tension and realign fracture fragments. Distraction across joints puts tension on the ligaments which may facilitate articular reduction by ligamentotaxis. A small amount of distraction with the DC frame typically facilitates early conversion to internal fixation. For intramedullary nails, the strut effect of the nail typically restores alignment and corrects translation and angulation. Rotation is within control of the operating surgeon, and the rotational reduction obtained intraoperatively can be maintained with static locking of the nail. For plate fixation of articular fracture, the initial maintenance of length may facilitate reduction of articular fragments. The frame may be maintained intraoperatively as a distractor to assist in disimpaction of articular fragments and visualization of the articular surface. For extreme comminution and potential instability after plate fixation, the fixator may occasionally be maintained postoperatively for additional stability.

Early conversion to internal fixation typically does not require removal of a lot of healing tissue at the fracture site. With intramedullary nailing, the periosteal callus that has formed may not be disturbed at all. Plate fixation is typically done with limited dissection and maintenance of most of any healing callus that has already formed. Locking plate fixation provides relative stability, and healing by periosteal callus is more pronounced than the primary healing reported for traditional compression plating. Although time to fracture healing is difficult to measure exactly in plated fractures, there is evidence that the ultimate time to union is no greater in patients treated with staged plating compared to immediate plating.

There are two major benefits to staged treatment: it causes a reduction in local and systemic complications. The soft tissue injury associated with fractures may be worsened by an early surgical approach with soft tissue dissection. After several days of healing, the soft tissue envelope may be better able to tolerate a surgical approach and heal more predictably. Another benefit of delayed internal fixation is declaration of wound status. Many soft tissue injuries heal, while others develop skin slough and infection. It is difficult to determine the prognosis for many limbs at the time of initial injury. Soft tissue loss that results in exposed internal fixation is particularly prone to infection. With staged internal fixation there is time for the wound to demarcate.

Secondary debridements can be done as needed and the ultimate soft tissue defect determined prior to internal fixation. If fracture blisters develop, these can be allowed to heal and the soft tissue swelling to resolve prior to performing the dissection of internal fixation. If a free flap or other soft tissue reconstruction is required, this can be determined prior to internal fixation with a reduction in the incidence of exposed implant and chronic infection. The contrarian view is that the initial debridement should be complete and that secondary sloughs are indication of failure adequately to cut out marginal tissue in the zone of injury. There is reliance then on plastic surgical procedures – free flaps, rotational flaps, fascio-cutaneous flaps – to reestablish the tissue envelope of the limb. The truth lies in between these extremes: early complete debridement with plastic surgery reconstruction and staged, serial wound care with late soft tissue procedures. Probably, new technology will assist decision making by providing parametric assessment of tissue viability. Experience and "big picture" thinking are indispensable to guiding therapy for complex limb injury.

Similarly, the patient's overall status may not tolerate early operative stabilization of all musculoskeletal injuries. After several weeks, the patient's general condition has typically recovered to allow safe intervention. It is also easier to prioritize secondary fixation, and this may require several sequential returns to the OR for conversion of various fractures to internal fixation one at a time.

In a recent survey conducted by the OTA [1], 255 members were asked about the time to definitive fixation after the placement of temporary external fixator for distal femur fractures. Most of the surgeons (70%) responded for 1–7 days, while 30% applied the external fixator for 8–14 days. For tibial plateau fractures, definitive reconstruction occurred at an average of 8–14 days according to 71.2% of respondents and 1–7 days according to 17.1% of respondents. Average time to definitive fixation after the placement of temporary external fixator for tibial plafond fractures was estimated at 8–14 days in 57.7% of responses and 15–21 days in 38.1% of responses.

13.3 Examples

I. Femur shaft fracture with CHI (closed head injury)
II. Distal tibia (pilon) fracture
III. Knee dislocation
IV. Floating elbow and wrist (ipsilateral humerus, radius, ulna fractures)

I. A 25-year-old male with multiple trauma after a car wreck. His injuries include a left femur shaft fracture (Fig. 13.1) and closed head injury with ISS (injury severity score) of 20 and GCS (Glasgow coma scale) of 4. His initial treatment includes a craniotomy and external fixation of his femur shaft (Figs. 13.2–13.4) with respiratory support on a ventilator. After 6 days, his neurologic status improves and he is weaned from the ventilator. On post-injury day 7 the external fixator is removed and an antegrade locked intramedullary nail is placed (Figs. 13.5–13.7). The patient begins ROM (range of motion) and ambulation. At 6 weeks he is ambulatory and has returned to work part time. At 4 months his fracture has healed. At 6 months he is back to normal activity and function.

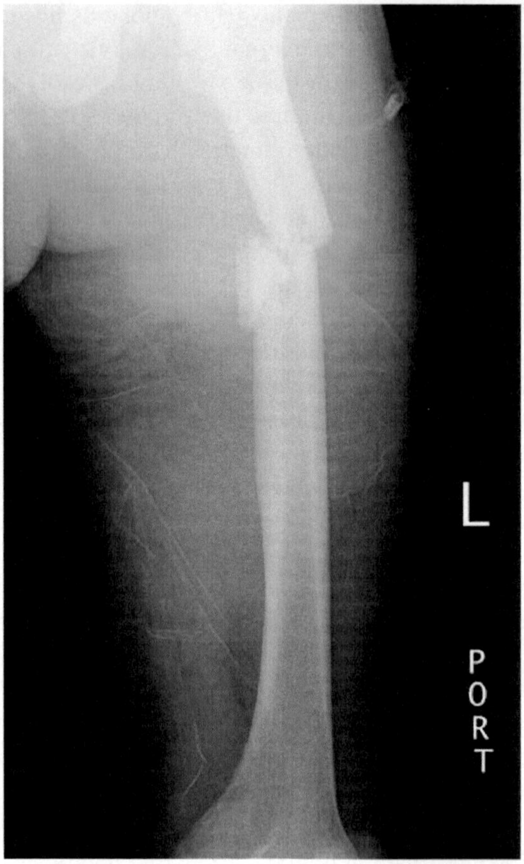

Fig. 13.1 Femoral shaft fracture

Algorithm for timing and strategies for conversion of external fixator to an intramedullary nail for femur shaft fractures.

A. Standard technique

1. Damage control frame is typically two 6-mm half pins in the proximal and distal fragments placed from laterally and connected with two connecting rods, making sure to achieve slight distraction to facilitate later passage of the IM nail.
2. If the femur shaft fracture is open, then debridement should be performed early.
3. If there are associated fractures (distal femur, proximal tibia, tibia shaft, etc.) then the frame can be extended with additional pins and connecting rods across the knee to the tibia.
4. The simple frames can be applied quickly with minimal blood loss or soft tissue damage, minimizing fat embolization, time in the operating room, or problems with hemodynamic instability or temperature control. The frame should be of sufficient stability to withstand the muscle spasms commonly associated with head injuries, and postoperative radiographs should be checked regularly.

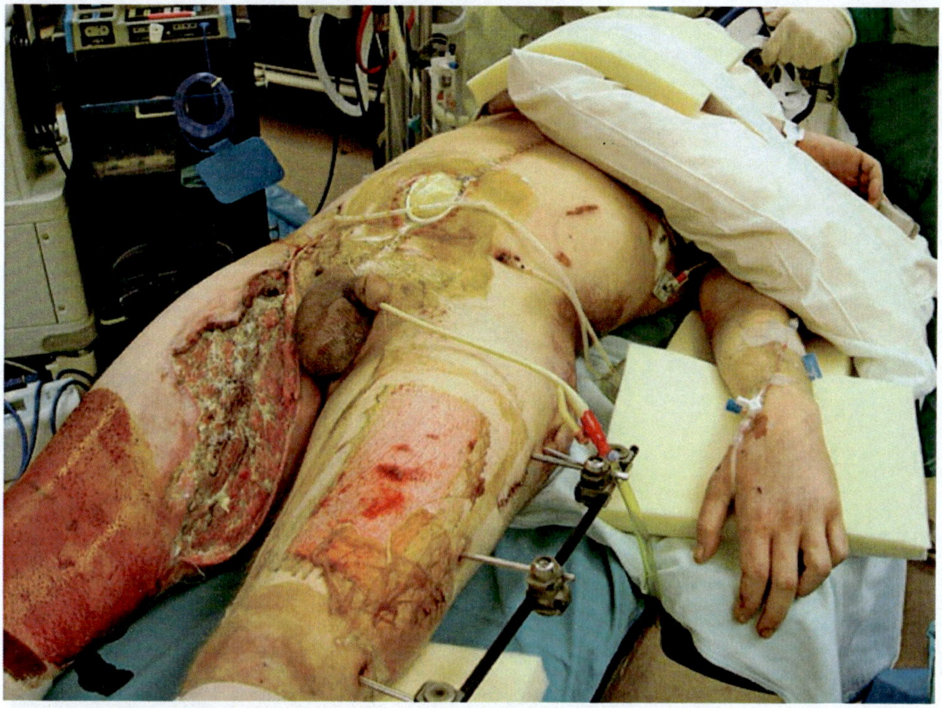

Fig. 13.2 External fixator placement

5. The frame should be supported by an external brace and the patient's limb should not be lifted by the fixator. This is a portable traction frame and not definitive fixation, and it should be treated as such.
6. The most common time for conversion to a nail is 1 week. The timing in an individual patient is primarily determined by resolution/stabilization of the neurologic status; the patient's overall condition and pulmonary status; and the number, severity, and priority of other skeletal injuries. The external fixator typically provides adequate stability to femur shaft fractures such that conversion to a nail is typically of secondary priority. Other injuries may need to be addressed before conversion. Similarly, if the patient's pulmonary or neurologic status remains unstable for a prolonged time, it is possible to safely make the conversion to a nail even 4–6 weeks after injury.
7. The frame can be removed as the initial step and standard IM nailing performed. In very unstable fractures, the frame may be maintained during positioning. The proximal pins can be used to manipulate the proximal fragment into an adducted position and remove unwanted flexion to facilitate proximal entry. The proximal pins can be removed and the distal pins utilized as a handle on the distal fragment to reduce the fracture and facilitate passage of the ball-tipped guide. The pins should be removed before reaming.

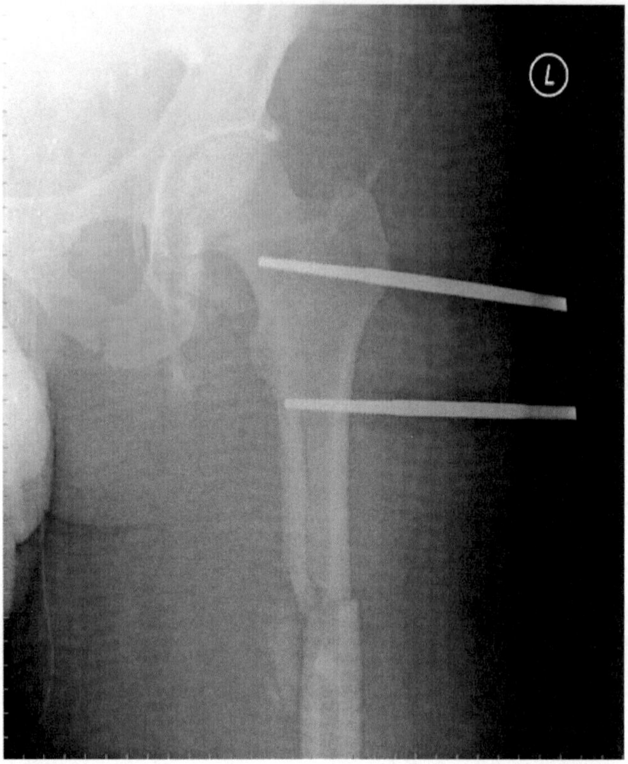

Fig. 13.3 Radiograph of external fixator pins in proximal femur

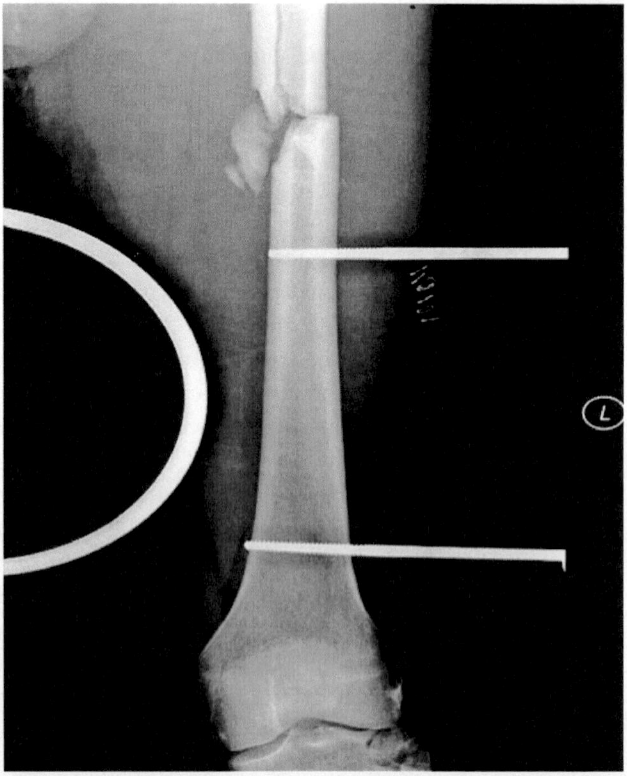

Fig. 13.4 Radiograph of external fixator pins in distal femur

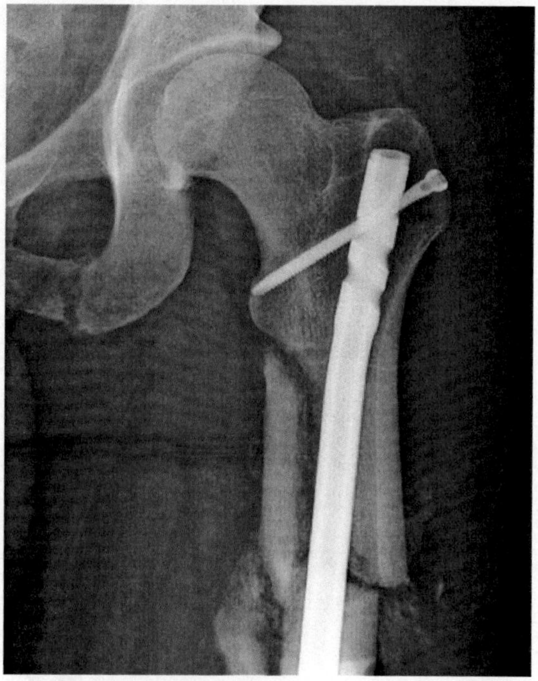

Fig. 13.5 AP radiograph of left hip at 4 weeks postoperative

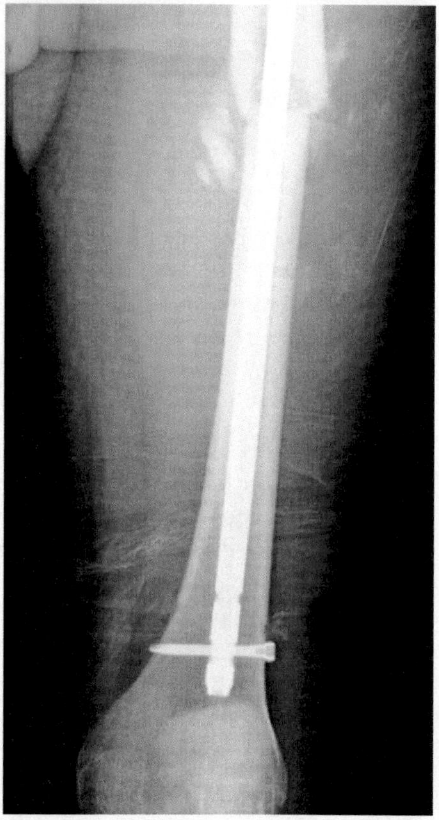

Fig. 13.6 AP radiograph of left femur at 4 weeks postoperative

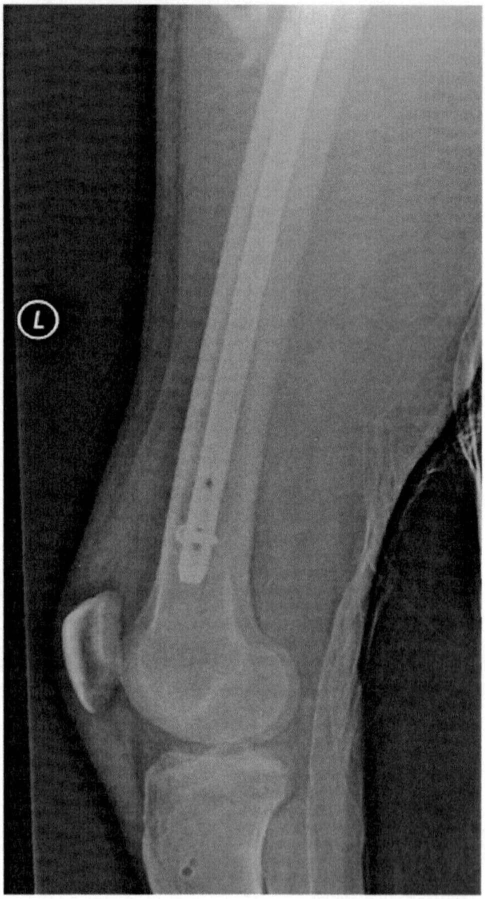

Fig. 13.7 Lateral radiograph of left femur at 4 weeks postoperative

8. If there has been a problem with pin track drainage or the pins have been in place for more than 2 weeks, overdrilling of the pin tracks after pin removal but before placement of the nail may debride the pin tracks and minimize the risk of subsequent infection.

B. Alternative strategy when early conversion is possible

1. In some situations, the patient stabilizes rapidly and conversion to an IM nail may be performed in a few days.
2. Care should be taken to avoid the "double hit" phenomena that has been associated with fat embolism syndrome. The theory is that pneumatocytes are stimulated by an initial exposure to medullary fat and are activated for several days. A second dose of medullary contents may produce a profound inflammatory response by these activated pneumatocytes and severe ARDS (Adult respiratory distress syndrome).

C. Alternative strategy when conversion is delayed more than 2 weeks

1. A staged conversion may be required in this situation to avoid an infected medullary nail.

2. At 4 weeks the external fixator is removed and the pin tracks are debrided and cultures obtained.
3. A traction pin is placed to maintain length and antibiotics are given.
4. If the cultures are negative a minimally reamed intramedullary nail is placed.
5. If cultures are positive, a repeat debridement and biopsy is performed and antibiotics are given for a longer period of time.
6. If the second cultures are negative, minimally reamed intramedullary nail is placed.
7. If the second culture is positive, a third debridement is performed, the medullary canal is reamed, and antibiotic beads or an antibiotic nail is placed.
8. If the culture is negative, an intramedullary nail is placed after 2 weeks.
9. If the third culture is positive, then treatment with an external fixator after more extensive debridement is performed.
10. Alternative, definitive fixation with a plate may be appropriate.

D. Alternative strategy when soft tissue coverage is difficult
E. Alternative strategy when there is segmental bone defect

1. A1 (shortening plus lengthening)
2. Shortening of the limb with primary wound closure
3. Application of distraction osteogenesis frame and lengthening back to normal. Regenerate forms at the corticotomy site while healing occurs at the fracture site.
4. A2 (bone transport).
5. Application of a distraction osteogenesis frame at normal length with bone transport to fill in the traumatic segmental bone defect.
6. Bone transport may fill the soft tissue defect, or coverage may be obtained by rotation or free flap.
7. A3
8. Either A1 or A2 may be accelerated by bifocal lengthening or transport. The soft tissue structures (nerves, vessels, muscle, etc.) are returning to their preinjury length and the rate of limited by formation of bone at each regenerate site of approximately 1 mm/day.

F. Alternative strategy when infection develops

1. More extensive and repeat debridement is typically required.
2. Implantation of antibiotic impregnated beads can be helpful at dead space management and to provide a high level of antibiotics at the injury site that may have poor circulation.
3. Conversion of the DC frame to a more stable and durable frame may allow treatment to healing in an external fixator.
4. The external fixator may be used until the soft tissue problem or infection is resolved. Staged conversion to internal fixation may then be used for delayed or nonunions of the bone.
5. Conversion of the DC frame to a stable and durable frame for bone transport may be useful in posttraumatic segmental bone defect cases.

G. Alternative strategy when pulmonary compromise is prolonged

1. In this situation, conversion to a plate may be indicated. Plating avoids extensive medullary manipulation and the potential for pulmonary compromise by fat embolism.
2. Healing rates and return of functional range of motion are nearly as good with plates as nails.
3. Prolonged limitation of weight bearing is typically advised until the fracture is healed (about 4 months) as the plate is a load-bearing device and early weight bearing is associated with a higher rate of fatigue failure of the plate or screws or screw–bone interface.
4. Locking plates are particularly attractive in this indication.

II. Distal tibia (pilon) fracture

A 30-year-old male falls from a roof sustaining a fracture of his right distal tibia. It is comminuted, intra-articular, and displaced with extension into the shaft (Figs. 13.8 and 13.9). The metaphysic is comminuted and the fibula is fractured 6 cm proximal to the joint. There are poke holes laterally and anteromedially.

A. Standard strategy

1. A DC external fixator is applied with half pins in the tibia shaft and a transfixation pin in the calcaneus with a triangular frame (Fig. 13.10) on the day of injury.
2. Restoration of length and axial alignment is provided by distraction (Figs. 13.11 and 13.12).
3. The wounds are debrided.
4. After several days, the extent of soft tissue injury will be clearer and the swelling will begin to resolve.
5. After 10 days, the soft tissue envelope is typically thought to be safe for internal fixation with a plate on the tibia and fibula.
6. Locking plates appear advantageous to avoid late angulation.
7. Percutaneous placement of plates appears advantageous as wound breakdown can still be a problem even after waiting until the soft tissue appears safe (Figs. 13.13–13.15).

B. Alternative with early fibula fixation

1. At the time of spanning XF application, the fibula may be plated in an anatomically reduced position. This incision is typically thought to be well tolerated by the soft tissue. Fibular reduction and fixation helps to reduce the tibial fragments and augment the stability provided by the DC fixator.
2. Care must be taken to avoid malreduction of the fibula as that will preclude later anatomic reduction of the tibia.
3. Early fibula fixation is associated with some problems. Wound healing may be problematic. Delayed union or varus angulation of the tibia may result if the XF is maintained until healing, as seen in a tibia shaft fracture with an intact fibula.

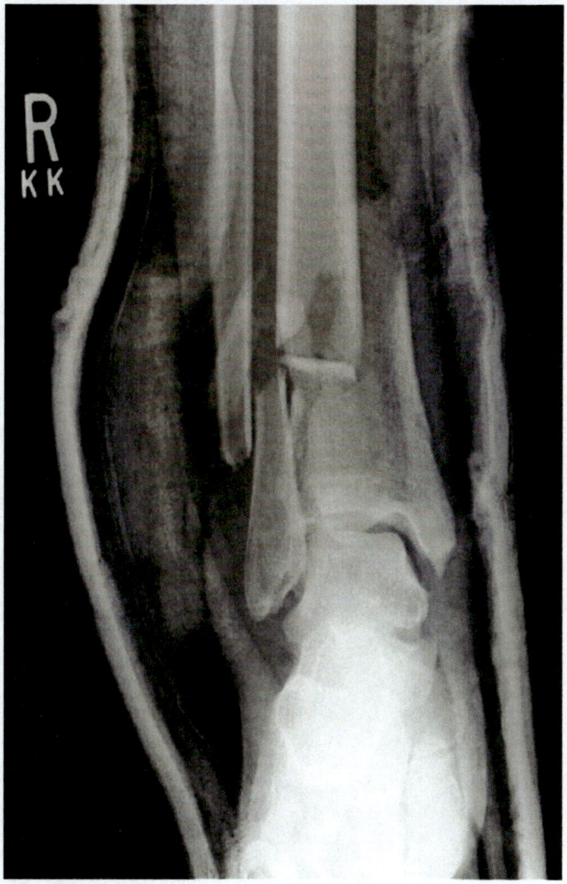

Fig. 13.8 AP radiograph of right comminuted pilon fracture

C. Alternative with articulated external fixation [2]

1. The injury can be treated to healing in an external fixation frame.
   (a) The frame is applied on the day of injury with half pins in the antero-medial tibia shaft.
   (b) Half pins are also applied in the medial calcaneus and talus spanning the posterior tibial neurovascular bundle and immobilizing the subtalar joint in a neutral position.
   (c) The talus pin is placed in the junction of the head and neck, halfway between the dorsal and plantar cortex, parallel to the dome of the talus, and perpendicular to the foot and tibia shaft.
   (d) Axial alignment is restored, and slight distraction is applied to effect an articular reduction by ligamentotaxis.
   (e) Open wounds are debrided and dressings applied.
2. The fibula is stabilized in a reduced position when indicated including
   (a) When there is gross instability after application of the XF
   (b) When there is lateral subluxation of the talus or distal tibia that cannot be controlled by the XF

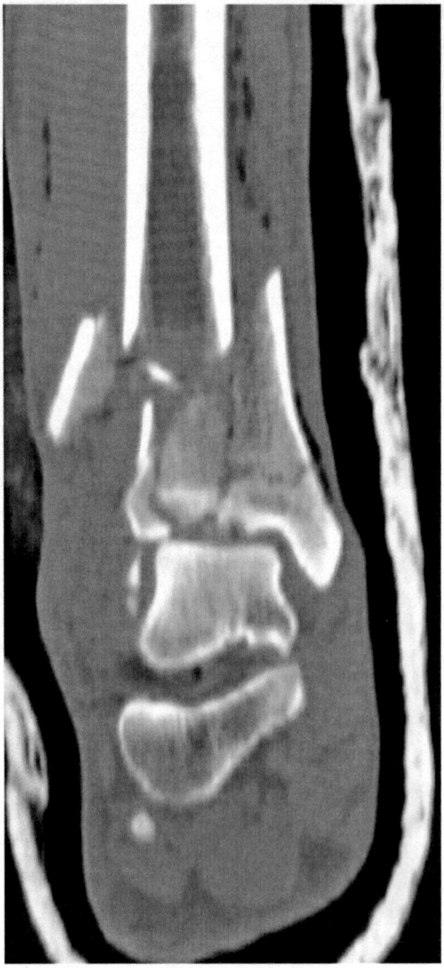

Fig. 13.9 Computerized tomography (coronal view) showing the intra-articular component of a right pilon fracture

(c) When there is a large tibia fragment that displaces with the fibula and does not reduce with distraction

3. A CT scan can be obtained in the frame to identify major fracture fragment location and displacement and allow development of a plan for articular reconstruction and internal fixation.
4. After several days, reduction and internal fixation of the articular surface is accomplished through fracture windows and percutaneous techniques. Extra distraction is temporarily applied, and the talar dome is used as a surface to guide articular reduction.
5. Midfoot equinus is prevented by a brace or early foot flat touchdown ambulation in compliant patients.
6. Ankle ROM with the articulated XF is begun after early healing has occurred after 4 weeks.
7. Partial weight bearing is allowed after 6 weeks in compliant patients and advanced about 20 lb per week.

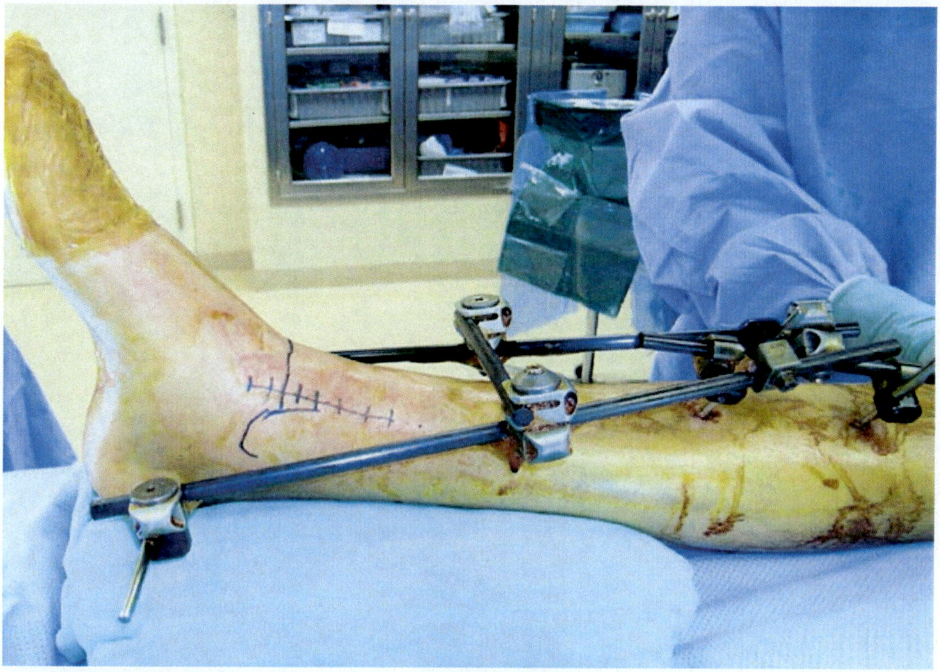

Fig. 13.10 Clinical picture of a bridging external fixator applied as a damage control frame on this right open pilon fracture

8. The external fixator is removed when the fracture appears radiographically healed at 12–14 weeks.
9. Orthotics and progressive increase in activity promote rehabilitation.
10. This treatment strategy is particularly effective in highly comminuted fractures (OTA type C) or those associated with severe soft tissue injury.

D. Alternative with ring fixator

1. The initial frame may be converted to a stable definitive treatment ring fixator.
2. The frame may be limited to the tibia and fibula or span the ankle joint with fixation into the foot.
3. Hybrid frames with half pins proximally and tensioned wires distally can be used.
4. At least three wires and four half pins in two planes should be used for adequate frame stability.
5. Tensioned olive wires are useful at reducing displaced fragments and stabilizing the fibula.
6. Articular fragment reduction may be done through limited or more extensive approaches with fixation by a combination of internal fixation screws and tensioned wires.
7. Partial weight bearing is allowed when early healing has occurred at 6 weeks.
8. The frame is removed in the OR after 12 weeks when radiographic healing is apparent.

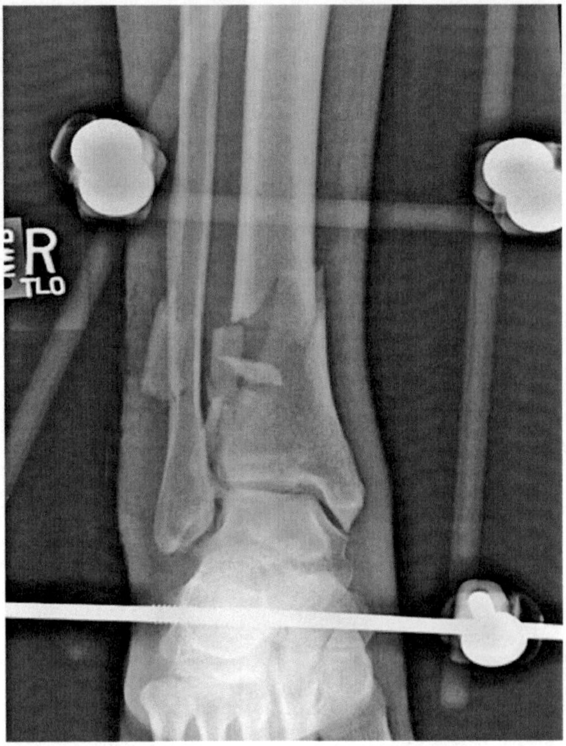

Fig. 13.11 AP radiograph following the closed reduction and application of external fixation

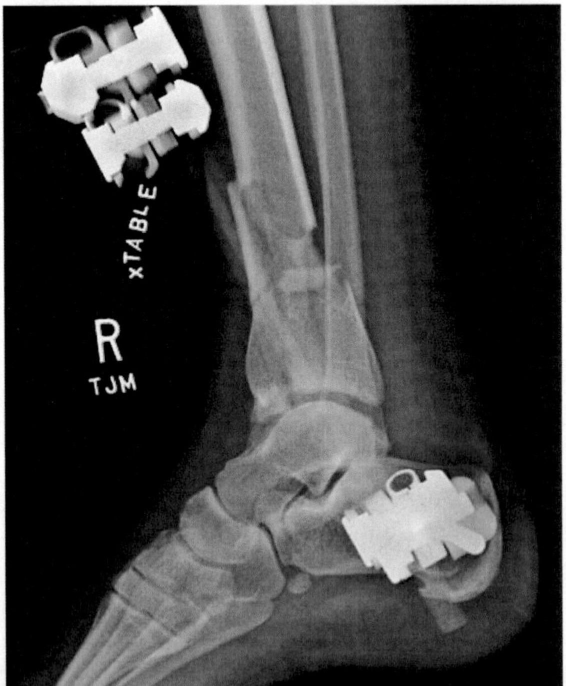

Fig. 13.12 Lateral radiograph following the closed reduction and application of external fixation

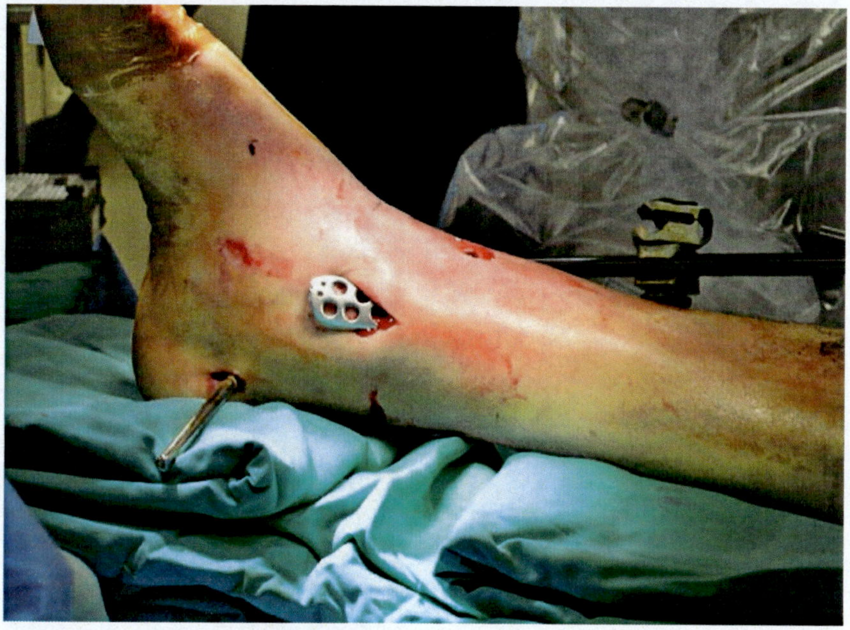

Fig. 13.13 Percutaneous insertion of locking plate

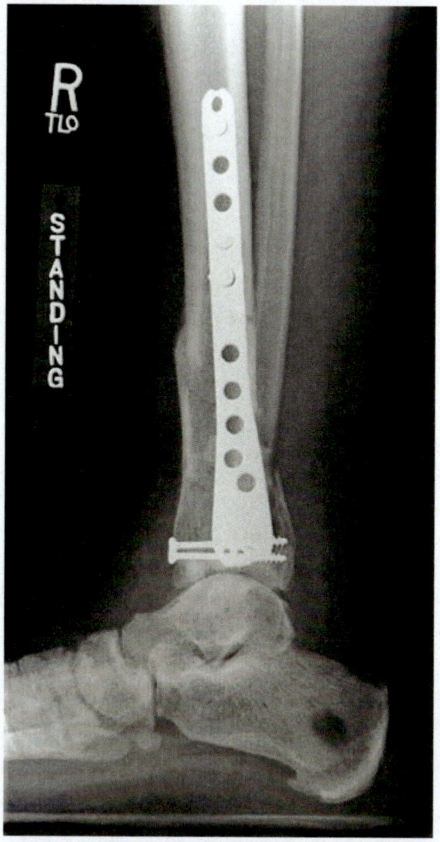

Fig. 13.14 Lateral radiograph at 10 days post ORIF

Fig. 13.15 AP radiograph at 10 days post ORIF

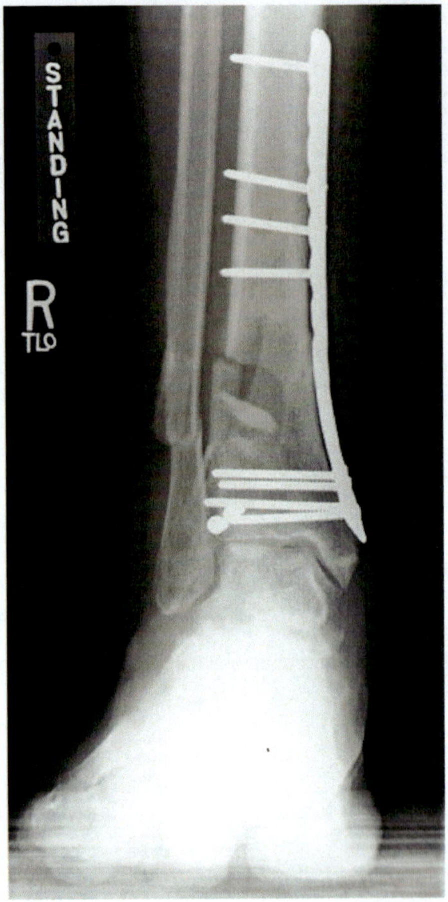

III. Knee dislocation

A 20-year-old male ejected from a car crash sustains multiple trauma including a head injury, right femur shaft open fracture and left knee dislocation (Figs. 13.16 and 13.17) with disruption of the popliteal artery.

a. Standard protocol [3].
b. The right femur is treated by damage control external fixator (Figs. 13.18 and 13.19), debridement of the open wound and staged conversion as noted previously.
c. Ligamentous assessment of the left knee is made under anesthesia.
d. The left knee is treated with arterial repair, four-compartment fasciotomies of the leg, and application of a knee spanning external fixator.
e. Half pins are placed anterolaterally in the femur and anteromedially in the tibia and a two connection rod frame constructed.
f. Care is taken to make certain the tibia is not posterior subluxated at the end of the case.
g. The fasciotomy incisions are closed or grafted when swelling allows after 1–2 weeks.
h. The fixator is removed after 10 weeks, the pin tracks are debrided and an exam under anesthesia is performed to assess ligamentous stability and ROM.

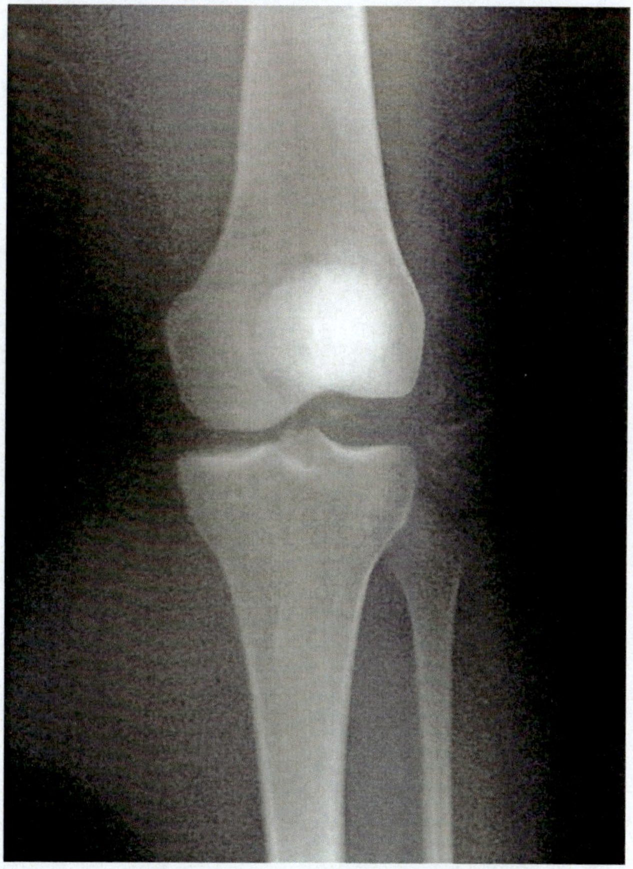

Fig. 13.16 AP radiograph of dislocated knee

i. Manipulation of the knee to regain ROM is performed, and a brace is applied.
j. After 3 months, the patient is reassessed and any functional instability is addressed by ligamentous reconstruction (Figs. 13.20 and 13.21).

A. Alternative with hinged fixator [4]

1. A hinged fixator may be utilized which allows stabilization and knee motion following or during the course of a ligament reconstruction.
2. The hinged fixator may be applied at the time of initial treatment in cases of isolated knee dislocation or as a conversion in complex dislocations or multiple trauma.
3. Hinged fixator application technique: it is important that the external fixator pin sites will not interfere with the ACL/PCL tunnel sites (during future ligament reconstruction).
4. Hinged fixator management: physical therapy regimen that featured early motion of the knee beginning with a range of zero to 30° in a continuous passive motion machine on postoperative day one. Motion was increased by no more than 10° per day, with a goal of at least a 90° arc of motion within 6 weeks. Approximately 6 weeks following the initial reconstruction, the external fixator is removed.

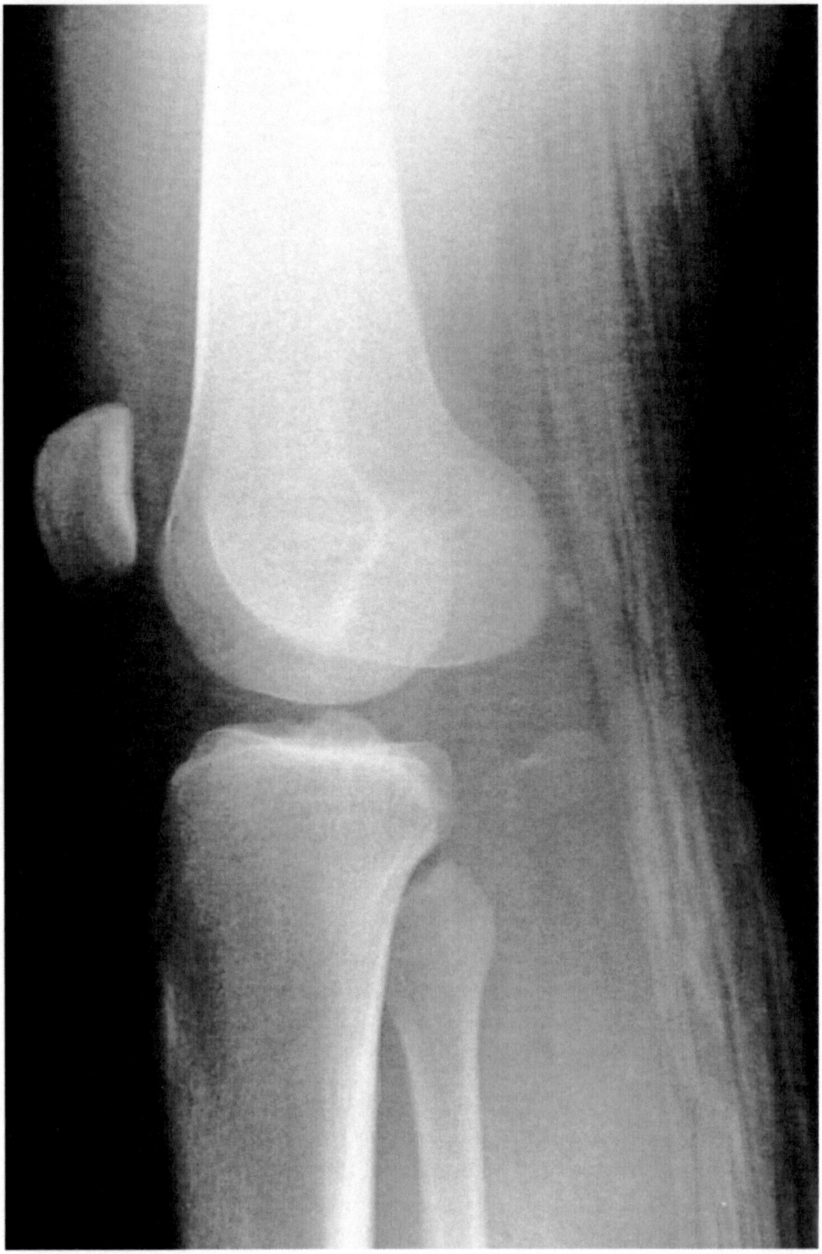

Fig. 13.17 Lateral radiograph of knee dislocation

Biomechanical studies have shown that the fixators were able to significantly decrease the forces in both the ACL and PCL in response to standard clinical stress tests, indicating a load-sharing protective effect of the fixator which may prove beneficial after multiple ligament reconstructions for knee dislocations.

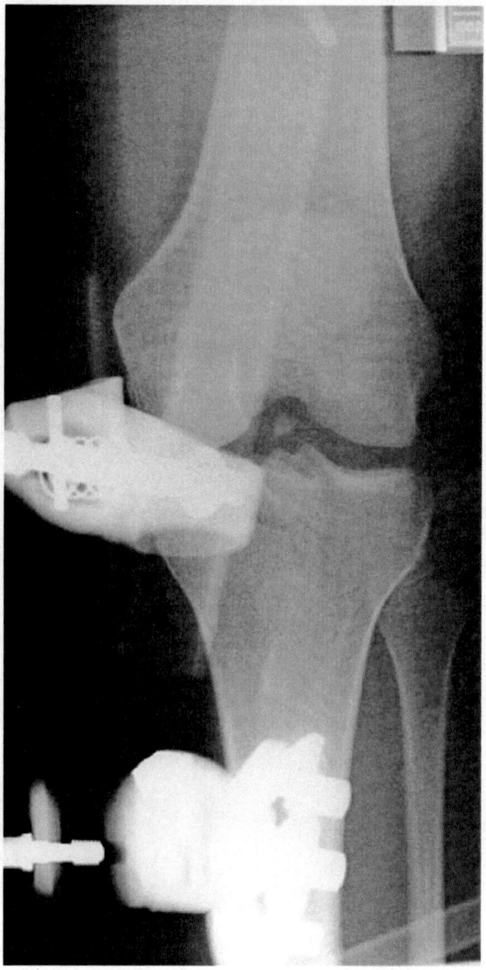

Fig. 13.18 AP radiograph of left knee post closed reduction and application of external fixator

B. Alternative with early conversion to ligamentous stabilization

1. Early conversion to ligamentous stabilization may be performed in compliant patients with high activity demand not afflicted by associated injuries or complications.
2. Most knee dislocations involve rupture of the ACL and PCL, and many have injuries to the MCL, LCL, PLC, or other knee structures.
3. A wide variety of combinations of ligamentous stabilization protocols have been utilized, including repairs and reconstructions.

    (a) Repair of collaterals and avulsions with

        (1) Allograft reconstruction of ACL and PCL (repair or reconstruct every injured structure)
        (2) PCL reconstruction
        (3) ACL reconstruction only

Fig. 13.19 Lateral radiograph of left knee post closed reduction and application of external fixator

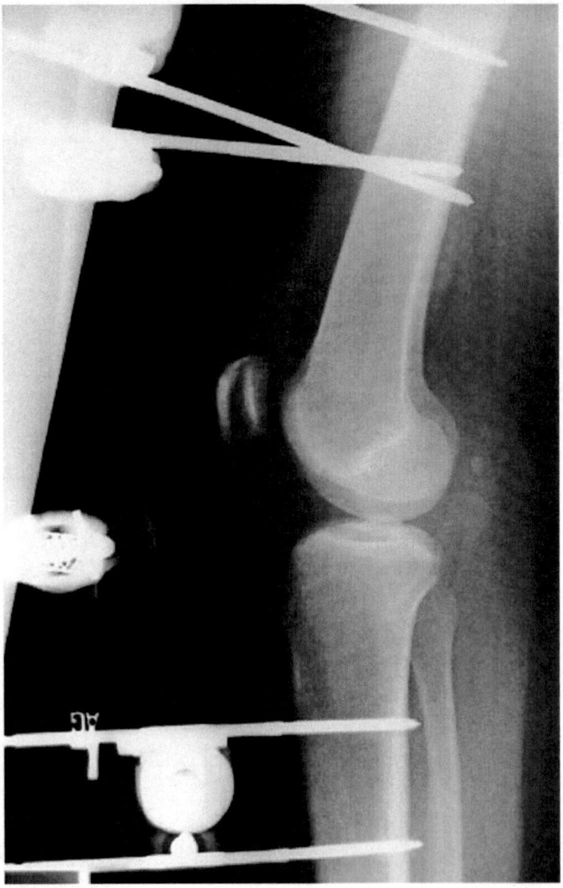

(b) Allograft reconstruction of cruciates only
   (i) Acute
   (ii) Delayed (after collaterals and other structures heal and knee motion regained)

(c) Staged reconstruction including one cruciate acutely and the other on a delayed basis

(d) Ligamentous repair and reconstruction augmented by hinged fixator for early controlled motion.

IV Monomelic injuries

A 30-year-old female involved in a T-bone car wreck with her left arm out the window sustaining fractures of the humerus shaft, the proximal ulna (open olecranon with shaft extention) and distal radius. She has an LCII pelvic ring disruption and a CHI. Sensation is diminished to the dorsum of the hand.

A. Standard strategy

1. External fixation of the pelvic ring and left upper extremity with irrigation and debridement of the open elbow wound on the day of admission (Figs. 13.22 and 13.23)

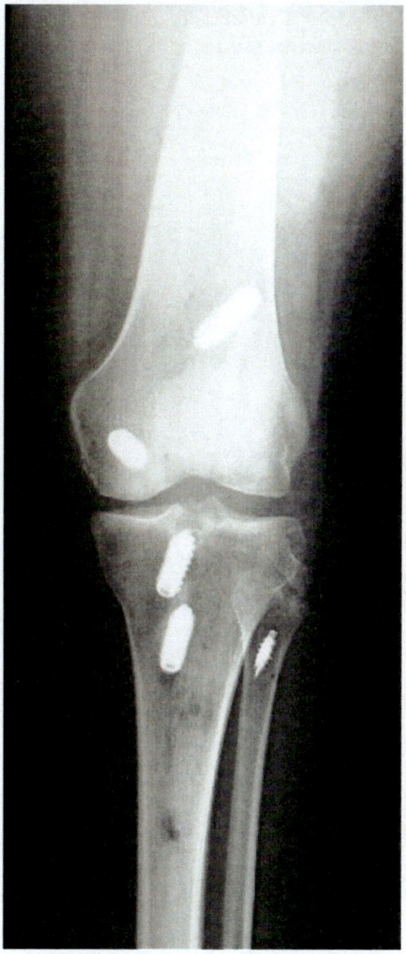

Fig. 13.20 AP radiograph of left knee post soft tissue reconstruction

2. Upper extremity frame configuration
   (a) Half pins in the lateral aspect of the proximal humerus with direct visualization of the bone
   (b) Half pin placement in the lateral aspect of the distal humerus with direct visualization of the bone staying posterior to the radial nerve
   (c) Two connecting rods to stabilize the humerus shaft fracture
   (d) Half pin placement in the subcutaneous aspect of ulna shaft
   (e) Two connecting rods to the humerus pins to stabilize the proximal ulna fracture and elbow
   (f) Half pins in the dorsoradial aspect of the radius shaft
   (g) Half pins in the dorsoradial aspect of the second metacarpal
   (h) Connecting rods to stabilize the distal radius fracture with slight distraction
3. Staged conversion to internal fixation as general condition allows (Figs. 13.24 and 13.25)
   (a) Anterolateral plating of the humerus shaft with fixator removal at 6 days. Radial nerve explored and in continuity

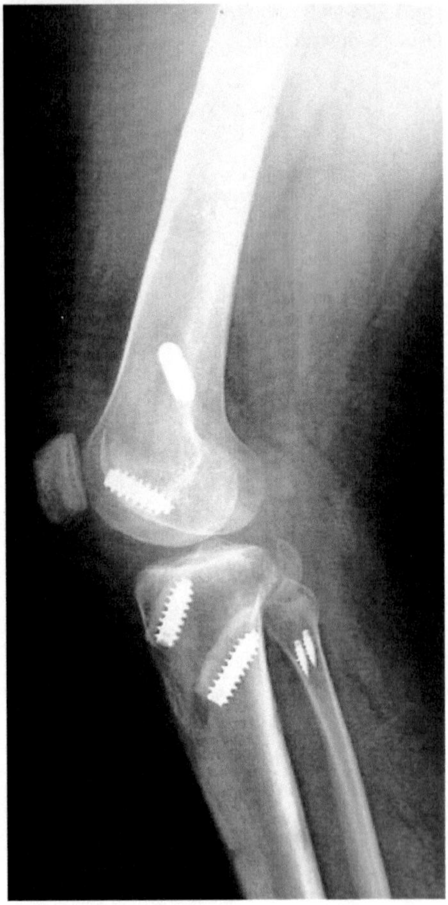

Fig. 13.21 Lateral radiograph of left knee post soft tissue reconstruction

(b) Proximal ulna plating with removal of the fixator and wound closure
(c) Elbow brace and ROM
(d) Volar locking plate for the distal radius at 10 days with removal of the fixator

4. Removal of pelvic fixator at 10 weeks

B. Alternatives

(a) Plating of the humerus, ulna, and radius at 10 days
(b) Plating of the humerus and ulna with treatment of the radius to healing in the external fixator
(c) If infection developed or elbow instability, then conversion to articulated external fixation of the elbow at 5–15 days

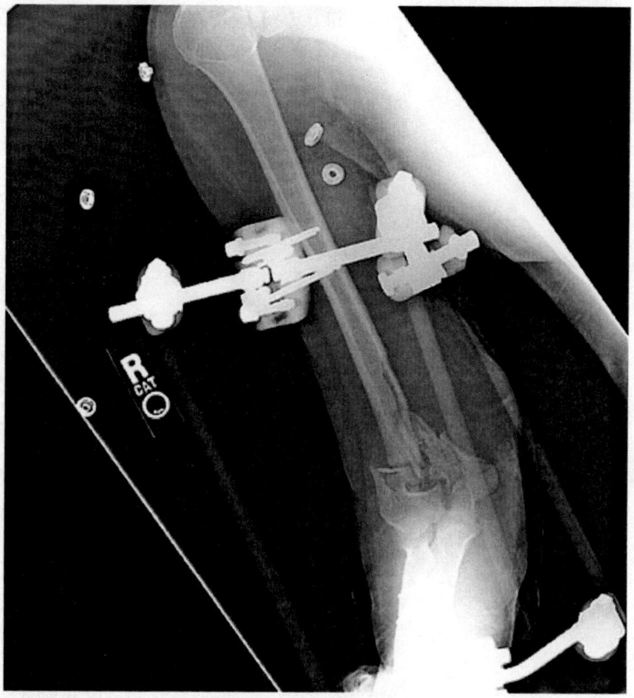

Fig. 13.22 AP radiograph of right elbow showing a comminuted fracture of the distal humerus

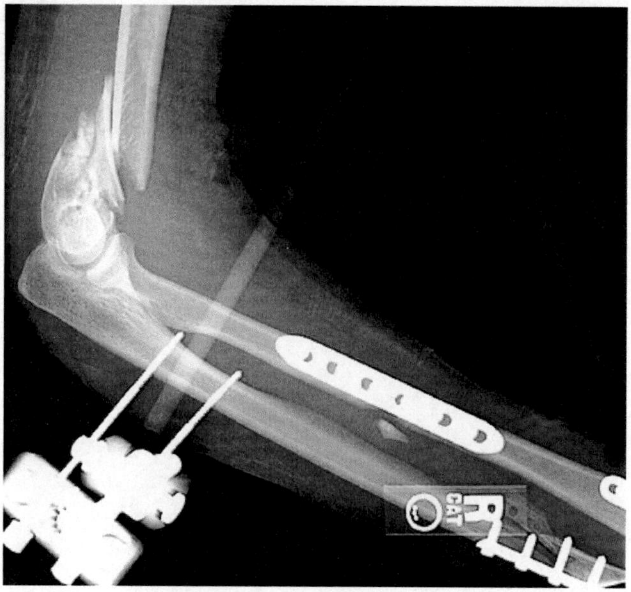

Fig. 13.23 Lateral radiograph following initial management with application of elbow bridging external fixation and fixation of ulna and radius fractures

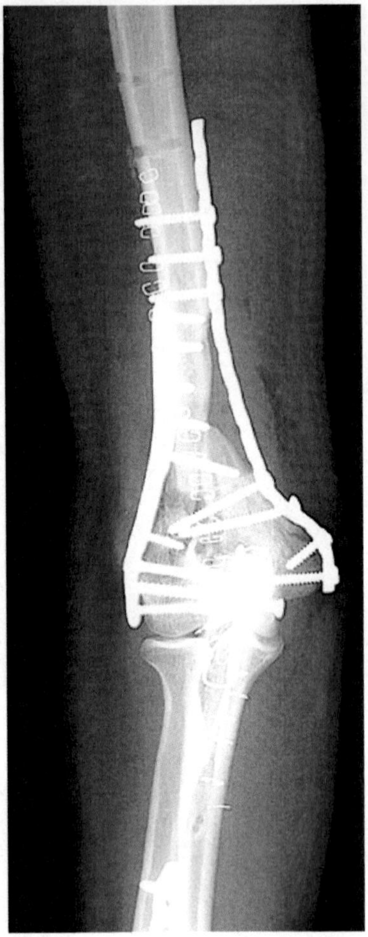

Fig. 13.24 AP radiograph of elbow post ORIF of distal humerus

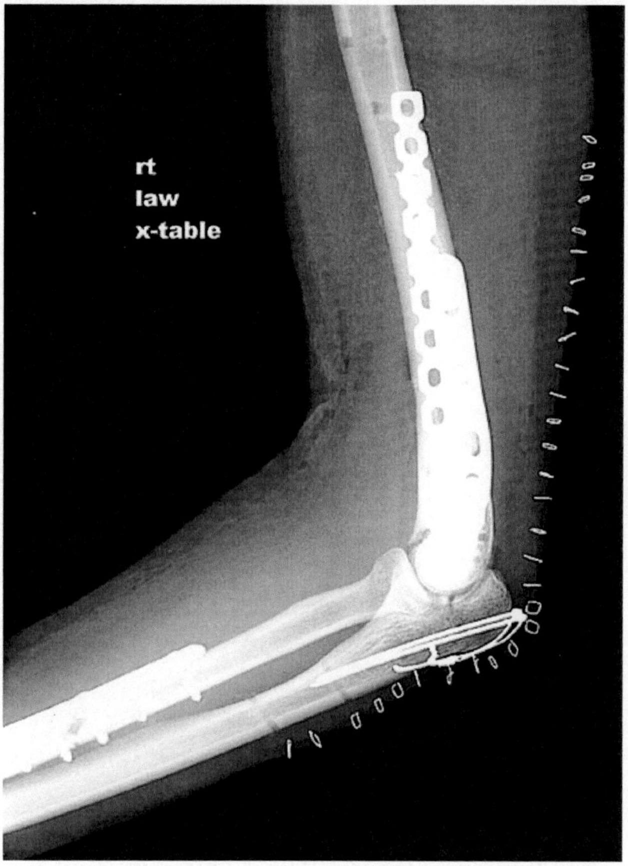

Fig. 13.25 Lateral radiograph of right elbow post ORIF of distal humerus

References

1. Collinge C, Kennedy J, Schmidt A. Temporizing external fixation of the lower extremity: a survey of the Orthopaedic Trauma Association Membership. Orthopaedics. 2010;33(4):239.
2. Marsh JL, Bonar S, Nepola JV, Decoster TA, Hurwitz SR. Use of an articulated external fixator for fractures of the tibial plafond. J Bone Joint Surg. 1995;77(10):1498–509.
3. Schenck Jr R. Classification of knee dislocations. Oper Tech Sports Med. 2003;11(3):193–8.
4. Stannard JP, Sheils TM, McGwin G, Volgas DA. The use of a hinged knee fixator after surgery for knee dislocation. Arthroscopy. 2003;19(6):626–31.

Chapter 14
Medico Legal Considerations Surrounding the Injured Patient

David Seligson and Charles Daniel Benson

14.1 The Situation

Injury creates a disruption in life. Not only is there the discomfort and inconvenience caused by trauma, but there is also loss. The loss of activities planned for the next day, the next week, and perhaps the next year. There is loss of income, loss of power, perhaps loss of relationships. The severity of a person's injuries can severely hamper fulfillment of previously made commitments. Mortgages, loans, and taxes are still due. The monthly bills have to be paid. The dog expects to be fed. Rarely do people have either the resources or the insurance to cover the whole contingency. Insurance policies written by lawyers protect the insurers, not the insured. The "weasel" words jump off the page. The insurer does not have the information needed to process the claim. Elaborate forms get sent out. The checks are not in the mail. The injured person's normal actions – having a drink at dinner, speeding slightly over the limit, failing to wear a seat belt – become "contributory negligence" and add to the financial burden of being hurt.

Injury involves loss, and loss causes grief. The process of grieving (grief reaction) is a well-known sequence. This sequence involves blame. First, the victim blames himself. Next, he questions what others could have done; finally, there is acceptance of the loss. How this process evolves depends upon many factors. The injured individual expecting, for example, to play basketball after work becomes a patient in a hospital bed. The patient is unable to escape the many people who come to the bedside to ask about anything and everything. The visitors at the bedside may ask not only appropriate questions about the recovery from injury but also personal

D. Seligson (✉)
Department of Orthopaedics, University Hospital Louisville, Louisville, KY, USA
e-mail: seligson@louisville.edu

C.D. Benson
Department of Orthopedic Surgery, Resident in Orthopedic Surgery, University of Kansas Medical Center, Kansas 66160, USA
e-mail: cdanbenson@aol.com

D. Seligson et al. (eds.), *External Fixation in Orthopedic Traumatology*,
DOI 10.1007/978-1-4471-2197-8_14,

and probing questions about relationships, finances, and the state of the bowels. The people that come may or may not be acceptable to the patient and may seem helpful or hostile depending on interpersonal factors that are sometimes difficult or impossible to discern.

14.2 Postoperative Follow-up

Coordination of the postoperative care of the polytraumatized patient may require several different services. If the patient has a head injury, laprotomy, or hand injury, he may appear in an office other than the orthopedic office after discharge from a rehabilitation facility. Often, the first post-hospitalization visit is in response to a perceived crisis – for example, drainage from the wound, swelling in the calf, or persistent headaches. The challenge of a trauma orthopedic practice is to create a system capable of responding to the perception of crisis with problem solving. The orthopedic traumatologist is fully prepared by training to care for the musculoskeletal injury.

However, the patient has a much more extensive and pressing shopping list. First, there are problems of discomfort and incapacity. Then, there are problems with medications. There are difficulties getting into other offices for care and difficulties arranging for ancillary services such as physical therapy. There is the need to obtain data from dysfunctional information systems. Where is the discharge summary? Where are the laboratory reports? Where are the radiographs? There is loss of income. Finally, there are a whole set of new problems imposed by insurers and other outside agencies. There are forms for insurance payments, forms for disability determinations, forms for the government, forms for medical leave, and forms for handicapped parking.

From the doctors' perspective, reimbursements for care of injured patients are not a certainty. The insurance industry will examine the claim and try to find a way to make some other party pay. The patient's activity at the time of injury goes under intense examination. Was the injured party where he was supposed to be? Does the equipment belong to the employer? Was the equipment defective? Did the employee fail to disclose a preexisting injury on the pre-employment medical questionnaire? Is the employee's health insurance responsible? Was the employee using proper protective equipment? The file will be set aside and a letter sent to the doctor's office requesting "more information." The request will ask again for the date of injury, diagnosis, dates of hospitalization, etc. All this information takes time and expense to acquire. The letter will probably contain a threat not to pay the claim and to delay the patient's reimbursement for lost wages until the insurer has received the information. Meanwhile, the doctor is accumulating out-of-pocket expenses for everything from wound dressings and energy bills for the lights in the office to technicians' wages and postage. Different insurance systems have different rules about coverage. In some States, the doctor cannot bill Workman's Compensation patients directly for professional services and other charges. How should the doctor proceed if a determination is not available as to who is actually to be responsible for bill? When accounts are closed, a good number of balances expire unpaid with notations from the billing office that the telephone number is "no longer in service" or post office stamps on unopened envelopes state that the party is "not at this address."

Several strategies are productive to organize postoperative care. These include the following:

14.2.1 Compulsive Information Management

There is no substitute for an accurate record of patient contacts with the office. This record should be permanent, in ink, and reviewed and initialed by the physician. When there are postoperative problems, there is a tendency to blame the provider. The office's failure to respond to a call can be cited as reason for an adverse outcome. In reality, the patient did call, but the office was unable to call back because the phone number was incorrect, the line was constantly busy, or the phone was on "voice mail." A contemporaneous, written phone log of the contact in the patient record is irrefutable documentation of what actually occurred. This record has authority over recollections of what happened. The written record takes precedence over "he said – she said." Therefore, any post facto attempt to alter the record must not be undertaken since these alterations will destroy the credibility of the written record. Other errors in follow-up include a failure to detect and screen an abnormal report received in the office. This could be a laboratory finding, x-ray report, or report from a therapist. Health providers must manage information so that if the doctor ordered a venous Doppler to "rule out" thromboembolism, the report from the vascular lab would be obtained and appropriate action taken.

14.2.2 Sharing Responsibility with Other Providers

As a successful trauma practice becomes more specialized and busy, the likelihood that the physician can manage comorbidities successfully decreases. There is simply not enough time to examine and treat a condition that is outside the traumatologist realm of expertise. It is important to work with colleagues in the care of complex, specialized posttraumatic conditions. Referral for consultation to other orthopedists with appropriate interests is a good strategy for dealing with difficult problems. Involve colleagues with, for example, spine interests in the treatment of a patient with significant compression fractures who is developing a kyphus deformity. Incontinence should be treated by either a urologist or a gynecologist, nightmare by the psychiatrist or neurologist, and so forth. A physician in Physical Medicine and Rehabilitation can help with the coordination of care for polytrauma patients. Similarly, an expert who regularly completes evaluation forms for disability determination, sets restrictions, and is accustomed to determining percent of permanent disability will have the time and expertise to do the job completely. These evaluations usually take several hours to complete, so it is unrealistic to do them "on the fly" in the context of a busy problem-focused orthopedic trauma practice which is geared to examining and treating twenty patients in a typical half day. Finally, most offices find that as they increase their referrals to other providers, so will consultations for good future problems increase.

14.2.3 Reasonable Administrative Fees

Lawyers expect to charge and receive payment for their time. Indeed, they carry diaries to enable them to account for every working minute spent during the day. Most people would do the same if their rate of reimbursement were several hundred dollars an hour. Doctors should think the same way. Our time is also valuable. Looking at a form, reviewing the medical record, forming an opinion, and sending out information all take time. Instead of complaining about the extra burden of administrative work, develop a system to charge for it. Reasonable charges for reasonable services are reimbursed most of the time. A physician's office is not expected to provide professional time, secretarial time, paper, envelopes, and even the postage stamps for the insurer questioning the medical office about the date of injury and place of treatment for a claim that has already been filed and re-filed. It is reasonable to ask the patient to pay some nominal fee for looking at the matter and getting the necessary forms in the mail.

14.2.4 Loss-Cutting

The provider's business practice should contain enough information to make decisions about continuing care for clients who default on payment. Orthopedic trauma doctors do not seek payment based on contingency. This is a sensitive area because of the liability issues surrounding care of the injured. The providers' patients can be closely in touch with the legal system. Lawyers and their associates are looking for sources of money to help the patient overcome the loss caused by the injury. Lawyers pay ultimately relates to how much revenue they can generate for their clients. These thoughts are not prejudiced against the legal profession; they are thoughts that reflect how our social system works. Patients who have loss of income and discomfort from injury tend to question their treatment. Is it normal to feel pain at the hip after a femur nailing? The treating physician who is insecure may allow that the nail is "a little long." This appliance, which is too long then, becomes a rationale to delay return to work. Even though for decades femur nails were placed with the extraction hole proximal to the greater trochanter. Fault for the increased economic damage may be assigned to the placement of the nail rather than the accident. X-rays confirm the offense for the layman. Understand that there is nothing normal about having a yard of surgical stainless steel pounded into ones femur through the buttock. Understand that the cause of discomfort lies in the injury and the patient's failure to get on with recovery. Dr. Tony Russell of Memphis has a sign in his office to tell his patients "You broke God's bone." This admonition helps the provider to expect fair wages for services rendered.

14.3 Disability and Return to Work Evaluation

None of us has the power of prophesy, yet we are increasingly being asked to provide opinions about the course and completeness of recovery. These questions arise even before major surgical interventions. Employers want their employees to be "100%" before they return to work. No one improves due to an injury, and no one will be as good tomorrow as he or she was yesterday. First, the traumatologist should find out enough about what the issues are, and the second, admonition is to stay out of the middle of an employer/employee confrontation. The issues may include what the patient does for work, how the injury occurred, and who will pay the bill. Not all of these matters may be easy to establish. The facts may change. Evaluation of the patient and medical documentation are the responsibility of the treating orthopedist. The patient may attempt to structure the medical record for his own perceived advantage. For example, the therapy notes state that the patient has level 10 pain on a scale of 0–10 where ten is terrible pain. The "nurse manager" wants to know "how can he ride motorcycles recreationally if his pain is 10/10" and "if he can ride motorcycles, why can't he work." Indeed the pain is not 10/10. Discussions about pain can take place with the patient, but this requires experience and skill. One can begin by accepting that the patient has pain. However, one can ask, is this pain really as bad as, for example, the pain of childbirth? "To be truthful," one patient then replied, "I did not tell the therapist that at all."

The employer can make accommodations, so the employee can return to work. Why any employer would want an employee who does not want to work yet on the job with a blowtorch is difficult to understand. A clue that the workplace situation is unfavorable will be a request to "place restrictions." The employer may ask, for example, for the doctor to determine "exactly how many hours can the patient stand." There are factors that influence this restriction beyond the ability of the doctor to ascertain in a follow-up visit. How far, for example, is the walk from parking to the place of employment? Are there steps? Where is the restroom located? The question indicates an unwillingness of the employer to use common sense or a desire of the employee/patient to make it difficult. These situations are impossible for the clinician to resolve. In practice, it is better not even to try. One major company had its injured employee return to work. The job was to sit in a plain room with nothing to do. In another situation, the patient had to walk slowly through the plant checking that the water bubblers were working. In both of these instances, the patients quit their jobs.

Indeed, simple, straightforward questions about work capacity and disability are manageable and are answerable directly. Questions about questions should be a tip-off to a "no win" situation. One strategy adopted in the past decade by insurers is to reduce surgical fees and use the money to hire "nurse managers." These nurses come with the patient to the office visit and intercede ostensibly on the part of the patient, or more accurately, on the part of the insurer. Usually, they understand musculoskeletal injury poorly, and invariably, they promote additional testing and outside consulting which actually delay the patient's return to work. As a general practice, these nurse managers can be regarded as taking time, at a reduced rate, from other patients who have come to the office for medical attention. It is not sensible to attempt to examine and treat the patient in their presence. The "case manager" can read the medical record after the encounter and can schedule a prepaid conference to get questions answered.

Most injuries lead to some degree of permanent disability. The published guidelines for the evaluation of permanent disability contain categories to account for chronic discomfort, functional losses, and condition specific ratings. Preparations of these guidelines are by a special group of professionals who are preserving their own professions by creating arcane schemes to place "objective" numbers on perceived illness. On the other hand, we are all familiar with hideously crippled arthritics that function incredibly well doing difficult and useful work in society. Work is tied to motivation, necessity, worldview, upbringing, and mindset, to mention a few of the variables.

14.4 Legal Matters

The interaction between injury, medical care, and the law is increasingly complicated. The system we had, functioned well when health care was less specialized, less costly and moved at a slower pace. Do not forget that at the end of the Second World War, the treatment of femur shaft fractures in the United States was nonoperative. The injured patient spent months in bed, never had surgery, and had a better than even chance of limping for the rest of their life. This has all changed. We are in a technological revolution. Not only are all the cases treated surgically, not only has the cost of the implants risen 20-fold, not only has hospitalization been reduced from months to days, but also the patient expects, no demands, a straight, strong, perfectly functioning extremity. Moreover, the patient has a right, legitimized by our government, to receive pain-free treatment.

The medical record is sentinel to the resolution of legal matters surrounding accident cases. Yet the medical record today is in a state of change. The government has mandated an electronic medical record. The concept is to reduce errors, increase legibility, and promote information exchange. In reality, hospital administration uses information control to control patient care. Instead of prescribing, one must select approved doses from "drop down" screens. The penalty for attempting to choose another medication with a different frequency of administration is loss of time working through a tedious computer routine or filling out special information forms. The physician signs a "face sheet" without real knowledge of the contents of the record. Review of computer-generated medical charts shows that they contain many incomplete fields. These records may further purport to show deficient physician response to calls from the hospital. For example, the nurse may attempt to call a physician but may be using the wrong phone number.

Today, the handwritten notes in the record are authoritative. Since writing of these notes is contemporaneous with events, these notes are the last word as to how care took place. It is unclear then how computer records, with entries by multiple providers, from multiple locations, at multiple times, are going to work in the legal process. Doubtless systems will evolve as flaws appear, and the process is improved. Doubtless, it will take more, not less, time to document patient care. Doubtless, the result will be more resources used up for administrative purposes and less care at the bedside.

In whatever form it appears, the physician should approach the record with caution. It is best for the doctor to enter notes about what is actually observed. It is realistic to provide simple explanations for planned actions. It is important to document patient and family contact – for example, "spoke with patient and his wife." Long notes are a "tip-off" to defensive behavior. Law offices have no qualms. They hire people to read the records and to look for irregularities. No record is perfect. No decision made about patient care is without alternatives that could possibly provide the chance for a better outcome. What keeps our system running is the fundamental trust between the physician and the patient's belief that the best will be done.

When an injury case moves from the bedside and the hospital, clinic, or office to the insurance office, the lawyer's office, or court, the paperwork changes. The physician is suddenly working in a foreign country and in a foreign language. One can learn to speak this language, but only incompletely. The doctor is not, and never will be, a native speaker. It is a particular language. Like a magician saying "abracadabra," the doctor must provide opinions "based on reasonable medical certainty" – i.e., more likely than not. Doctors deal in hunches, intuition, suspicion, and also experience and training. Can one really ascertain within 51 of 100 chances that the articular damage to the knee will lead to arthritis?

There are different levels of interaction with the legal profession. These include reports, sworn statements, and depositions. In a report, one writes answers to specific questions. Here, a physician must get together the documentation he or she needs, write straightforward answers, review the document, and send it all out. It is more difficult with the sworn statement. In a sworn statement, a lawyer with a court reporter will ask questions for the purpose of getting specific information "on the record." Doctors want to please, and doctors are defensive. We may not understand what exact words the lawyer requires in the sworn statement – the "open sesame!" Be certain, however, that all this unusual activity aims at getting something from the doctor for obtaining a bigger prize. Approach sworn statements with incredulity, listen carefully to the questions, go off the record if necessary, and be certain to provide only the facts. In a deposition, the physician is in the proverbial "hot seat." The format is adversarial; both sides are present. There are two kinds of depositions – depositions in malpractice cases where the doctor giving the deposition is the defendant, and all other depositions. Malpractice depositions are a special problem to be discussed later. All other depositions are discussed now.

A deposition is a fact-finding exercise. Historically, the form has varied. Information can, for example, be extracted with torture. Today, questions and answers are dutifully recorded or videographically documented. The deponent has a duty to answer only the questions that are asked and a sworn duty to tell the truth. Approach questions like approaching a railroad stop, look, listen, and sign. Listen to the whole question, think, and then speak. The most frequent problem is a mismatch between the language of the examining lawyer and the physician's conceptual framework. The question, for example, may ask, "Isn't pain 'subjective' as opposed to 'objective'?" The lawyer will try to establish then that the patient's perception of pain is altered by the possibility of increasing dollars received in settlement. From a medical standpoint, the visual analogue pain scale is a reproductable measure of pain and is "objective" parametric data. One can only answer questions that one understands. In this setting, the lawyer may seek to restrict answers to yes or no only. If a deposition takes an adversarial, as opposed to a fact-finding, tone, the deponent is advised to request that the hostility cease or seek relief from the judge in the case under whose auspices the deposition is being taken. In general, lawyers do not want to take inordinate time for a deposition, and just when it seems that the questions will not end, the lawyers end the matter.

On the other hand, in depositions in which the physician is a defendant in a malpractice action, the deposition will be hostile. The lawyer will use questions to find out how the doctor will respond under pressure. Depositions may run over several days. Judges who are part of this arcane legal process will provide no relief for the accused. The object is usually not trial, but settlement. The vast majority of medical malpractice actions never come to court because they are either dropped or settled. If a case goes to trial, defense will spend at least $60,000, which is enough to manage unimportant claims. The big cases can come close to trial. Here, one must budget time; here, one must be patient; here, one must not become a career victim of legal process. The bright spot in this picture is that the overwhelming majority of cases that go to the jury are won by the doctor.

14.5 The Future

Our present system of compensating the injured by an adversarial system of assigning fault and rewarding dysfunction cannot long survive. It is making us sicker as a society. As the insurance industry and the health provider cartel grow in economic power, it will become liable for misadventures in the provision of care for injury. What will be required is social solidarity to guarantee services and livelihood for those with disabilities following trauma. Today, employers do not usually hire the handicapped. They want workers who are 100% healthy. The Federal Disability Acts are unfunded mandates. What is legal and what actually happens are not the same. Our citizens have demonstrated that any entitlement program, no matter how modest or well intended, will be abused. The number of citizens who will not work after expensive back surgery and who expect compensatory disability income is astounding. Today's program of using doctors' malpractice payment as a source of income for the injured cannot long persist. There exists widespread pessimism in traumatology circles that the best and brightest will join a profession increasingly burdened with unrealistic patient expectations, rising administrative tasks, falling compensation, and increasing malpractice premiums. The system will finally implode when less bright minds attempt to do more difficult tasks with less resources and system support.

There will emerge, finally, a better, more logical way of organizing the care of the injured and providing the wherewithal to do the job properly.

Index

D. Seligson et al. (eds.), *External Fixation in Orthopedic Traumatology*,
DOI 10.1007/978-1-4471-2197-8, © Springer-Verlag London Limited 2012